Stoma Care and Rehabilitation

For Elsevier

Associate Editor: Dinah Thom
Project Manager: Joannah Duncan
Designer: Stewart Larking
Illustration Manager: Bruce Hogarth
Illustrators: Paul Richardson and Richard Morris

Stoma Care and Rehabilitation

Edited by

Brigid Breckman BA(Hons), RGN, RNT, JBCNS Certificate in Stoma Care, Diploma in Counselling Skills, Master Practitioner in Neurolinguistic Programming (NLP)

Freelance Writer, Workshop Leader and Counsellor, Hornchurch, Essex, UK

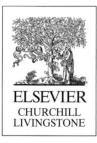

ELSEVIER
CHURCHILL
LIVINGSTONE

EDINBURGH LONDON NEW YORK OXFORD PHILADELPHIA ST LOUIS SYDNEY TORONTO 2005

ELSEVIER
CHURCHILL
LIVINGSTONE

First published 2005

ISBN 0 443 10091 8

British Library Cataloguing in Publication Data
A catalogue record for this book is available from the British Library

Library of Congress Cataloging in Publication Data
A catalog record for this book is available from the Library of Congress

Notice
Knowledge and best practice in this field are constantly changing. As new research and experience broaden our knowledge, changes in practice, treatment and drug therapy may become necessary or appropriate. Readers are advised to check the most current information provided (i) on procedures featured or (ii) by the manufacturer of each product to be administered, to verify the recommended dose or formula, the method and duration of administration, and contraindications. It is the responsibility of the practitioner, relying on their own experience and knowledge of the patient, to make diagnoses, to determine dosages and the best treatment for each individual patient, and to take all appropriate safety precautions. To the fullest extent of the law, neither the publisher nor the editor and contributors assume any liability for any injury and/or damage.

The Publisher

ELSEVIER your source for books, journals and multimedia in the health sciences

www.elsevierhealth.com

The publisher's policy is to use **paper manufactured from sustainable forests**

Printed in China

Contents

Illustrations and patient scenarios

Patient scenarios

Contributors

Barbara Borwell MA(Ed), RGN, ENB(216, 980), NDN Certificate, FETC 730, Diploma in Counselling, Certificate in Counselling and Psychosexual Therapy
Visiting Lecturer in breast, stoma, and psychosexual care, Bournemouth University, UK

Brigid Breckman BA(Hons), RGN, RNT, JBCNS Certificate in Stoma Care, Diploma in Counselling Skills, Master Practitioner in Neurolinguistic Programming (NLP)
Freelance writer, workshop leader and counsellor, 29 Mansfield Gardens, Hornchurch, Essex RM12 4NL, UK

Rachel Busuttil Leaver BSc(Hons), PGCE, RGN
Lecturer Practitioner – Urological Nursing, London South Bank University and Department of Urology, University College London Hospitals Foundation Trust, UK

Sharon Fillingham MSc, BSc(Hons), RGN, Diploma in Counselling, ENB(216, 980, 978)
Clinical Nurse Specialist in Urinary Diversion/Psychosexual and Gender Therapy, Department of Urology, University College London Hospitals Foundation Trust, UK

Helen Johnson BSc(Hons), RGN, RSCN, ENB(216)
Clinical Nurse Specialist in Stoma Care, Hospital For Sick Children NHS Trust, Great Ormond Street, London, UK

Wendy Pringle BSc(Hons), RGN, Enterostomal Therapist, HVCert
Colorectal Nurse Consultant, University Hospital Birmingham NHS Foundation Trust, UK

Ann Richards MSc, BA(Hons), RGN, RNT
Senior Lecturer in Pharmacology and Physiology, Department of Allied Health Professions, University of Hertfordshire, UK

Maddie White BSc(Hons), RGN, ENB(216, 980, 998), Certificate in Counselling
Colorectal Nurse Specialist, University Hospital Birmingham NHS Foundation Trust, UK

Preface

As stoma care has developed during the past thirty years awareness of the extent and complexity of care which patients require has grown. Feedback from patients and nurses about their experiences of stoma care and their needs has influenced the style and content of this book considerably. Informal discussions and research findings have both highlighted the need for a style of stoma care that will enable patients to rehabilitate as well as manage their practical stoma care.

Classification of what constitutes normal stoma care and what is defined as specialised problem-solving care is changing. In part this is due to sufficient patients telling us they need certain aspects of care in order to cope with their surgery and learn to live with their stoma. It is also due to the collective knowledge of growing numbers of nurses who have specialised in stoma care for long enough to recognise the breadth and depth of care that patients and their families generally require. This greater understanding has led to the 'twin track' approach to stoma care being described in this book. It shows how care can be given in current situations in a manner that also promotes long-term rehabilitation.

Identifying what stoma care components are required, and why, does not automatically enable us to provide them. Therefore there is also a major focus in this book on *how* a style, depth and quality of stoma care can be provided which will support and promote patients' physical and psychological rehabilitation. Much of the emphasis is on how skills can be used strategically to follow the principles of stoma care, and to achieve goals that you and your patients want to achieve.

Effective communication and collaboration are central in successful stoma care. On courses ways of achieving these are often presented through 'live' demonstrations. These enable people to gain more sense of what these approaches can be like in action, discuss their relevance, and consider how they will use or adapt them. We provide *patient scenarios* here to serve a similar purpose for readers. We hope they contribute to our overall aim of providing a realistic mental map of stoma care which healthcare team members can share and use flexibly to provide a patient-centred style of care.

In addition to seeking to reflect current knowledge and effective practice, this book has a further key aim. That is to describe stoma care in ways that enable readers whose levels of skill development may vary from novice to expert to be able to draw on it to extend their expertise. This means that you and your colleagues may find different sections of the book, and particular aspects of stoma care, match your interests and learning needs at different times. Hopefully this will be a book you find useful to revisit as you extend your practice.

The scope of this book and, in particular, the aim of ranging from basic to advanced practice in the care described, has meant that the feedback sought from colleagues has been substantial. It is impossible to acknowledge all the people who have provided advice, information and thought-provoking comments as this book progressed to its present form. However, special thanks are due to Heather Gillanders, Stoma Care Nurse, Luton and Dunstable NHS Trust; Heather Hill, Clinical Nurse Consultant in Stomal Therapy and Wound Management,

Concord Repatriation General Hospital, Australia (now retired); Elaine Swan, Advanced Nurse Practitioner in Colorectal Nursing, Walsall Hospitals NHS Trust; and Jane Winney, Clinical Nurse Specialist in Colorectal Nursing, Hereford Hospital NHS Trust.

Thanks are also due to David Exon, Consultant General Surgeon, Tayside University Hospitals NHS Trust (Ninewells), for his feedback and suggestions on Chapters 3 and 5. I would also like to acknowledge the generosity with which contributors have provided specialist information which has enhanced the book as a whole in addition to their own chapters. Finally, thanks from all of us go to family, friends and colleagues who have supported us in many ways as we have completed this book.

Brigid Breckman
Hornchurch, Essex 2005

Introduction

Brigid Breckman

I believe that caring for patients who are undergoing surgery and learning to live with a bowel or urinary stoma is both exciting and challenging. It is exciting because each person reacts to their situation and its implications for their life and sense of themselves differently. These differences give us the opportunity to work flexibly and creatively with each patient and their family. Matching the information and care we give to their particular situation and needs so there is a 'good fit' between what is needed and what is provided is exciting. Contributing to patients' immediate wellbeing and longer-term rehabilitation can be immensely satisfying.

Patients acquire substantial amounts of information on separate occasions from a variety of staff. They need to coordinate what they learn into a level of knowledge and skills that will enable them to live with their stoma competently and confidently. This requirement is challenging for patients and nurses to fulfil. It invites us to provide care in ways that help patients to learn, organise and use information well. It can be useful to think of this process as helping patients to complete a jigsaw or picture puzzle. When patients are actively encouraged to slot into place in their mind the different bits of information and self-care skills and link one with another they connect them up into a whole picture of their situation, and the ways in which they can manage their stoma care and rehabilitation. The *patient scenarios* throughout the book give you examples to consider of patients being helped to coordinate what they are learning into their own personal jigsaw.

As members of the healthcare team we can also think of our system of collectively providing information and care as making a professional jigsaw for each patient. Doing this helps us monitor whether there are any missing pieces in the care we are providing. It reminds us to explicitly link information and care given by our colleagues and ourselves into a connected, holistic system of care for each patient.

Collaboration and coordination are much easier to achieve when all members of the healthcare team share a mental map of *what* stoma care entails, *why* different elements are necessary, and *how* they can be provided. Using the same vision of overall care helps us identify:

- how the care we individually give fits into the whole system provided by the team
- which elements of stoma care can be provided by most team members and which elements are best provided by colleagues with particular expertise
- when to draw on colleagues' expertise in order to provide the level of information and care particular patients require
- whether the care being given is coherent and comprehensive enough to meet the needs of particular patients and their families
- aspects of stoma care in which, individually and/or as a team, we could acquire greater expertise.

This book provides a description of stoma care which individuals and the whole team can use as a mental map of the care through which, collectively, you help patients rehabilitate following stoma surgery. In order to provide this perspective of stoma care all the chapter authors asked:

- What information and care do people who have, or are going to have, a stoma need in order to rehabilitate physically and psychologically?
- What skills and experiences will most effectively help patients learn to look after their stoma and incorporate it into their lifestyle?
- How can we work with patients to identify what their particular situations and needs entail, and respond to them in ways that promote their well-being and rehabilitation?
- How, when and why should particular information, skills and care activities be used?
- How can we help people move from experiencing themselves as 'a stoma patient' to 'being a person who happens to have a stoma'?

In answering these questions we have drawn on ideas, research and approaches used in various fields, including:

- *stoma care*, e.g. research and other literature including patients' reports of living with a stoma and problems that needed resolving, colleagues' accounts of effective care
- *related nursing fields*, e.g. cancer care
- *related medical and other fields*, e.g. physiological research; studies of loss, bereavement, communication and counselling
- *models of helping processes*, e.g. goal-setting; problem-solving.

Thinking widely about patients and stoma care has helped us describe the kind of care most patients require in order to rehabilitate physically and psychologically. This is a mixed blessing. It increases awareness of the levels of skill development that nurses can achieve, and the benefits these bring to patients and their families. However, it can also increase discomfort and frustration when we notice gaps between what patients need and what we are currently capable of providing, individually and as a team.

Patients also often describe their sense of gaps in their skill development. For example, they may compare their knowledge and skills to those demonstrated by experienced nurses. They may be aware they want to achieve particular goals, but not know how to do so.

In such circumstances nurses and patients may decide it is not possible for the necessary levels of skills to be gained and used. This is rarely true. What many people do not have is knowledge of:

- what different levels of skill entail
- what lengths of time are generally needed for skill acquisition at different levels
- how to promote and develop skills.

With this information you, your colleagues and patients can have realistic expectations, and a sense of achievement as knowledge and skills are gained. This is important because most patients will require much of the stoma care described in this book. However, this does not mean that every nurse should be able to provide all of these aspects of care. We describe care requiring different levels of expertise and approaches from a variety of fields of knowledge. You may find that, like many nurses, you feel informed and skilled in some areas and less competent in others. This is entirely normal as opportunities to acquire information and skills in the many different elements that can make up 'stoma care' will vary. It is easier to enjoy broadening and deepening our knowledge if our expectations of what we 'should' know and be able to do at different stages in our professional development are realistic. Unrealistic expectations can lead us to feel uncomfortable when we cannot meet patients' particular needs. Unrealistic expectations make it harder to recognise and value the competencies we do have, and to feel comfortable asking for colleagues' help in situations where patients need more advanced care than we can so far provide.

In the rest of this introduction I am therefore drawing on the work of Patricia Benner and her colleagues (Benner 1984, Benner et al 1996). Their research and descriptions of how nurses develop and demonstrate various levels of skill provide us with practical ideas as well as theoretical knowledge. They clarify the levels of skill nurses can acquire, relating them to the learning experiences and time that will need to be spent with patients undergoing similar treatment and care for those skills to be acquired.

Key points from their research are included here so you can use them when considering your own development and the stoma care described in this book.

Benner (1984) suggests that *expertise is contextual*. It is acquired as time is spent nursing patients who have similar conditions and treatments, and who describe similar experiences, concerns and problems. Nurses develop knowledge of normal events and progress to be expected with these patients, likely problems and how these can be recognised at an early stage, and effective ways of minimising or resolving them. Expert nurses know what information and care is generally required by their specific group of patients, when different elements of care will be relevant, and how they can enhance patients' physical and psychological wellbeing.

This level of expertise can take five or more years of working with the same kind of patients to develop. Benner (1984) and Benner et al (1996) used the Dreyfus model of skill acquisition to identify the stages of skill development that nurses go through as they pass from novice to expert practitioner. These five levels of proficiency are:

- novice
- advanced beginner
- competent
- proficient
- expert.

Nurses using this model may initially find they have some difficulty in reconciling the names given to the different levels of skill acquisition and the roles and responsibilities of the nurses who are demonstrating them. This is partly because we may use these terms or labels of competency differently in our everyday language to the specific ways in which Benner and her colleagues use them. Their work also invites us to revise some of the links we have assumed to be present between nurses' roles and their levels of expertise. Traditionally, if patients required specific levels of nursing expertise it has been assumed that the staff employed in particular roles would be able to provide it: patient need and staff capability would match. However, what the research shows is that there is often a gap between the levels of expertise patients require and the expertise that nurses can provide *in view of their length of experience and opportunities for skill acquisition with patients in this kind of situation.*

This means that nurses employed, for example, as staff nurses, sisters/ward managers and community nurses will not necessarily have been in a position to acquire stoma care expertise (because it requires specific and sufficient experience *in the context of nursing patients with stomas*). Likewise, stoma care nurses may not have been in a position to acquire a particular element of stoma care expertise (e.g. because the need for this aspect of stoma care rarely arises in their clinical area).

Recognising these implications of Benner et al's (1996) research is very liberating. Firstly, it enables us to understand, without feeling guilty, why we might not have acquired levels of expertise that patients need. Secondly, it encourages us to stop assuming there is something intrinsically wrong with us if we have not yet acquired the same expertise as colleagues employed in the same role, and put our energies into acquiring it. Thirdly, it encourages us to work as a team to deliver to patients the levels of skilled care they require. This increases both the effectiveness and the satisfaction with care experienced by all concerned.

Throughout this book, when particular levels of skill are being described, it is the following concepts of skill levels that are meant. Becoming familiar with them helps us use this research as a map to identify what aspects of care we can provide well and what greater expertise we can acquire individually, and collectively with colleagues (see Ch. 23).

STAGE 1: NOVICE

Nurses, patients and relatives who have no experience of stoma care will initially operate at this level because they will be unfamiliar with what should be done and how to do it. Novices need to be taught about stoma care in ways that support them as they acquire experience and skills. This includes:

(a) through rules or guidelines on how to act; e.g. the steps that need to be taken to empty or change an appliance (see Ch. 4)
(b) through fulfilment of tasks they can learn to do outside the clinical context or as steps related to practical stoma care; e.g. practising preparation of new equipment; learning to match items of stomal equipment with items on their list of equipment they will require at home
(c) through descriptions and indications of elements of a situation that can be explained without prior exposure to real situations; e.g. at what stage to order more equipment in order to maintain adequate supplies; at what level of fullness to empty a urostomy bag.

It is important to remember these rules do not tell people which are the most relevant tasks to perform in actual situations and they do not have the experience to guide them. However, they enable novices to begin to get enough experience which in time they will be able to use to guide more flexible actions.

STAGE 2: ADVANCED BEGINNER

These are people who can demonstrate marginally acceptable performance. They have had enough experience to be able to note (or have pointed out to them) the recurrent meaningful components of situations because this prior experience enables them to recognise what characteristics or cues look like. See, *for example*, Patient scenario 7.2 in Chapter 7, where Mr Patel has had enough experience to be able to use feedback given to him by Mrs Reid.

Advanced beginners can be helped to utilise principles or guidelines that indicate which actions could or should be taken in certain situations. For example, see the differences in Chapter 4 between the basic steps of changing equipment which would be taught to novices and the principles of self-care which patients and nurses with some experience could understand and learn to follow.

It is important to remember that advanced beginners will not yet have enough experience to recognise the relative importance or unimportance of various elements of a situation. They therefore need help to:

(a) recognise different aspects of a situation and set priorities from amongst these various elements
(b) recognise which patient needs are more important.

In order to safeguard and promote fulfilment of patients' needs advanced beginners need to have colleagues who have acquired at least the competent level of skills available to work with them; for example, to help them gain and apply knowledge of different appliances and skin care aids when considering the needs of specific patients (see Chs 4 and 6).

STAGE 3: COMPETENT

Nurses operating at competent level are likely to have been working *in the same or similar situations for 2–3 years*. During this time they have built up expertise with patients having similar types of surgery and/or alternative treatments and the kinds of needs and problems that are likely to arise. These nurses are consciously aware of the need to plan care that is congruent with patients' current needs and will promote their future rehabilitation, and use analytical skills to do so. They lack the speed and flexibility of nurses at proficient level, but they do have a feeling of mastery and the ability to cope with, and manage multiple aspects of clinical care. *For example*, Nurse Beech's work with Mr and Mrs Earl in Chapter 8 (Patient scenario 8.5).

Nurses who have gained a competent level of expertise benefit from practice in planning and coordinating multiple, complex care demands. It is therefore important that these nurses (and their managers) assess whether the level of expertise that particular courses seek to promote is congruent with their needs. Learning activities such as using case studies and simulations should be built in to courses and study days they attend so they are encouraged to expand the complexity of patient situations and types of care they can manage, and develop flexible ways of evaluating the outcomes of their practice.

STAGE 4: PROFICIENT

At this level nurses perceive situations *as a whole* rather than in terms of aspects of the situation. They know from experience what typical events to expect in given situations, can recognise changes from the norm, and how their actions need to be modified in response. This perspective is generally not consciously 'thought out' but rather presents itself as a holistic sense of the situation and key responses that are needed. Proficient level nurses use *maxims* or cryptic descriptions of skilled performance as guides. Maxims reflect nuances of a situation and can provide direction as to what must be taken into consideration but, as their meaning can change in different situations, their use may be limited for all but equally skilled colleagues. However, proficient performers will regress to a competent analytical level if this is required in the particular situation (e.g. to teach less advanced colleagues or to clarify the basis on which their responses are being made) or if they are in a new or unusual situation and need to consciously work out what is required.

Benner (1984, p 31) suggests that this level of performance can usually be found in nurses *who have worked with similar client groups for about 3–5 years*. Proficient performers can frequently recognise deterioration/problems/early warning signals in patients prior to explicit changes in their vital signs. For example, an experienced ward sister or stoma care nurse might recognise subtle changes in a patient's condition either because they had substantial experience of how that patient normally 'came across' or because they could compare this with their experiences of many other patients in similar circumstances.

STAGE 5: EXPERT

Expert performers no longer rely on analytical principles (e.g. rules, guidelines, maxims) to connect their understanding of a situation to appropriate action. Their substantial experience in their particular field gives them an intuitive grasp of situations, enabling them to zero in accurately on the problem area and/or key aspects of care that are needed without spending time consciously considering a range of possible alternatives.

Experts are strongly influenced by the context and meanings or implications inherent in situations. Their evaluation of what is, or could be, needed is shaped by the particular elements that make up an individual situation as a whole rather than by generalised context-free principles; *for example*, Mrs Reid's work with Mr Fletcher, particularly in Chapter 22 (see Patient scenario 22.2). However, Benner also points out that experts will need to use analytical problem-solving skills in situations where they have not had previous experience, or they have grasped the situation wrongly and events and behaviour are not turning out as expected.

Patients and their families can benefit hugely from this kind of informed, perceptive and personalised expert care. However, its intuitive nature may leave less expert nurses unable to identify how their colleague knew what to do and how to do it. Likewise the elegant combination of the skills they used may make it hard for less experienced nurses to recognise what they were and how and why they were combined. Expert nurses should also acquire both the commitment and ability to 'unpack' or describe their practice in ways that enable the knowledge and judgements inherent in it to become visible to their colleagues, and thus able to be learned and utilised (e.g. Grey 2004, Salter 1998; see also Ch. 23). Examples of such 'unpacking' are shown in the *patient scenarios* and level of detail used to describe aspects of care throughout this book.

As you will see from the above descriptions these different levels reflect changes in three general aspects of skilled performance. Firstly, there is a movement from reliance on abstract principles to the use of past concrete experience as paradigms (models, patterns, examples). Secondly, the learner's perception of situations where care is required changes, being seen less and less as made up of equally relevant bits, and increasingly becoming viewed as a complete whole, in which only certain parts are relevant. Thirdly, the person moves from being a 'detached' observer to an 'involved' performer. They no longer stand outside the situation but are engaged in it.

Skilled performance involves both interventions and clinical judgement, including how we interpret situations, the intentions that direct our actions, and what we do or do not do. This is as true for stoma care as a whole as it is for some of the smaller strands that help to make it up. You can use this model of skill acquisition to consider your development in stoma care as a whole, or in particular aspects of it. *For example,* you could reflect on your levels of practice in physical aspects of care and psychological aspects separately. You may have major competence in working with patients with conventional stomas but minimal experience with those who have internal pouches and want to extend your abilities with this second group. You might identify that your counselling skills are at advanced beginner level and that now you want to gain further expertise in order to provide some of the more advanced approaches described in the book.

Likewise you can use this book to consider specific aspects of stoma care, or review it as a whole. Chapter 1 provides an overview of rehabilitative stoma care. It will give you a sense of the breadth and depth of care that can be provided. Subsequent chapters have been grouped in sections to enable you and your colleagues to develop your expertise in particular aspects of stoma care. The first section, on physiological and surgical aspects and practical care, has the relatively narrow focus that most nurses use when first learning stoma care. Each of the following sections moves to a wider and deeper view of stoma care. This will help you and other readers move through the levels of development that Benner et al (1996) describe, expanding your perspective of the care that patients may need, and the knowledge and skills with which to provide it.

As you consider the information in the various chapters you will find there is a major focus on *how* care can be given as well as what care is needed. This will enable you and your colleagues to add to the skills you already use, as well as your knowledge. However you may be unfamiliar with some of the approaches (particularly those from non-nursing fields) that have been described. You may initially wonder whether they are relevant and possible to include in your own practice. Over the years I have found that, at the beginning of courses I have run in communication, counselling, loss and bereavement, and neurolinguistic programming (NLP), colleagues have regularly asked me whether the models, skills and approaches I would be teaching them could realistically be used to inform and enhance patients' care. Equally regularly, as the courses continued, feedback from those colleagues (in all branches of nursing) indicated that the skills and approaches were indeed learnable, usable, and enabling them to respond more helpfully in a wide range of situations. I have used this feedback plus other colleagues' comments and suggestions, as well as my own training and experience in these fields, to make sure that the approaches included in this book are ones that can be used by many nurses as part of their normal care.

References

Benner P 1984 From novice to expert. Addison-Wesley, Menlo Park, CA

Benner P, Tanner C A, Chesla C A 1996 Expertise in nursing practice. Springer, New York

Grey A 2004 Meeting the diverse needs of urological cancer patients. Cancer Nursing Practice 3(1):19–26

Salter M 1998 If you can help somebody (Nursing interventions to facilitate adaptation to an altered body image). In: World Council of Enterostomal Therapists congress proceedings. Horton Print Group, Bradford, West Yorkshire, p 229–235

Chapter 1

What is rehabilitative stoma care?

Brigid Breckman

In this book the term *stoma* refers to an artificial opening created surgically for patients in order to allow their urine or faeces to leave their body by a new route: through this spout or outlet on their abdomen. The term *stoma care* is used to describe two things:

- the components of patients' overall nursing care which they need because they have, or will have, a stoma
- a style of nursing care, which informs and supports patients pre- and postoperatively for the purpose of helping them achieve the kind of lifestyle, self-image and experience of being physically and psychologically rehabilitated that they define as normal and acceptable to them (Breckman 1991).

This style of nursing therefore includes helping patients handle any areas that are relevant to their wellbeing and ability to rehabilitate. These include:

- *tasks*, such as management of their stoma and appliance
- *issues*, such as whether their surgery is likely to be curative or affect sexual function
- *experiences*, such as discovering they have cancer, handling questions about their operation at work and socially.

Many patients go through at least three main stages on their road to rehabilitation. Firstly, they learn to basically look after their stoma and manage their equipment. This requires some thought and careful actions initially, but gradually becomes more automatic, and achieved without much conscious thought or concern by the majority of patients. The next main stage depends to some extent on the degree of physical health and strength regained by the patient. At this stage the patient, complete with stoma, engages in the kinds of activities they regard as part of their normal lifestyle. The presence of this physical rehabilitation does not necessarily mean that the patient's emotional or psychological rehabilitation has also occurred: this often takes longer. In the third stage patients report thinking of themselves, and feeling 'back to normal' or 'being myself again'. The stoma by now is experienced as an integral part of the person rather than separate or added onto them. This psychological rehabilitation is not achieved by all patients (Wade 1989, White 1999).

Our perception of what rehabilitation entails, and the length of time it takes patients to achieve it, influences the components of stoma care we think we should provide and the length of time over which we believe our care should be affecting patients. Stoma care is generally most helpful when it enables patients to achieve each of the above rehabilitative stages. Our care must therefore be relevant to patients' needs at the time we provide it *and* of a type that will also promote their longer-term physical and psychological rehabilitation.

The ability to provide 'care for now which is also care for later' is a key component of rehabilitative stoma care. It is similar to using a camera with a zoom lens. Every time we provide care we zoom in to get a close-up focus on what our patient needs now. Then we retract the zoom in order to see the larger picture. This perspective reminds us of the patient's individual circumstances and rehabilitative goals as a whole. We use the information from both positions to identify and provide care that meets their current needs and supports their longer term recovery. Acquiring the ability to provide care in this way is not only beneficial to patients and their families. The sense of being actively involved in promoting their long-term rehabilitation is rewarding for staff also.

The question of how long a time we should be thinking of when we plan care for ongoing rehabilitation is difficult to answer precisely. Research indicates that sizeable numbers of patients can still be experiencing major problems one year after surgery (Wade 1989, Pringle & Swan 2001). Discussions with patients and stoma care nurses over the past thirty years indicate that patients generally seem to fall into two groups.

Patients who gain relief from long-standing symptoms which have significantly curtailed their lives

often appear to rehabilitate within 6–12 months of surgery. Achievement of this rehabilitative timespan seems higher in patients who have had less extensive surgery from which to recover.

Patients who have had more extensive surgery (e.g. abdomino-perineal excision of rectum, cysto-urethrectomy) can take up to two years to achieve their maximum rehabilitation. This longer period of time seems more common when patients have had shorter periods of illness and incapacitating symptoms prior to surgery.

Accepting that this length of time may be needed to rehabilitate becomes easier when we consider two major processes which patients will usually be undergoing during this time. Firstly, this type of surgery leads most patients to experience varying degrees of loss and change and they need to come to terms with these experiences. Much of the research into people's experience of bereavement and loss found periods of up to two years were required for their recovery (e.g. Parkes 1998, Worden 2003). Secondly, patients need to acquire sizeable amounts of information and a range of skills with which to manage their stoma care and living with a stoma and the effects of their surgery. Research into nurses' acquisition of skills has shown that it was only after 2–3 years of working with the same patient group that nurses developed competent level skills which included feelings of mastery and the ability to cope with, and manage, multiple aspects of clinical care (Benner 1984, Benner et al 1996). Since patients have, of necessity, to manage living with their stoma daily this amount of experience may speed up their acquisition of relevant knowledge and skills if these are built up from an adequate foundation. However, it is reasonable to accept that it could still take them 1–2 years to acquire that sense of mastery and confidence in themselves and their ability to live normal lives which they want 'being rehabilitated' to include.

In the light of these research and anecdotal reports it seems useful to think of our rehabilitative care as needing to inform and support patients over a 2-year period. However, the time in which hospital staff can help patients acquire an adequate foundation of knowledge and skills is shrinking as the time patients generally spend having surgery and recuperating before discharge is being reduced. The availability of stoma care and community nurses to support and advise patients through home visits is also changing. Anecdotal evidence suggests that the financial goals that managers are required to meet are leading to constraints on the number of home visits clinical nurses can carry out. These circumstances mean we must be able to:

- grasp opportunities to provide information and care in the time available
- enable patients to identify their rehabilitative goals and organise our care so it maximises support for their achievement
- identify specifically how information, care and teaching is linked to patients' wellbeing and rehabilitative goals, so we can highlight their relevance and necessity to colleagues as well as patients and their families
- help patients acquire a foundation of knowledge and skills which will enable them to continue their rehabilitation without being dependent on extensive ongoing input from the healthcare team
- create sufficient rapport and collaboration in our relationship with patients to enable them to initiate contact with us if they require additional help in the future when appointments with the healthcare team may be minimal.

The style of care we provide has important implications for patients' experiences and development of expertise. Obviously patient care includes completion of tasks that need to be done in order to manage aspects of their situation, treatment, and physical and psychological wellbeing. However, if we mainly perceive care as a series of tasks to be done, we can end up judging whether care was successful or appropriate by focusing solely on whether those tasks were completed. This distracts our attention from the effects of our care on patients and whether the outcomes they experience from our activities meet their needs or help them achieve their goals.

In rehabilitative stoma care our focus is primarily patient-centred rather than task-centred. Initially healthcare staff start with a mental map of the care patients, with a particular condition and treatment, generally need. This map influences the information and care we assume will be needed. Each patient's goals, which they want to achieve as they undergo surgery and rehabilitation, should be identified and documented so they are available to all the healthcare team. When this is done we can adapt elements of care so they are congruent with, and supportive of, patients' individual goals. This practice encourages us to monitor whether what we are doing, and how we are doing it, is promoting desirable goals and experiences for individual patients. In addition

to looking for evidence that we have successfully completed a task, we seek evidence that the patient's experience is as it should be.

For example, patients experiencing nausea usually want it relieved or minimised. Our goal should therefore also be to have relieved their nausea. The task of giving appropriate medication is a strategy (a means to an end) through which we hope to relieve their nausea. Evaluation of success involves asking the patient about their experience: has their nausea been relieved and, if so, is the relief they are experiencing at a level that is satisfactory for them?

Patients' rehabilitative goals are likely to include psychological aspects as well as physical ones. For example, they may say they want to feel confident when changing stomal equipment as well as to be competent in doing so. In the past it has been assumed that if patients regained or developed the ability to physically do what they wanted (e.g. go to work; meet friends; go on holiday), then their psychological experiences (e.g. how they felt/ thought about themselves and their ability to handle such situations with confidence and enjoyment) would automatically develop in line with their physical capability, enabling their psychological wellbeing to also be successfully achieved. There is growing research evidence that this does not necessarily occur (e.g. Wade 1989, Pringle & Swan 2001, White 1999).

Key assumptions underpinning the style of care described in this book are that:

- each time we provide any stoma care we have an opportunity to make it 'care for now plus care for later' and thus assist long-term rehabilitation
- any stoma care provided will have both a physical and a psychological element to it, which will lead to patients experiencing physical and psychological outcomes; we must therefore plan and provide our care so that it actively fosters psychological as well as physical outcomes which are helpful for individual patients
- patients and their families generally welcome care that actively helps them promote their psychological wellbeing as well as physical rehabilitation
- the quality of the communication and collaboration in our practice affects the levels of wellbeing and rehabilitation patients experience.

Research underpinning this last assumption will be discussed in more detail in later chapters so it can be linked to useful communication skills. Key points to remember here are that:

- the levels of information we give patients must be congruent with the levels of information they think they need; a mismatch of too much or too little can lead to dissatisfaction and depression (Pringle & Swan 2001)
- new patients who engaged in collaborative discussion when making decisions about their colostomy management have reported higher levels of satisfaction than patients who had less collaborative decision-making approaches used with them (Thompson 1998).

The care described in this book will help you work in a collaborative manner. This includes providing information and involving patients in decision-making at the levels they individually require rather than imposing them. Such care falls into five main areas, which overlap to some extent. We can use these as a framework to consider how we can recognise patients' needs and help them achieve their goals in each area.

These areas are:

- care that helps patients prepare for surgery
- care in the initial postoperative period
- care that helps patients become knowledgeable about living with their stoma
- care that helps patients become adept at their own stoma care
- care that promotes and supports continuation and further development of patients' physical and psychological rehabilitation.

Throughout the book there are *patient scenarios*. These give *examples* of how various collaborative approaches can be used to help patients achieve goals and increase their wellbeing in each of these care areas. They are *not* meant to be prescriptive. They give you opportunities to consider what such approaches might be like in action and whether you and your colleagues could use or adapt them in your own practice. The issues in them have all been raised by real patients, relatives and nurses. However, the descriptions of people in the scenarios are composites, each based on several people, in order to protect individuals' confidentiality. Likewise the stoma care nurse in the scenarios, Mrs Reid, is not based on one particular nurse but demonstrates values and capabilities shown by many expert colleagues. I hope the descriptions of her work with various patients will give a sense of the range of issues that specialist nurses seek to address, and the depth and diversity of practice that can be involved.

Generally, if we ask patients what their lives are normally like, or were like before illness curtailed them, we will acquire a wealth of information which can shape our care and help us identify rehabilitative goals patients want to achieve. Often these are relevant to more than one area of care. It is useful to get in the habit of specifically making a mental note of information we recognise we may want to use in subsequent interactions with patients as this aids recall later.

In the rest of this chapter I am providing two *patient scenarios* featuring the same patient to help you get a real sense of what 'rehabilitative stoma care' can be like in action. You may like to make a note of information you think you and your colleagues would want to use, either when it was given or later, if you were looking after this patient. This will also help you make the most of later scenarios involving the same patient.

PATIENT SCENARIOS

In an ideal world all patients would be seen by a stoma care nurse before they were admitted for surgery so that they would have the maximum time in which to acquire relevant information and have help to deal with concerns. However, such pre-admission care does not always occur. Nurses and patients then need to be able to use the limited time between admission and operation to maximum advantage. I have therefore deliberately used a situation where the patient has not seen the stoma care nurse before his admission. For clarity I am basically using scenarios with one patient, Mr Fletcher, and two nurses: Mrs Reid, who is a stoma care nurse, and Staff Nurse Linden, who works on a surgical ward. The two scenarios highlight some aspects of pre- and postoperative care, and how it is shaped by John and Mary Fletcher's particular concerns and needs.

PATIENT SCENARIO 1.1: Staff Nurse Linden has been working on a busy surgical ward for the past 18 months. Patients are frequently admitted here for stoma surgery, and she enjoys looking after them. Today she has admitted John Fletcher, a 55-year old married man who has rectal cancer. He is due to have his rectum removed and a colostomy formed in a few days time. Nurse Linden has already looked at his medical notes, so she knows that his rectal cancer was only diagnosed very recently in the outpatients department, following an urgent referral from his GP. In addition, she has gained general background information from Mr Fletcher about himself as part of her admission procedure. He tells her he prefers to be called John.

Nurse Linden already has a general understanding of the care that patients usually require to help them prepare for stoma surgery. She combines this with the specific information John has now given. This enables her to assess whether her initial concept of his situation and the care he might require needs to be adapted. When Nurse Linden was admitting John she gave him a certain amount of information about how the ward functioned, when his doctor was likely to come and see him, and told him a specialist stoma care nurse would be coming to see him.

Later that day, while Mary Fletcher is visiting her husband, the stoma care nurse, Mrs Reid, arrives on the ward. Before she goes to see them she gathers background information about John from the nursing and medical notes, and by talking to Nurse Linden. This enables Mrs Reid to start adapting her general mental map of the components of stoma care required to create a specific concept of the care John may need. She continues this adaptation process throughout her discussions with the Fletchers. Both John and Mary have read the booklet about living with a colostomy, given to them earlier by Nurse Linden, and found the information helpful. From her conversation with the Fletchers Mrs Reid discovers that they are anxious about the amount of time he will be off work. John and a friend run a small house decorating business. His income largely depends on the work he and his partner can complete. Mary mentions that John is very independent and will not ask for help with anything. She does not want him to return to work too soon after his operation. She thinks they can manage on her wages from her part-time job for a while. Mrs Reid checks with John and Mary that she has correctly understood that an important rehabilitation goal for them is that John will return to work full-time at his business, but only when he is really fit enough to do so.

Mrs Reid also enquires about the Fletchers' understanding of his condition, what the surgery will include, and how a colostomy generally appears and functions. Both of them know he has cancer, and have a good understanding of the planned surgery and what the stoma could look

like. Mrs Reid learns that the Fletchers generally handle difficulties by dealing with them when they occur, rather than worrying about them beforehand. Mary says they are not going to even think for a minute that John's operation might not be successful and that, if it interferes with his sexual ability, they will sort that out when they have to. Mrs Reid notices John looks upset at this point, and mutters that he will be like an old man soon. She decides that she will clarify with the doctors how extensive the surgery might have to be and what degree of sexual impairment they think might occur before she next sees John, in case he wants to discuss these areas in more depth or express his feelings more openly. She knows patients often welcome this kind of psychological support. She tells John and Mary that she wants to do this, and also to begin to discuss his rehabilitation plans with the other nurses, so that everyone is working in the same direction. They think this is a good idea.

As Mrs Reid continues to talk to John on other visits, her understanding of the physical and psychological style of rehabilitation that John wants becomes more detailed. Information gained now, such as John's difficulty in asking for help, gets used throughout the rest of his planned care in the form of physical and psychological strategies for helping John get any help he needs at each stage. Since Nurse Linden is familiar with the care most stoma patients generally require she and Mrs Reid can use that as a shared mental map with which to discuss the actual style and components of care John needs, and the rehabilitative goals that John and Mary have identified at this point.

Their next step is to discuss John's goals with other staff involved in his care. This step is essential so that any conflicting ideas regarding his care can be identified and resolved. Nurse Linden outlines John's goals and the reasons for them at report time. Care that will help John achieve his goals is beginning to be identified and Nurse Linden will use this information when writing his care plan.

At this point an event occurs that is quite common. Some staff question the inclusion of particular topics in discussion with John and Mary. They express concern over the depth of information they feel they will be expected to provide on normal sexual function and how this could be affected by John's surgery. Sister Stone, the ward sister, uses this opportunity to show how teamwork can be used to help John achieve his goals *and* identify and meet goals held by various members of staff. She asks Mrs Reid to join the discussion to provide more information on John's needs and goals. She also encourages her colleagues to clarify the goals they want to achieve whilst looking after John. This open discussion enables several *staff goals* to emerge, including:

- two nurses want to avoid discussing sexual issues with John without upsetting him
- two nurses want to gain more information about possible sexual impairment after abdomino-perineal excision of rectum, and to be able to give the kind of advice that would be helpful for John and Mary Fletcher
- Mrs Reid and Sister Stone are able and want to encourage the Fletchers to talk about any sexual concerns, and to give appropriate basic information, advice, and counselling in response
- Nurse Linden can give some basic information about possible sexual impairment, but wants to be better able to help the Fletchers express feelings and needs if they want to do so
- the registrar and house officer are willing to answer questions about possible physical impairment if John asks any
- the consultant generally prefers his registrar to deal with any discussion about sex.

The nurses and junior doctors take account of these goals as well as John's goal of knowing now what possible impairment there might be after his operation, plus Mary's stated strategy of not thinking about any possible problems until they have turned into actual ones. The strategies used to meet these goals include the following:

- Mr Spender, the registrar, and Sister Stone run a joint ward teaching session on the sexual impairment that may occur with different kinds of stoma surgery.
- Mrs Reid encourages nurses to identify and try out helpful ways of accepting and acknowledging a patient's need to gain information and/or express feelings, and combine this with referral to a colleague who is willing and able to provide the desired care.
- During her lunchtime teaching reports Sister Stone promotes discussion on the kind of information and advice on sexual function patients on the ward might need. She wants staff to become more aware of, and comfortable with these areas of care, and include them in the care they plan and give those patients.

- Mrs Reid takes Nurse Linden with her to observe how she introduces the topics of changing body image and sexual function when working with John, and the strategies and skills she uses to help him voice fears and feelings and handle the uncertainty about the outcomes of his surgery. This first step to help Nurse Linden achieve her goal also encourages John to believe that his concerns are viewed as important by nurses providing his care.

Discussing what care John Fletcher needs, and what care the nurses feel able to give, has encouraged them to identify ways of expanding and becoming more confident in their practice. It has also helped the team looking after John to identify some resources they do have: staff who have relevant background knowledge, and staff who are skilled in appropriate methods of communication, all of which can be utilised by the team. It is highly likely that John will get more skilled, informed care as a result of this initial discussion on goals, and strategies for achieving them. The time has therefore been well spent.

I suggested earlier in this chapter that the components and style of stoma care that we give should aim to meet both the patient's immediate physical and psychological needs, *and* promote his long-term physical and psychological rehabilitation. In Patient scenario 1.1 Mary mentioned that her husband is very independent, and will not ask for help. In the next scenario, that information is being used to help John and Mary make plans for his first few weeks at home.

PATIENT SCENARIO 1.2: A few days postoperatively Mrs Reid is beginning to teach John Fletcher how to look after his stoma. He still gets easily tired, and seems rather concerned when she tells him it will probably take at least a couple of months before he regains much energy, although he will notice a gradual improvement in what he can do without getting overtired. Given John's reluctance to ask for help, and the reality that his wife will need to continue working when he comes home because of their financial situation, it is important to consider how he will get help and avoid overdoing things in his early days at home when Mary is out at work.

Mrs Reid has quite a lot of information by now about the kind of physical and psychological rehabilitation John wants to achieve, gained through discussions with both John and Mary. However, the plans for how John will move from how he is physically and psychologically now to achieving his rehabilitated state are still too vague to help him successfully move from one to the other. While John is learning to manage his own stoma care, and increasing his knowledge about living with his colostomy, he can also be helped to work out how he can bridge that gap between now and being fully rehabilitated.

Firstly, she asks John to tell her what he thinks his day will generally be like in the first week at home, and what Mary's day will be like. Next she asks John what he would like to achieve, or be able to have done, during that first week, and also how he would like to be feeling in himself. His answer begins to provide her with the information they will both need to identify:
- *goals* that promote his rehabilitation
- *components of care* that will support those goals (including self-care)
- *processes* through which the relevant care might be provided in the context of his home, and to fit in with the reality that Mary will be at work for four days each week.

Mrs Reid gives John information about suitable levels of activities for his first month at home, and the importance of also planning and getting adequate periods of rest. She uses specific goals, such as fixing up an easy method of obtaining his supply of stomal equipment, to encourage John to see this detailed planning as a really worthwhile aid to achieving a gradual return to his normal lifestyle, and fitting his stoma into it.

Mrs Reid notices that John does not seem to be planning much psychological support for himself. Since he dislikes asking for help she thinks it could be particularly important for him to build into his rehabilitation plan specific, regular supportive measures which will enable his psychological rehabilitation to take place. She starts this process by giving John and Mary some information about the kinds of processes many patients go through as they come to terms with the alterations in how they look and how their bowels function, and any changes in sexual function. She also stresses that it takes time for most people to come to terms with having had surgery for cancer. She continues with the information that many patients find it useful to take time to consider which friends, relatives, etc. they would enjoy being with, or who could provide some kind of supportive contact which would help them as they learn to believe they are acceptable human beings, complete with stoma, and resume social and other activities. Actively building contact with a variety of suitable people into the planned rehabilitative routine helps prevent any one person getting overloaded with responsibility for giving emotional support. It also increases the likelihood that people who value and care for the patient will be readily available if he needs a listening ear to hear about problems or support his expression of feelings.

By presenting this concept of psychological rehabilitation as 'information about strategies which other patients have found useful' Mrs Reid gives the Fletchers the opportunity to consider it without pressure to adopt it wholesale. It opens the door for them to explore their feelings and needs with each other, with support from the staff as appropriate. By the time John goes home he is more likely to have expanded his original set of physical goals and strategies to complete his rehabilitation to include psychological goals and strategies as well.

References

Benner P 1984 From novice to expert. Addison-Wesley, Menlo Park, CA

Benner P, Tanner C A, Chesla C A 1996 Expertise in nursing practice. Springer, New York

Breckman B 1991 Communicating stoma care. Unpublished teaching manual, BA (Hons) submission, University of East London

Parkes C M 1998 Bereavement: studies of grief in adult life, 3rd edn. Penguin Books, London

Pringle W, Swan E 2001 Continuing care after discharge from hospital for stoma patients. British Journal of Nursing 10(19):1274–1288

Thompson J 1998 Patient participation in decisions about longterm colostomy management. In: World Council of Enterostomal Therapists congress proceedings. Horton Print Group, Bradford, West Yorkshire, p 167–172

Wade B 1989 A stoma is for life. Scutari Press, London

White C A 1999 Psychological aspects of stoma care. In: Taylor P (ed) Stoma care in the community. Nursing Times Books, London, p 89–109

Worden J W 2003 Grief counselling and grief therapy, 3rd edn. Brunner-Routledge, Hove, UK

SECTION 1

Practical care for patients with 'conventional' stomas

Chapter 2

Intestinal physiology and its implications for patients with bowel stomas

Ann Richards

We all have our own favourite foods which may or may not be 'healthy'. Between cultures, diets vary enormously, and our own diet may differ greatly from day to day. Whatever we actually choose to eat and drink, our digestive system ensures that all is broken down to the simplest components which can then be absorbed into the bloodstream and used for energy, growth and repair. Any indigestible remains are eliminated as faeces. The gastrointestinal tract thus provides the body with a constant supply of water, electrolytes and nutrients. Normally we take this very much for granted. It is not until we experience problems with the system that we realise how vital its smooth functioning is to our daily existence.

Stoma care takes place in situations where patients' normal system of digesting and absorbing foods is surgically altered through gut resection and/or through diversion of faeces out of the body before they have passed through the complete gastrointestinal system. It is that reality with which patients require our help. The ability to use physiological knowledge in order to plan and provide information and care and monitor patients' conditions is a key part of expert stoma care. As you will see, much of the practical care described in the following chapters is derived from applying the information in this chapter but detailed explanations of how, precisely, physiological effects and implications are being responded to in the practical care described are not spelled out in those chapters to avoid repetition. It is from this chapter that you can get a useful overview of digestive function with which to make sense of patients' situations, physiologically, and on which you can base the information and care you provide. Since most stomal diversions primarily affect digestive processes that occur in the small intestine to anal bowel section the main focus in this chapter is in this area.

As you read this chapter you will enhance your ability to use the information in it if you apply it to a patient you know, remembering the operation they had and in what part of the bowel their stoma was created. For example, if your patient had her colon removed and an ileostomy formed out of terminal ileum, use the information in this chapter to answer the following questions:

- What physiological functions would she still have with which to digest and absorb food and drink?
- What physiological functions might she have lost, or reduced, and might these be temporary or permanent?
- As a result of the answers to the last two questions, what advice would you give her as to what she can, and should, eat and drink? Are there foods you think she should avoid, and why?
- Based on your answers to the first three questions, what would you expect her stoma effluent to be like (e.g. amount passed, consistency, frequency)?
- Given the above information, what type of appliance would she probably need to use?
- Would she need to protect her skin from stomal effluent? If so, why? What level of skin protection might you advise her to use (e.g. minimal, moderate, substantial)?

These questions can also be used when thinking of patients who have had other types of resection and/or diversion. As you become more skilled in applying your physiological knowledge in this way you will find it easy to do so when you are making sense of patients' notes (e.g. their condition and operation) and identifying the specific information and care they individually need.

More comprehensive information on the whole digestive system, i.e. the alimentary canal (mouth, oesophagus, stomach, small and large intestines, rectum and anus) and the accessory organs of digestion (salivary glands, pancreas, liver and gall bladder) is provided in physiology texts (e.g. Guyton & Hall 2000, Marieb 2003, Montague et al 2005).

Food is ingested at the mouth and, after swallowing, moves along the digestive tract being mixed and churned as it progresses (Fig. 2.1). Digestion is the process of breakdown of this food into a form that can be absorbed into the bloodstream. It is both

mechanical and chemical in nature. Mechanical digestion includes such processes as chewing, churning and grinding of food which all aid its breakdown. Chemical digestion ensures complex nutrients are split into simpler molecules by the action of secretions containing enzymes.

- Carbohydrates, which include sugars and starches, are broken down to simple sugar molecules such as glucose.
- Fats and oils are broken down to fatty acids and glycerol.
- Proteins are broken down to amino acids.

These simpler molecules can now be absorbed into the bloodstream or lymphatics to be used by the body for the production of energy or for growth and repair. The absorption of these nutrients mostly occurs in the small intestine and any disordered functioning here may lead to poor digestion and absorption of food products.

For digestion to occur, the time the food spends in each part of the tract is critical. The need for propulsion and mixing of the food changes as it is processed and for these to occur at the optimal rate both nervous and hormonal control is necessary. The time taken for nutrients to pass along the digestive tract (transit time) depends on the type of food eaten (see Table 2.1 for approximate times). Fatty foods stay in the stomach longest and so give a feeling of satiety.

From the oesophagus through to the anus the basic structure of the tract follows the same pattern, with some functional adaptations throughout its length. Structure is always related to function. To understand how both the healthy and the disordered gastrointestinal tract function, a basic knowledge of its structure is needed.

STRUCTURE OF THE GASTROINTESTINAL TRACT

The wall of the tract generally consists of four layers: (1) the mucosa; (2) the submucosa; (3) the muscularis; and (4) the serosa (adventitia).

Table 2.1 Approximate length of time spent by food in areas of the digestive tract

Oesophagus	4–8 seconds
Stomach	4–5 hours
Small intestine	3–6 hours
Large intestine	8–15 hours

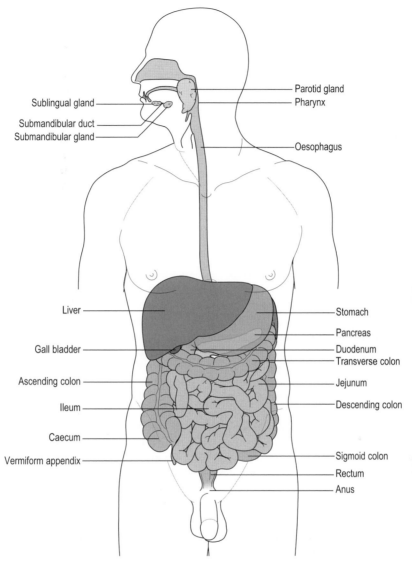

Figure 2.1   The gastrointestinal tract. From Smith (2005).

THE MUCOSA

This is the lining of the tract and is made up of three layers – a surface epithelial layer, a connective tissue layer and a thin muscular layer. Throughout the gastrointestinal tract these three layers vary in thickness and glandular development.

The main functions of the mucosa are:

- secretion of mucus, digestive enzymes and hormones
- protection – there are patches of lymphoid tissue in this layer
- absorption of digestive products into the blood.

In inflammatory conditions of the bowel there is often an increased production of mucus, which can be seen in the stools.

THE SUBMUCOSA

This layer lies beneath the mucosa and consists of connective tissue containing a rich supply of blood vessels, lymphatic vessels, nerve fibres and elastic fibres.

Its nerve supply is called the submucosal plexus and it is part of the autonomic nervous system, which is important in regulating the secretions of the mucosa.

Parasympathetic nerves usually increase secretion and thus aid digestion, whilst sympathetic nerves decrease secretion.

THE MUSCULARIS

This layer is formed of muscle fibres and mixes and propels food along the gastrointestinal tract. There is an inner circular layer and an outer longitudinal layer of smooth, involuntary muscle which is not under conscious control.

In several parts of the tract the inner circular layer thickens to form sphincters which prevent back flow of food and also control its passage from one part of the tract to the next. The external anal sphincter is striated muscle and thus under voluntary control, enabling continence to be maintained.

Between the circular and longitudinal muscle layers is the myenteric plexus. This is another autonomic nerve supply controlling motility which is increased by parasympathetic activity and decreased by sympathetic activity.

Peristalsis is the main movement of the gastrointestinal tract and consists of contraction above a section of bowel, and relaxation below, ensuring the passage of food substances along the tube in one direction. There are other gut movements which all appear to be adaptations of this mechanism. Examples are segmentation and mass movement, which occur in the colon and will be described later.

A stoma is formed from part of the intestine and so will be seen to move or wiggle as peristalsis is still taking place. This may be quite a surprise for clients with a new stoma, or inexperienced student nurses, who should be informed of this aspect of physiology.

THE SEROSA (ADVENTITIA)

This is the protective outer layer and is composed of a serous membrane made up of connective tissue covered with a single layer of epithelial cells. The peritoneum is the largest serous membrane in the body.

BLOOD SUPPLY

The arteries supplying the gastrointestinal tract with oxygenated blood are branches of the abdominal aorta. They include the coeliac artery, which gives rise to the gastric, splenic and hepatic arteries, and the superior and inferior mesenteric arteries, which supply the small and large intestines. Nutrient-rich venous blood from most of the tract drains into the hepatic portal vein and is taken to the liver, which is involved in the metabolic processing of these nutrients.

DIGESTION

The mechanical digestion of food begins in the mouth where the teeth grind and crush the ingested food and mix it with saliva containing the enzyme salivary amylase which begins chemical digestion. Food is formed into a bolus in the mouth and is swallowed, passing down the oesophagus by waves of peristalsis. On entering the stomach, the food is mixed with gastric juice and pepsin, which contribute to chemical digestion, and is churned to form a thick paste called chyme that passes through the pyloric sphincter into the duodenum. Very little absorption occurs in the stomach – some water is absorbed here but in addition, only alcohol and some acidic drugs such as aspirin are absorbed to any extent. Intrinsic factor, necessary for the absorption of vitamin B_{12} and thus the prevention of pernicious anaemia, is secreted here.

Gastric contents may start to enter the duodenum 30 minutes after eating a meal and about 6–10 ml of chyme enter the duodenum every minute. The stomach usually empties completely within 4–5 hours of eating a meal although the rate of emptying depends on the type of food eaten. The larger and more fluid the meal, the more rapid the stomach emptying.

The small intestine is a convoluted tube of about 2.5 cm (1 inch) diameter and about 6 metres in length at autopsy. In the living body it is maintained substantially shorter by muscular tone and measures about 2 metres. It is the main organ of both digestion and absorption, consisting of the:

- duodenum – the first part of the small intestine – a C-shaped portion extending from the pylorus for about 25 cm (10 inches) and curving around the head of the pancreas
- jejunum – about 2.5 metres (8 feet) long
- ileum – about 3.6 metres (12 feet) long and joining the large intestine at the ileocaecal valve.

The wall of the small intestine is made up of the same four layers as the rest of the gastrointestinal tract but the mucosa and the submucosa are modified in the following ways to increase digestive and absorptive powers.

(a) The intestinal mucosa is thrown into many folds, which increase the surface area available for absorption about three-fold and also force chyme to spiral around the lumen; this ensures mixing with intestinal juices and slows its passage to allow maximum absorption to occur.

(b) From the mid-duodenum onwards there are millions (20–40 per mm^2) of finger-like projections, projecting about one millimetre from the surface of the mucosa, and covering the entire surface of the small intestine. These are the villi and increase the absorptive powers another ten-fold. Digested foodstuffs are absorbed through the epithelial cells and each villus has its own capillary blood supply to carry the absorbed nutrients into the portal circulation. It also has a central lymph vessel or lacteal into which digested fats, as triglycerides, are absorbed. The villi are largest in the duodenum and decrease in size along the small intestine.

(c) Each epithelial cell (enterocyte) in the small intestine has a brush border of about 600 microvilli protruding into the chyme. This increases the surface area another twenty-fold. If you imagine spreading the intestinal contents over the area of a tennis court, that is equivalent to the total surface area of the small intestine, i.e. 200–250 square metres.

In starvation the enterocytes shrink and this may decrease the height of the villi by up to half. This decreases the absorptive powers of the small intestine. Mucosal hypoplasia may also occur during prolonged parenteral feeding but this is fully reversible when enteric feeding is recommenced.

Damage to enterocytes may occur in coeliac disease, Crohn's disease or due to radiation or cytotoxic therapy. Such damage is likely to result in a loss of intestinal enzymes for digestion and surface area for absorption. This may necessitate dietary changes. In coeliac disease a gluten-free diet should result in the villous architecture in the small bowel returning to normal. In other cases, a bland diet with adequate protein, calories, vitamins and minerals may be needed and small, frequent meals may need to be taken.

THE DUODENUM

The duodenum itself does not secrete any enzymes but pancreatic juice enters and contains an enzyme-rich secretion which aids the digestion of carbohydrates, fats and proteins. Bile is manufactured in the liver and stored in the gall bladder. It is released into the duodenum and helps to emulsify fats, so making their digestion easier. There are glands in the submucosa of the duodenum that secrete alkaline mucus to neutralise stomach acid and to prevent self digestion.

THE JEJUNUM AND ILEUM

The mucosa of the small intestine secretes about 2000 ml of intestinal juice daily. This watery and slightly alkaline secretion (pH 7.5–8.0) is rapidly reabsorbed by the villi and acts as a vehicle for the absorption of nutrients from the chyme. If loss from an ileostomy is excessive, bicarbonate can be lost from the alkaline solution and metabolic acidosis can occur. Symptoms include deep, rapid breathing in an attempt to eliminate excess acid from the body.

People with a stoma require protection of their peristomal skin from stomal effluent. Skin is slightly acidic and is less likely to be damaged by effluent that is slightly acidic or neutral in nature. Strongly acidic or alkaline effluent will be more damaging but even non-caustic effluent can be damaging due to pooling in the peristomal area (Meadows 1997).

Enzymes involved in the completion of digestion of carbohydrates, fats and proteins are released by the brush border of the intestinal cells. In this part of the small intestine carbohydrate is broken down to glucose and other simple sugars. Protein digestion is completed to individual amino acids. Both simple sugars and amino acids are then absorbed into the bloodstream via the intestinal mucosa. Fats are hydrolysed into fatty acids and glycerol which are transported as small, spherical globules (micelles) for absorption.

MOTILITY IN THE SMALL INTESTINE

Although true peristalsis does occur it is after the absorption of most nutrients when waves of contraction pass the length of the intestine to ensure all digestive products and bacteria are moved along through the ileocaecal valve. The main muscular activity in the small intestine is called segmentation and is initiated by pacemaker cells in the longitudinal muscle layer. The intestinal contents are moved backwards and forwards a few centimetres at a time by the alternate contraction and relaxation of rings of smooth muscle. This allows a steady movement along the tract to ensure adequate time is allowed for absorption to occur. Contents take 3–6 hours to pass the length of the small intestine and, coupled with the time food is in the stomach, this means that people with an ileostomy are likely to pass food residue 7–10 hours after meals are eaten (Table 2.1).

THE LARGE INTESTINE

This extends from the ileum at the ileocaecal valve to the anus and is approximately 1.5 metres in length. It is attached to the posterior abdominal wall by visceral peritoneum (the mesocolon) and frames the small intestine. Its divisions are the: caecum, appendix, colon (ascending, transverse, descending and sigmoid), rectum, anal canal and anus.

The mucosa of the colon is simple columnar epithelium with numerous goblet cells. These produce large amounts of mucus that lubricate the faeces in their passage along the remainder of the gastrointestinal tract and also protect against bacterial products which may be acidic and irritating. There are no villi as the products of digestion have been absorbed in the small intestine and the absorptive surface of the large intestine is only about 3% of that of the small intestine.

The longitudinal muscle layer forms three thickened bands called the teniae coli. These run the length of the large intestine and give the colon a puckered appearance, gathering it into a series of pouches.

MOTILITY IN THE LARGE INTESTINE

Segmentation is the commonest type of movement seen in the large bowel. This results in mixing movements (haustrations), arising from contraction of the circular muscle fibres, and facilitating absorption. Peristalsis does occur in the colon but at a slower rate than in the rest of the tract, propelling the faeces towards the rectum. After a meal there is a gastrocolic reflex when signals from the stomach cause contractions in the terminal ileum, relaxation of the ileocaecal valve and colonic peristalsis. This leads to mass movements in the colon which are a modified form of peristalsis and only occur a few times daily. They are usually strongest for about 15 minutes during the first hour after breakfast.

DEFECATION

Elimination of faeces or flatus via the rectum is normally voluntarily controlled by using our sphincter muscles. However, a stoma does not have sphincter muscles. Patients are therefore not able to control elimination of faeces or flatus via their stoma. Some people with a sigmoid colostomy report their stoma is 'controlled' to act at particular times. This routine is actually due to regular mass movement of faeces after certain meals.

When patients have a Hartmann's procedure or 'loop' stoma they retain their distal bowel and rectum. They may pass mucus or faecal material rectally as well as via their stoma. Patients should be alerted to this possibility.

BACTERIAL ACTION IN THE COLON

Bacteria ferment some of the remaining indigestible carbohydrates and in doing so release carbon dioxide, hydrogen and methane gas. About 500 ml of these gases (flatus) may be expelled daily but this increases when foods with high carbohydrate (fibre) content are eaten, e.g. baked beans, onions and pulses. Some of the gases produced, such as hydrogen sulphide, have an unpleasant odour. This has implications for people who no longer have a sphincter to control flatus passage, and is often of concern to them. Dietary considerations are discussed in Chapter 16 and management of flatus with stomal equipment is discussed in Chapter 5.

Gases can also enter the gastrointestinal tract from swallowed air or by diffusion from the blood. Most swallowed air is usually expelled by belching and only small amounts of gas are present in the small intestine. The amount of gases entering or forming in the large intestine daily averages 7 to 10 litres, the majority of this being absorbed through the intestinal mucosa and only about 500 ml being expelled as flatus (Guyton & Hall 2000).

The characteristic odour of faeces is given by two substances arising from bacterial decomposition.

These are indole and skatole. The bacteria in the colon also synthesise some of the B complex vitamins (thiamine, folic acid and riboflavin) and vitamin K. The latter is needed for normal blood clotting and bacterial synthesis is an important source as there may be insufficient vitamin K in the diet to maintain blood coagulability.

ABSORPTION IN THE SMALL AND LARGE INTESTINE

Most absorption of water, salts and nutrient products occurs in the upper part of the small intestine. With the evolution of surgery, metabolic complications in patients with an ileostomy are becoming less common (Fumi et al 1996).

WATER

The total quantity of fluid that must be absorbed daily is equal to that ingested (approximately 2000–2500 ml), plus that secreted into the gastrointestinal tract (7000 ml). Of this, all but 1.5 litres is absorbed in the small intestine, the remainder passing into the colon. Most of this remaining fluid is absorbed in the proximal colon, leaving the distal part for storage. After total colectomy, as much as 400–1000 ml of ileostomy fluid may be excreted, resulting in chronic salt and water depletion which is compensated for by the activation of the renin-angiotensin-aldosterone system (Christl & Scheppach 1997).

After 3–10 hours in the colon the chyme has become semi-solid and is now known as faeces. The longer the faeces remain in the colon, the more water will be absorbed. Approximately 70% of the food residue is excreted within 72 hours of digestion and the remaining 30% may remain in the colon for a week or longer in those without a stoma. The wide lumen of the large intestine (diameter 5–6 cm) gives the capacity to store food residues until defecation is appropriate.

Although on average less than 10 litres of fluid enter the gut each day, 20 litres a day could be processed without the development of diarrhoea. This water absorption occurs passively, by osmosis and does not require energy.

Most water is absorbed in the jejunum, about 5–6 litres daily. About 2 litres daily are absorbed in the ileum. The remaining 1.5–2 litres are absorbed in the colon.

It follows that, usually, the more proximal a stoma the more fluid the effluent is, although other factors may have an influence on the output such as the amount of bowel resected and diet. Thus a transverse colostomy will emit a semi-fluid stool whilst a colostomy created from the sigmoid colon may well emit formed faeces (Black 2000).

Both the consistency and volume of output from a stoma will vary, dependent on the type of stoma. Output from a jejunostomy is likely to be fluid and from an ileostomy or ascending colostomy output is rather like porridge. From a transverse colostomy it will be semi-formed and from a descending or sigmoid colostomy, output may be semi-formed to formed (Meadows 1997).

SALTS

The secretions of the gastrointestinal tract contain salts as well as water. Each day 20–30 g of sodium are secreted and also have to be reabsorbed. Sodium ions are actively reabsorbed in the jejunum, ileum and colon, with chloride ions following passively. Potassium ions are passively absorbed from the ileum and colon but active absorption may also occur. In terminal ileostomies there is a tendency towards sodium and water depletion with both potassium and magnesium depletion also having been described (Fumi et al 1996). Active absorption of magnesium occurs in the jejunum and ileum. If there is any fat malabsorption this can increase any magnesium deficiency due to the fat binding the magnesium. If a low fat diet is eaten, the absorption of magnesium improves (Spiller 1993).

Calcium ions are passively absorbed in both the small intestine and the colon and also actively absorbed in the proximal small bowel, especially the duodenum. The rate of active absorption is partly controlled by parathormone and vitamin D and is dependent on the body's needs. Retention of at least half the large bowel increases the absorption of calcium. In one study (Walters 1993) 30% of patients with inflammatory bowel disease were found to have osteoporosis. However, most of these patients had had intestinal resections and had also had high lifetime doses of steroids, which would increase the risk of osteoporosis. Intestinal absorption of vitamin D is a less important source than synthesis in the skin. Kennedy et al (1983) studied calcium metabolism in 39 subjects living with a permanent ileostomy after proctocolectomy, and in a control group of 39 healthy volunteers. No significant differences were found in plasma levels of calcium, phosphate, magnesium or vitamin D.

Zinc absorption in the small intestine is facilitated by glucose. Only 15% of ingested zinc is absorbed and most is excreted in the faeces. Crohn's disease is commonly associated with a low zinc level – probably due to excessive losses of gastrointestinal secretions which have a high zinc content. Zinc supplementation has been found to be helpful in healing eczematous skin lesions in such patients (Spiller 1993).

Iron is actively absorbed from the upper part of the small intestine. Ostomists should not experience problems with iron absorption unless there is chronic blood loss such as may occur in ulcerative colitis or Crohn's disease, which could lead to iron deficiency anaemia. Only about 5–10% of total dietary iron intake is normally absorbed from the gastrointestinal tract and this appears to be partly dependent on the body's needs because in a deficiency the absorption is increased (Fairbanks & Beutler 1994).

The large intestine can absorb still more water and ions although virtually no nutrients. It is able to absorb sodium more completely than the small intestine. This active absorption of sodium aids the absorption of water. The large intestine can absorb between 5 and 7 litres of fluid and electrolytes daily but should the amount of fluids entering the colon exceed this, diarrhoea will result.

NUTRIENTS

The products of digestion are absorbed alongside the fluid in the small intestine and several hundred grams of carbohydrate, fat and protein are absorbed daily. However, the absorptive capacity of the small intestine is much greater than this. Several kilograms of carbohydrate, 500–1000 grams of fat, 500–700 grams of protein and 20 or more litres of water could be absorbed per day (Guyton & Hall 2000). This excess capacity means that about 50% of the small intestine can be removed surgically before there is an appreciable effect on digestion and absorption. Most nutrients are absorbed within the first 150–200 cm of the jejunum, fats being the exception (Wood 1996). Fat digestion is normally completed in the jejunum but the intestine has enormous reserves and the process is easily displaced downwards if the jejunum is removed (Zentler-Munro & Northfield 1993). Absorption of fats occurs throughout the small intestine.

Amino acid absorption is faster in the distal jejunum than in the ileum. Small intestine enterocytes show active, energy-dependent uptake of glucose and galactose with an absorptive capacity well in excess of any quantity likely to be ingested. Maldigestion of lactose, sucrose or fructose leads to extra fluid entering the small intestine and symptoms of flatulence, abdominal colic and diarrhoea.

VITAMINS

Vitamin B_{12} combines with the intrinsic factor secreted in the stomach and is actively absorbed from the terminal ileum attached to a co-transporter. Resection of more than 60 cm of ileum almost always leads to B_{12} deficiency (Hoffbrand 1993) and so B_{12} therapy may be started postoperatively in these cases. Deficiency would not show for 2–3 years when liver stores of B_{12} run out.

Water-soluble vitamins (B group and C) are absorbed passively with water and by active transport throughout the small intestine and so failure of absorption is rare except after massive intestinal resection. The usual cause of deficiency is inadequate intake (Spiller 1993).

Absorption of folate takes place exclusively in the small intestine (Gregory 1995), mostly in the duodenum and jejunum. Absorption from the lower small intestine is substantially less and folates are not absorbed from the large intestine. However, many colonic bacteria are capable of synthesising folate and this ability is lost following colectomy, sometimes necessitating supplementation. Folate is an increasingly important vitamin, not only to prevent neural tube defects in pregnancy but also to reduce plasma homocysteine levels which are associated with an increased risk of cardiovascular disease (Riddell et al 2000).

Absorption of the fat-soluble vitamins A, D, E and K is dependent on the production of bile and the absorption of fats. In the presence of bile approximately 97% of fat is absorbed in the small intestine. In the absence of bile acids, only 50 to 60% is normally absorbed. The fats are absorbed into the central lacteal of the villi and thus into the lymphatic system. They are carried in the lymph to eventually join the venous system in the great veins of the neck. Fat malabsorption can accompany massive ileal resection due to a reduction in the absorptive surface and the bile acid pool (Wood 1996).

STONE FORMATION

The distal ileum is the active site of bile salt reabsorption. Resection or disease of a major length of distal ileum (100 cm or more) can interrupt the enterohepatic circulation to such an extent as to decrease the bile acid pool size and reduce bile salt concentration. Gastric acid secretion increases, probably as a result of a hormonal reflex and both disturbances combine to aggravate steatorrhoea (Zentler-Munro & Northfield 1993). The presence of increased bile acids in the colon leads to enhanced oxalate absorption which, combined with a low urinary output, may lead to the formation of calcium oxalate kidney stones. In resection of the colon there is also an increased tendency to form uric acid stones. Total colectomy presents a different picture and lack of bacterial colonisation in the large bowel may lead to malabsorption of bile acids that may result in an increased incidence of cholesterol gall stones (Christl & Scheppach 1997).

CONSEQUENCES OF BOWEL RESECTION

These depend on the extent and region of the resection, the state of the residual gut, the integrity of the terminal ileum and whether the ileocaecal valve is preserved. Resection of short segments is usually well tolerated. Specific nutritional disturbances occur if more than 50% of small bowel is resected and resection of 70% may need parenteral nutrition (Obermayer-Pietsch & Krejs 1993). To absorb sufficient fluid, salts and nutrients to survive without parenteral support, with an end-jejunostomy, approximately one metre of jejunum is needed (Nightingale et al 1992). Jejunal resection alone may not result in diarrhoea because the ileum can adapt and bile salts are absorbed lower in the terminal ileum. Resection of the ileum, or ileocaecal area alone may induce severe diarrhoea and malabsorption due to loss of special transport functions, even though less than 30% of the small intestine is removed (Obermayer-Pietsch & Krejs 1993). Bile acid malabsorption and fat malabsorption lead to diarrhoea. The ileum can normally act as a functional reserve if items escape absorption but if the ileum is resected there is no equivalent reserve area to take over. In ileostomy patients, loss of bacterial fermentation in the large bowel leads to a significant loss of energy in the ileostomy fluid (Christl & Scheppach 1997).

Following resection, disease of the remaining small intestine may lead to severe problems and short bowel syndrome occurs when there is a reduction in the capacity of the small intestine to digest and absorb adequate amounts of nutrients. Excessive quantities of fluid and electrolytes may also be lost (Wood 1996). This may occur following massive resection but may occur due to extensive inflammation. Wood (1996) suggests that the term 'intestinal failure' may be a better one to use.

ADAPTATION OF THE SMALL BOWEL

After total colonic resection ileostomy outputs reach 800–1000 ml (Table 2.2) but malabsorption of nutrients is not evident. The diarrhoea diminishes with time as the intestine adapts (Chadwick 1993). After extensive resection the remaining bowel dilates (Pokorny & Fowler 1991). Radiographic studies have shown a several-fold increase in length of the remaining bowel. Increase in absorption per unit length of intestine has also been shown to occur for glucose and amino acids. The mucosa adapts by cellular proliferation and so increased enterocytes. The transit time for the chyme, which is shortened post-

Table 2.2 Daily loss of water and salts in faeces

Loss of water and salts per day	Normal faeces	Recent ileostomy	Established ileostomy	Recent colostomy	Established transverse colostomy
Water (ml)	50–150	500–1000	400–450	200–800	300
Sodium (mmol)	5	130	35–90	80	50
Chloride (mmol)	3	110	45–60	50	40
Potassium (mmol)	4	20	10	20	10

The above are approximate figures and will vary according to the exact type of stoma.

operatively, becomes prolonged perhaps due to hormonal influences. Gastrin may not be cleared adequately due to loss of small bowel and this may lead to increased stimulation of hydrochloric acid production and hyperacidity. Increased intestinal blood flow due to increased vessel size may also occur and facilitate absorption. All these adaptations help the digestive and absorptive powers of the ostomist to move in the direction of normality with time.

Especially in a new stoma, intestinal secretions rich in sodium and potassium may be lost and the client may develop extracellular fluid volume deficit, hypokalaemia, hyponatraemia or metabolic acidosis. Loss of skin turgor and a dry mouth may be signs of dehydration. Weakness, confusion and cardiac arrhythmias may be due to low potassium levels, although clinical symptoms may not develop until the potassium level is down to 3 mmol/litre. It is best to prevent this by ensuring an adequate intake of foods containing potassium. Even in an established stoma there is going to be more loss of both fluid and electrolytes from this route. The body will attempt to compensate by adaptations discussed above and by altering the composition of urine. When more fluid and salts are lost from the stoma, aldosterone is released from the adrenal cortex, leading to salt and water reabsorption and production of concentrated urine that has a lower sodium content.

When caring for clients with a stoma we need to be very aware of all the possible changes that may occur following a loss of part of the bowel which will have an effect on the body's normal physiology. We need to look for any signs of dehydration or electrolyte loss as well as those of possible malabsorption of both macro- and micronutrients.

References

Black P K 2000 Holistic stoma care. Baillière Tindall and RCN, Edinburgh

Chadwick V S 1993 Mechanisms of malabsorption and diarrhoea; clinical investigation of patients with malabsorption and diarrhoea. In: Bouchier A D, Allen R N, Hodgson H J F, Keighley M R B Gastroenterology, Volume 1, 2nd edn. W B Saunders, London, p 459–467

Christl S U, Scheppach W 1997 Metabolic consequences of total colectomy. Scandinavian Journal of Gastroenterology Supplement 222: 20–24

Fairbanks V F, Beutler E 1994 Iron metabolism. In: Williams W J, Beutler E, Erslev A J, Litchman M A Hematology, 5th edn. McGraw-Hill, New York

Fumi L, Berntsson I, Aberg K et al 1996 Water and electrolyte losses in ileostomy patients: evaluation of a new oral rehydration solution. In: World Council of Enterostomal Therapists congress proceedings. Hollister Incorporated, Libertyville, IL, p 105–107

Gregory J F III 1995 The bioavailability of folate. In: Bailey L (ed) Folate in health and disease. M Dekker, New York, p 195–235

Guyton M D, Hall J E 2000 Textbook of medical physiology, 10th edn. W B Saunders, London

Hoffbrand A V 1993 Digestion and malabsorption of haematinics. In: Bouchier A D, Allen R N, Hodgson H J F, Keighley M R B Gastroenterology, Volume 1, 2nd edn. W B Saunders, London, p 420–432

Kennedy H J, Compston J, Heynan G et al 1983 Calcium metabolism in subjects living with a permanent ileostomy. Digestion 26(3):131–136

Marieb E N 2003 Human anatomy and physiology, 5th edn. Benjamin Cummings, CA

Meadows C 1997 Stoma and fistula care. In: Bruce L, Finlay T M D (eds) Nursing in gastroenterology. Churchill Livingstone, New York, p 85–118

Montague S E, Watson R, Herbert R 2005 Physiology for nursing practice, 3rd edn. Baillière Tindall, Edinburgh

Nightingale J M D, Leonard-Jones J E, Gertner D J et al 1992 Colonic preservation reduces need for parenteral therapy, increases incidence of renal stones, but does not change the high prevalence of gall stones in patients with short bowel. Gut 33:1493–1497

Obermayer-Pietsch B M, Krejs G J 1993 Short gut syndrome. In: Bouchier A D, Allen R N, Hodgson H J F, Keighley M R B Gastroenterology, Volume 1, 2nd edn. W B Saunders, London, p 672–682

Pokorny W J, Fowler C L 1991 Isoperistaltic intestinal lengthening for short bowel syndrome. Surgery, Gynaecology and Obstetrics 172:39–43

Riddell L J, Chisholm A, Williams S, Mann J L 2000 Dietary strategies for lowering homocysteine concentrations. American Journal of Clinical Nutrition 71(6):1448–1454

Smith G 2005 The acquisition of nutrients. In: Montague S E, Watson R, Herbert R Physiology for nursing practice, 3rd edn. Baillière Tindall, Edinburgh

Spiller R C 1993. Digestion and malabsorption of nutrients: carbohydrate, protein, minerals, vitamins. In: Bouchier A D, Allen R N, Hodgson H J F, Keighley M R B Gastroenterology Volume 1, 2nd edn. W B Saunders, London, p 386–420

Walters J R F 1993 Absorption and malabsorption of calcium and vitamin D. In: Bouchier A D, Allen R N, Hodgson H J F, Keighley M R B Gastroenterology, Volume 1, 2nd edn. W B Saunders, London, p 433–444

Wood S 1996 Nutrition and the short bowel syndrome. In: Myers C (ed) Stoma care nursing. Arnold, London, p 81–89

Zentler-Munro P L, Northfield T C 1993 Digestion and malabsorption of fat. In: Bouchier A D, Allen R N, Hodgson H J F, Keighley M R B Gastroenterology, Volume 1, 2nd edn. W B Saunders, London, p 393–341

Chapter **3**

Types of bowel stoma and why they are created

Barbara Borwell and Brigid Breckman

Surgical advances are increasing the types of bowel diversion available to patients. Operations initially only performed in specialist centres become more generally available as their benefits are established, and the necessary surgical expertise becomes more widespread. For example, some internal bowel pouches described in Chapter 10 are now perceived as lying at the 'mainstream' end of the spectrum of operations. In contrast, the gracilis neosphincter operations (see Ch. 11) are performed in specialist centres and are relatively low in number. These developments mean nurses must also gain sufficient understanding of the expanding range of operations so that we can give knowledgeable care to patients. This chapter should therefore be read in conjunction with Chapters 10 and 11.

In this chapter the group of operations often termed as 'conventional' stoma surgery are considered. They entail surgical diversion using ileum (ileostomy) or colon (colostomy) and often bowel resection. Stomas may be temporary or permanent. In order to understand which of the various bowel diversions may be appropriate for particular patients, and why, we must look at several aspects of their situation:

1. diseases/conditions of the lower gastrointestinal (GI) tract whose treatment may include stoma formation
2. operations that include stoma formation
3. types of stoma
4. points to consider.

These components can be considered separately, as we do here, to aid clarification. However, in multidisciplinary team discussions these components are often combined because they are interrelated.

DISEASES/CONDITIONS OF THE LOWER GI TRACT WHOSE TREATMENT MAY INCLUDE STOMA FORMATION

ULCERATIVE COLITIS

Forbes (2002) provides an overview of medical aspects of ulcerative colitis (UC). It is an inflammatory disease which affects the more superficial layers of the bowel. It usually starts in the rectum and spread is continuous into the proximal colon, affecting varying amounts of bowel. Cohen et al (2002) suggest the peak ages for ulcerative colitis are 20–40 years. This relatively young age is important because of the long-term risk of cancer. Sufferers who have had the disease for over 10 years with the inflammatory process active in the entire left-sided colon and rectum appear to be at most risk (Acheson & Scholefield 2002). Indications for surgery are only for chronic UC and include:

- unsuccessful medical treatment
- growth failure in children
- cancerous changes.

Surgical options will vary depending on whether a patient's condition allows elective surgery or when emergency treatment is required (see later). As ulcerative colitis generally does not affect the small intestine (backwash ileitis can occur) surgical resection of the colon, rectum and mucosa of the upper anal canal can remove both the diseased portion of bowel and tissues in which further disease could occur. Key areas for discussion include whether the anus and sphincteric function can be preserved, and the degree to which different operations can affect frequency and control of evacuation (Nicholls & Williams 2002).

The occurrence of ulcerative colitis or cancer in residual tissue after surgery does not always give rise to symptoms that would signal the need for investigation and treatment. Regular long-term endoscopic monitoring is therefore essential for these patients. Where patients are unlikely to undergo such monitoring this may influence decisions as to whether they should be left with any residual tissue.

CROHN'S DISEASE

Crohn's disease is a very different kind of inflammatory disease to that of UC. Inflammation can involve the whole thickness of bowel wall, giving rise to ulceration and fistula formation. Any part of the GI tract can be involved and generally Crohn's disease does *not* occur as a continuous inflammatory process. This means that surgery removing severely affected portions of bowel may well improve the patient's condition but further disease can still occur within the remaining GI tract.

The choice of operation will be determined by the position and severity of the disease. Rectal and anal involvement is likely to necessitate excision and stoma formation. If the colon is free of disease then a colostomy may be performed but where colonic disease is also present then proctocolectomy and ileostomy formation will usually be required.

FAMILIAL ADENOMATOUS POLYPOSIS (FAP)

FAP is a genetically inherited disease that affects the whole body. Patients develop numerous adenomatous polyps in their colon and rectum. These are significant because cancerous transformation in these adenomas occurs if they are left untreated (Cole & Sleightholme 2001).

FAP is caused by a mutation of the APC gene, which lies on the long arm of chromosome 5. It is an autosomal dominant condition: every child of a parent with FAP has a 50% chance of inheriting it. Neale & Phillips (2002) provide a useful overview of the possibilities and difficulties of screening for FAP genetic mutations. If DNA is available from an affected family member then mutation detection is possible in about 70% of families. In these families, first degree relatives should be offered predictive screening with appropriate genetic counselling (Cole & Sleightholme 2001).

Ongoing surveillance is necessary in order to identify extra-colonic manifestations including non-adenomatous gastric polyps, desmoid tumours and adenomatous duodenal polyps. Treatment is more likely to be effective when any cancerous changes in polyps are detected early. Neale & Phillips (2002) suggest this normally involves families with FAP in:

- annual rigid sigmoidoscopy from 14 years of age

- colonoscopy at age 20, subsequently repeated every 5 years
- updating of the family tree to identify new members.

Older patients who are not known to have family with FAP may present with symptoms and/or polyposis. Their parents and siblings should be offered screening.

Cole & Sleightholme (2001) report that the mean age for colorectal cancer occurrence in people with FAP is during their mid thirties, often with synchronous tumours. It is not always necessary for these patients to have a permanent ileostomy with proctocolectomy (Neale & Phillips 2002). However, a permanent ileostomy is indicated for patients who have developed a low rectal cancer. If polyps are occurring, surgery to remove potential or actual cancers will be required. This may entail either:

- colectomy with ileorectal anastomosis (and subsequent 6-monthly examination of the rectal stump for dense rectal polyposis, adenomas or cancer) or
- restorative proctocolectomy with an ileo-anal pouch (see Ch. 10).

Patients undergoing either operation may require a temporary ileostomy to facilitate healing.

HEREDITARY NON-POLYPOSIS COLON CANCER (HNPCC)

This is an autosomal dominant condition where cancers more often arise in the right colon as well as in extra-colonic locations (e.g. gynaecological, small bowel, urinary tract). The situation regarding genetic testing and treatment of people with family histories of HNPCC is complex, with more genetic mutations being identified. Ruo & Guillem (2002) suggest that genetic testing may assist in identifying gene mutation carriers in at-risk families before they develop cancer. HNPCC cancers can be multiple. They tend to occur in the proximal colon, although right-sided cancers and other sites including endometrium are possible (Brown & Bishop 2000). Prophylactic surgery includes subtotal colectomy with ileorectal anastomosis or restorative protocolectomy. Ongoing surveillance is required with 2-yearly colonoscopy and gastroscopy (Cairns & Scholefield 2002). The mean age for cancer diagnosis in patients with HNPCC is 42–49 years.

COLORECTAL CANCER

Colorectal cancer usually occurs as a result of a series of changes known as the adenoma-carcinoma sequence, whereby the adenoma becomes dysplastic. Small benign adenomas develop and may enlarge, with some eventually undergoing malignant changes. Metastases to local lymph nodes can then occur with further spread to additional sites (Northover et al 2002). However, Hardy et al (2001) suggest that the sequence of events where cancer arises from ulcerative colitis may differ, and likewise the period of time cancers take to develop.

Colorectal cancer is the second most common cancer in the UK (Cancer Research UK 2003), usually occurring at ages 60–70 and killing about 20 000 people a year. Knowledge of how and why colorectal cancer occurs, both in families with hereditary conditions and in the general population, is growing. Genetic and other factors are described in a number of publications (e.g. Kerr et al 2001, Pemberton 2002).

Treatment of colorectal cancer varies to some extent in different countries. In most instances surgery will be used if it is thought possible either to remove the cancer with sufficient surgical clearance of the tumour and surrounding tissue to minimise the risk of recurrence, or to reduce its effects on the bowel and other tissues. Explanation about the kind of treatment relevant to each patient and whether this is palliative or curative is given by the surgeon, based on information determined by the colorectal cancer multidisciplinary team (MDT), which includes nursing representatives (NHSE 2004). However, other healthcare members should understand the rationale for treatment options and decisions to ensure explanations and further discussion (often requested by patients and their families) are informed and consistent.

A range of investigations will be carried out in order to identify what the patient's situation entails (Knowles 2002). Normally, sufficient information should be gathered to answer the following questions:

- How widespread is the cancer overall?
- How extensive is the local bowel cancer?
- How can that local bowel cancer best be removed?
- What bowel will that leave with which to create a new faecal pathway?
- Which operation(s) will give this patient the best functioning bowel system with their remaining bowel?

- Will a temporary or permanent stoma be required with this new bowel system?
- What are the implications (positive and negative) of the operation(s) for this patient's quality of life, including bowel, bladder and sexual functions?
- If this patient requires radiotherapy or chemotherapy in addition to surgery are there differences in how these might affect the patient if they had different operations?
- Given the stage of this patient's disease and their overall condition, what prognosis is thought likely? Would this be likely to differ if one operation was performed rather than another?
- Does this patient, the surgeon, and/or the MDT overall think a particular operation would be preferable? If so, why?

Patients differ in the depth to which they want to be informed about their situation, and the degree to which they want to influence the choice of treatment. Discussions with patients and, where appropriate, their family must be sensitively conducted and supportive in manner.

The above questions indicate key factors that inform the reasons for, and choices of, treatment.

The extent of the disease generally

The purpose of the various examinations, tests and scans which patients undergo is not only to diagnose whether they have colorectal cancer or other conditions. It is important to establish the local extent of any cancer and whether liver or lung metastases are present. The contribution that the various tests can make in providing information for this *staging process* is discussed in the Association of Coloproctology of Great Britain and Ireland (2001) guidelines for management of colorectal cancer (see Ch. 24).

To enable the healthcare team to have a common understanding of the extent of each patient's disease it will be *classified* using both the tumour, node and metastases (TNM) classification and a modification of Dukes' (1937) classification (Knowles 2002). This classification may change. Preoperatively a classification is tentatively allocated, based on the information available from the tests and assessments. Once the pathological specimen has been examined a postoperative final classification is generated: the TN stage is prefixed by the letter 'p' (e.g. pT3 N1). These classifications are used to consider whether additional treatment should be offered, and to gain some indication of the patient's likely prognosis. The percentage of patients who survive for 5 years following diagnosis of colorectal cancer differs between the stages. Survival figures quoted by different authors vary, depending on factors such as the quality of pathological reporting and whether figures are adjusted for age. The figures shown in Table 3.1 are drawn from Blackley (2004), Hardy et al (2001) and Steele (2001).

The extent of localised disease

The level of the tumour is described in terms of distance from the anal verge and is generally expressed as lying within specific areas or levels of bowel:

upper third of rectum: 12–15 cm from anal verge
middle third of rectum: 8–11 cm from anal verge
lower third of rectum: 4–7 cm from anal verge
anal canal itself: 3 cm.

In order to minimise the likelihood of residual or recurrent tumour a 2 cm margin of normal tissue and lymph nodes should be resected beyond the distal palpable tumour. The extensiveness of the

Table 3.1 Five-year survival in colorectal cancer by TNM or Dukes stage

TNM classification	Modified Dukes	Five-year survival
Stage 0: carcinoma in situ		
Stage I: no nodal involvement; no metastases; tumour invades submucosa (T1, N0, M0)	A	85–100%
Tumour invades muscularis propria (T2, N0, M0)		
Stage II: no nodal involvement; no metastases; tumour invades into subserosa (T3, N0, M0)	B	67–85%
Tumour invades other organs (T4, N0, M0)		
Stage III: regional lymph nodes involved (any T, N1, M0)	C	30–40%
Stage IV: distant metastases	D	Below 5%

operation required to achieve this *distal clearance* and conservation of anal sphincters is determined by several factors including the cancer type and distance from the anal verge or dentate line. According to Phillips (2002, p 100) in practice this measure is mainly irrelevant as the amount of bowel removed is determined by guidelines for performing a total mesorectal excision for mid and low rectal tumours (NHSE 2004). Tumours in the lower third of rectum do require a 2 cm clearance for management by anal sphincter-saving techniques (Phillips 2002, p 100). The realistic possibility of achieving a leak-free anastomosis of bowel and competent anal function following tumour resection depends on:

- whether preoperative radiotherapy was given
- the expertise of the surgeon
- the availability of sufficient bowel to make an anastomosis (with or without a pouch) and preserve adequate sphincteric function.

The advent of stapling devices and other techniques now enables bowel anastomosis at a lower level to be performed successfully. In some instances the tumour may be bulky or look as if it would be difficult to resect. Preoperative radiotherapy can be used to shrink rectal tumours so that surgery becomes possible, but appears of no benefit with colonic cancers (Midgley & Kerr 2001). Preoperative staging of cancer with magnetic resolution imaging

(MRI) has enabled patient selection for either neo-adjuvant radiotherapy alone or combined with chemotherapy. This information guides decisions on the mode and extent of surgery which should be performed. This is particularly important for rectal cancer as it helps indicate whether, when the tumour and a surrounding margin of normal tissue is resected, it will be possible to:

- maintain bowel sphincter function
- preserve the autonomic nerves and plexuses required for normal sexual and bladder function.

There is now more agreement on the ways in which rectal cancer should be removed surgically. Detailed descriptions are available (Cohen 2002, Enker & Martz 2002, Phillips & Williams 2002, Association of Coloproctology of Great Britain and Ireland 2001), from which the following points are drawn.

Cancer is likely to spread into the mesorectum as well as within the rectum. Complete removal of the mesorectum (Fig. 3.1), which includes the entire rectal mesentery and 'en bloc' dissection of involved lymphatic tissue and potential satellite nodules, will greatly reduce the risk of local recurrence of the disease. In order to carry out this total mesorectal excision (TME) procedure incorporating adequate distal clearance, sharp dissection should be used. The use of skilled sharp dissection is important as it

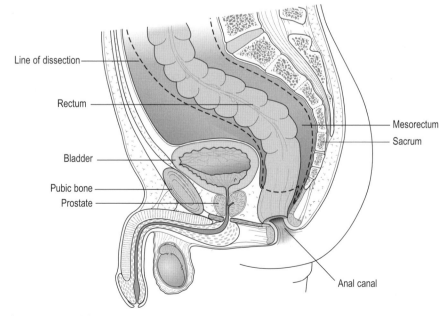

Figure 3.1   Total mesorectal excision.

reduces the risk of sexual and bladder dysfunction from nerve and plexus damage as well as rectal or mesorectal perforation and possible spillage of cancer cells.

The presence of regional lymph node metastases

Surgical management will be influenced by patient factors and tumour site within the rectum. Comparison between the outcome of resection and anastomosis and abdomino-perineal excision of the rectum (APER) concluded that there is no evidence that sphincter conservation impairs survival, but APER has a continuing morbidity and complications (NHSE 1997).

Tumour histology

Tumours that are histologically defined as poorly differentiated or anaplastic indicate a poorer prognosis than those that are well differentiated.

ANAL CANCER

These tumours are uncommon: specialist skills from a designated MDT are recommended for their management to achieve optimal patient outcomes (NHSE 2004, p 98). An overview is provided by Young-Fadok (2002). They are normally assessed using endorectal ultrasound as well as biopsy in order to stage the disease. Concurrent chemoradiation is the primary recommended treatment in most instances, with abdomino-perineal excision of rectum being reserved for the minority of patients whose disease proves resistant to it (Bernick & Wong 2002). However, Young-Fadok (2002) suggests that local excision of small lesions at the anal margin is the best treatment because it avoids drawn out adjuvant therapy.

OPERATIONS THAT INCLUDE STOMA FORMATION

It is generally helpful for the patient and the healthcare team to consider three main aspects of their situation when identifying the best surgical options:

1. The general type of operation which they require. This will largely depend on their disease: its extent at the time of surgery; its potential to re-occur; and whether or not it is, or has the potential to become, cancerous.

2. The effects that any potentially suitable operations could have on that person's subsequent quality of life.
3. The degree to which that person is physically and psychologically fit enough to go through particular operations and manage their probable effects.

Postoperatively surgeons will have a more concrete idea of the changes that their surgery has created for the individual patient. However, additional factors at the time of surgery, such as the presence of adhesions or difficulty in ascertaining whether all diseased tissue has been removed, may make precise assessment of long-term effects of the surgery difficult. Both patient and staff may have to wait and see how the body heals and settles into its new way of functioning.

Detailed descriptions of the diseases, operations and points to consider are available elsewhere (e.g. Pemberton 2002, Keighley & Williams 1999). Situations likely to warrant stoma formation include those where:

(a) Removal of diseased bowel and surrounding tissue leaves insufficient bowel, rectum and anus to function adequately and continently. *For example*:
   - abdomino-perineal excision of rectum, including creation of a permanent colostomy, for cancer
   - where there is trauma to the lower rectum and/or anus.
(b) Faecal diversion is required above a mechanical or functional bowel obstruction in order to rest the affected bowel portion. *For example*:
   - to prevent faecal flow through rectovaginal or rectovesical fistulas so cleanliness and healing can be promoted
   - to rest bowel in acute inflammatory conditions such as Crohn's disease
   - to enable decompression of bowel to take place after emergency surgery for total bowel obstruction, as a prelude to subsequent treatment. Treatment of left-sided large bowel obstruction has been superseded in some centres with self-expanding metal colonic stents (Godber 2004).
(c) A temporary diversion of faeces is needed above an anastomosis following resection to enable effective healing of the joined bowel to take place. *For example*:
   - low and ultra-low anterior resections carrying a 'significant' risk of anastomotic leakage.

OPERATIONS INCLUDING ILEOSTOMY

Generally ileostomies are created when the condition of a patient's colon requires it to be removed, or effluent diverted from it. The extent of the surgery and whether a temporary or permanent ileostomy will be required varies depending on the patient's overall situation. Loop stomas are discussed in Chapter 4.

Panproctocolectomy or conventional proctocolectomy with permanent ileostomy

This operation is performed less often for patients with ulcerative colitis now that restorative proctocolectomy is more widely available. It involves removal of the whole colon, rectum and anal canal, leaving the patient with a permanent terminal ileostomy. Patients will also have a perineal wound. In this operation close rectal dissection is normally combined with inter-sphincteric and perimuscular removal of the anal canal. This means that pelvic nerve dysfunction (which could lead to difficulties in getting and maintaining an erection, or bladder problems) can usually be avoided (Sagar & Pemberton 2002).

This surgery is not entirely problem free. Farthing (1996, p 101–102) suggests that about 25% of patients still have an unhealed perineal wound 6 months after surgery. The cumulative surgical revision rate of the terminal ileostomy is between 20% and 30% at 5 years; and the rate of intestinal obstruction due to adhesions is 10–20% during that period. However, there are also advantages in that the surgery is curative for ulcerative colitis. Patients with poor anal sphincter control or those who do not want to cope with the unpredictable function of a restorative proctocolectomy may attain improved bowel management through having a stoma and achieving really adept care of it.

Colectomy with ileorectal anastomosis

Where patients require emergency surgery this may entail colectomy with formation of a temporary ileostomy and preservation of the rectal stump. This enables the patient's condition to be improved and decisions can then be made as to whether an ileorectal anastomosis can be performed and the stoma closed. Ongoing monitoring of the rectal stump for recurring ulcerative colitis, FAP or malignant changes will be necessary. This operation is performed less frequently for ulcerative colitis now that the various pouch operations are widely established (see Ch. 10). However, it can be the operation of choice for patients who have colonic Crohn's disease or FAP without rectal or anal involvement.

Restorative proctocolectomy

In this operation a total colectomy is performed and small bowel is used to create an internal pouch or reservoir anastomosed to the anal canal (see Ch. 10). Some patient situations will warrant a covering temporary end ileostomy whilst in other cases the surgeon may not deem this necessary.

Creation of a pouch may be thought more suitable than an ileorectal anastomosis for older patients with FAP as the risk of rectal cancer rises from 8% at age 50 to 30% at age 60 (Neale & Phillips 2002).

This operation is contraindicated for patients with Crohn's disease as recurrent small bowel inflammation and anal fistulas give a high failure rate (Nicholls & Williams 2002, p 75).

Sagar & Pemberton (2002, p 85) suggest the quality of life of patients with a pelvic ileal reservoir (restorative proctocolectomy) is better than that of patients with a Kock pouch or medically treated colitis. However, it should be remembered that this operation is only indicated for permanent avoidance of a stoma. Williams & Nicholls (2002) describe those problems that can occur, and the importance of careful patient selection, support and management.

OPERATIONS INCLUDING COLOSTOMY

Generally colostomies are created as part of treatment for two main types of situation:

1. The presence of bowel impairment which requires diversion of faeces above (proximal) to it, enabling the condition either to resolve or be treated. In most of these situations the stoma will be created as a temporary diversion. Its position will depend on which segment of bowel is being treated, and where in the bowel pathway an easily managed stoma can be created. Historically, many stomas were created from transverse colon in order to leave the maximum amount of bowel to function before effluent diversion. In order to facilitate subsequent closure many of these were loop colostomies. However, their size and posi-

tion made adherence and management of stomal equipment difficult. More loop ileostomies are now being created when temporary stomas are required as their abdominal position and smaller size can aid stoma care management. Loop stomas are discussed in Chapter 4.

2. Rectal and/or anal disease is being removed and it is not possible to reconstruct a bowel pathway with sphincteric control. A permanent end colostomy will be created as far along the bowel pathway as possible to retain maximum bowel function.

Abdomino–perineal excision of rectum

Enker & Martz (2002) suggest this is the procedure of choice for:

- invasive carcinoma of the distal rectum
- persistent or recurrent epidermoid carcinomas of the anal canal
- rare lesions of the anorectum (e.g. melanoma)
- sarcomas arising from the levator ani involving the anal canal
- patients with resectable recurrent cancer.

This major operation entails removal of the rectum and anus and creation of an end colostomy. There will also be a perineal wound. The principles of total mesorectal excision with autonomic nerve preservation should be followed as most regional rectal cancer is contained within the mesorectum (Association of Coloproctology of Great Britain and Ireland 2001, NHSE 2004). Where there is no tumour involvement of the vagina, the sharp dissection of TME enables a non-violated full thickness wall of the vagina with intact blood supply to be left (Enker & Martz 2002, p 265). Where there is adjacent organ involvement en bloc resection, and reconstruction if possible, will be necessary to avoid cutting across tumour.

Until quite recently a blunt dissection and wider resection, including removal of the upper third of the vagina in females, was used in abdomino-perineal excision and may still be used in some countries (Northover et al 2002). This wider excision can result in damage to men and women's pelvic nerves which supply the bladder and sexual organs. Information about potential nerve damage preoperatively, and actual or probable damage postoperatively, must be based on the surgical approach used for the particular patient.

It is important to understand that, if physical impairment does occur, it is not the formation of a stoma that damages the relevant nerves but the procedure of widely excising the rectum. Sexual impairment, and how people experiencing it can be helped, is discussed in Chapter 5.

Anterior resection with temporary colostomy

This major operation may be carried out in conjunction with colo-anal pouch formation (see Ch. 10) or colo-anal anastomosis. The rectal section containing the cancer is removed while retaining the anal sphincters. Total mesorectal excision is used to achieve adequate tumour clearance whilst minimising nerve damage which could impair bladder and/or sexual function (Northover et al 2002).

Anterior dissection in men can be problematic, particularly with an anterior placed tumour where control of bleeding during dissection may expose the seminal vesicles and nervi erigentes to potential damage, leading to erectile dysfunction. The presacral nerves that control ejaculation are usually conserved.

The advent of stapling devices and increased training in surgical techniques now means that much lower rectal excisions and anastomoses can be achieved (Cohen 2002). In some situations achieving a secure leak-proof anastomosis can be difficult so a *temporary defunctioning stoma* may be created. This diverts faeces from the body above the anastomosis so it can heal without effluent passing through it. Although a transverse loop colostomy may be created, many surgeons raise a loop ileostomy. It avoids traction on the anastomosis, and blood supply to the descending colon is not compromised (Penna & Parc 2002). In addition, the site and size of loop ileostomies make them easier to manage than transverse colostomies (Black 2000).

Creating a colo-anal anastomosis after resection results in a bowel pathway without a faecal reservoir or storage facility. Phillips & Williams (2002) suggest that a colo-anal anastomosis (i.e. without a stoma or a pouch) can result in many patients having four to six bowel actions during the day plus nighttime actions a year postoperatively. However, they also report that pouch surgery can result in evacuation problems. Careful consideration therefore needs to be given to the overall effects of the various 'anterior resection' operations and their implications for a patient's bowel function and quality of life.

Hartmann's procedure

This involves removal of sigmoid colon and upper rectum, and creation of an end colostomy from the remaining colon while leaving the rectal stump closed inside the patient. This leaves open the possibility of a later operation to reconnect the bowel to the rectal stump and close the colostomy.

Devine's colostomy

A Devine's, or divided colostomy is raised in cases where it is essential to avoid spillage of faeces into the distal section of bowel. The two ends of divided bowel are brought out onto the patient's abdomen at some distance from each other. The outlet from the functioning digestive tract is the *colostomy*. The distal portion of bowel which opens onto the abdomen is called a *mucous fistula* (see Ch. 14). Subsequent rejoining of the bowel and closure of the colostomy will depend on the patient's general condition and situation regarding their disease. This diversion can be easier to close than the more commonly performed Hartmann's one.

Pelvic exenteration

Total pelvic exenteration for extensive pelvic cancer is relatively rare. It is performed jointly by colorectal and urological surgeons, leaving patients with a colostomy and urostomy following clearance of all the pelvic organs.

In *men* it may be offered where rectal cancer has spread to involve the seminal vesicles, prostate, or base of the bladder, requiring their removal as well as an APER (Phillips 2002). Phillips suggests preoperative radiotherapy should be given to promote tumour shrinkage and facilitate the surgery.

Patients and their partners may wish to consider banking sperm before treatment (Salter 1996, p 210). Once patients have fully recovered discussions about options such as penile implants may be helpful (see Ch. 6).

In *women* it may be utilised where tumour recurs in the central pelvic area after radiotherapy for cervical cancer. This operation essentially combines: APER, hysterectomy, salpingo-oophorectomy, cystectomy, and excision of the vagina and upper third of the urethra (Blackley 2004, McCartney 1986). Vaginal reconstruction may be possible later for some women (Blackley 1986, McCartney 1986).

In some instances less extensive operations may be suitable (Blackley 2004).

Anterior exenteration involves excision of:

- reproductive organs, including vaginal resection
- bladder and upper third of the urethra.

An ileal conduit or continent urinary reservoir is created. The bowel system is retained.

Posterior exenteration involves excision of:

- rectum and anus
- reproductive organs including vaginal resection.

A colostomy or colo-anal pouch is created. The urinary system is retained.

Diversion during treatment

Ileostomies and colostomies can sometimes be used to protect the distal bowel during intensive chemoradiation or radiotherapy alone.

TYPES OF STOMA

Stomas are usually identified according to one or more of the following:

- their position in the bowel tract (e.g. ileostomy; descending colostomy; Fig. 3.2)
- their proposed function (e.g. temporary or permanent)
- the nature of their formation (e.g. loop ileostomy; end colostomy)
- the surgeon who developed the technique (e.g. Hartmann's procedure).

The way in which the stoma is fashioned is determined by the purpose of the stoma, the nature of the operation as a whole, the extent and nature of the disease necessitating surgery, and the patient's physical condition to withstand a major operation.

An *end* or *terminal* ileostomy or colostomy entails one end of bowel being used to create the stoma. Generally, any bowel beyond the diversion is removed, and the stoma is permanent.

A *loop* ileostomy or colostomy is formed when a loop of bowel is brought onto the anterior abdominal wall and usually supported by a temporary rod or bridge so that the stoma does not retract. The stoma has two openings: a *proximal* opening (in an ileostomy the stoma is spouted) through which faeces from the functioning digestive system will pass, and a *distal* opening which leads to the redundant bowel (see Ch. 4, Fig. 4.2). The bridge/rod is

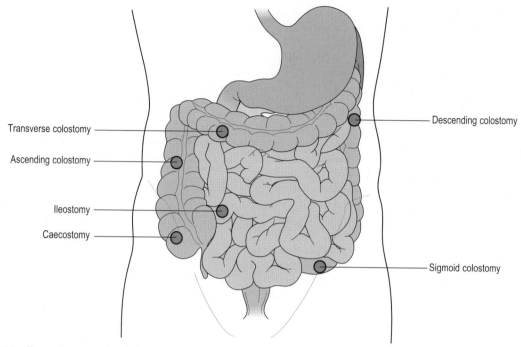

Transverse colostomy

Ascending colostomy

Ileostomy

Caecostomy

Descending colostomy

Sigmoid colostomy

Figure 3.2   Types of stoma and typical sites.

removed after 5–8 days when the spur of bowel between these two openings should be sufficiently established, and preventing spillage from the active proximal end into the distal one. Usually a loop stoma will be temporary. Sometimes a loop stoma is created in patients whose general condition or disease does not permit further surgery and/or subsequent stoma closure. This palliative procedure helps maintain bowel function (e.g. in advanced cancer). Functional implications and management of loop stomas are discussed in Chapter 4.

POINTS TO CONSIDER

The diseases leading to surgery including stoma formation are complex, as are the factors to consider when patients' treatment is planned. The time between patients' initial consultation with their doctor and operation is often quite short, especially with colorectal cancer where specific guidelines are in place (NHSE 2004). During that time patients have to deal with questions, examinations and tests. Their results can have substantial implications and, quite reasonably, they and their family may seek to

discuss these with members of the team engaged in their care. We can prepare ourselves for such occasions by reflecting on issues and questions commonly raised and regularly updating and expanding our background knowledge. In this final section several factors which may be of concern are outlined.

STOMA SITING

The presence of any stoma, whether temporary or permanent, affects patients' lives. If there is any possibility that a stoma might be created it is essential that this is discussed preoperatively with patients. Appropriate siting for all stomas is necessary for two reasons. Firstly, it can make the difference between patients having a stoma that is easy to manage or one where the site causes substantial management difficulties. This is important for patients whether their stoma is for a short or long period of time. Secondly, stomas originally planned as short-term measures can sometimes be required for a substantial period of time or permanently. The quality of preoperative preparation can contribute substantially to the quality of life and acceptance of their stoma that these patients achieve.

BALANCING THE EFFECTS OF SURGERY AGAINST THE COST OF ITS EFFECTS ON PATIENTS' LIVES

Unfortunately people with colorectal cancer often do not realise that changes in their bowel habits can be an early symptom of this disease so they do not seek medical help promptly. Many people already have some disease spread by the time a surgeon sees them. Given the 5-year survival figures listed in Table 3.1, people may question whether major surgery which can include temporary or permanent stoma formation will produce an outcome in which benefits outweigh physical and psychological 'costs'.

The effects on patients' lives of major surgery and learning to live with a stoma are indeed considerable. In their study of patients who had surgery for colorectal cancer, Pringle & Swan (2001) found that, one year after surgery, more than half of the patients who had survived for that length of time were reporting fatigue and/or problems with flatus, almost one in ten were experiencing severe pain, and a third had concerns about odour. Other problems were reported and, one year postoperatively, only one in three patients had resumed the kind of social lives they had led before their illness.

Patients who experience relatively low levels of problems from their disease preoperatively may find it particularly difficult to accept surgery that can disrupt and reduce the quality of their lives for many months, or possibly the remainder of their lives. However, patients do not have the option of their cancer remaining static. When surgery is discussed the choice for patient and surgeon is not between whether that patient should accept surgery or live with their current level of symptoms. The question is whether the surgery can prevent or reduce the problems that could arise if the colorectal tumour was left in situ. Problems can include intestinal obstruction, bowel perforation, tumour fungation and the invasion of surrounding structures such as the genitourinary system. These can give rise to substantial and distressing symptoms which are arguably more difficult to control and manage than the after-effects of stoma surgery (Finlay 1997).

Patients who have been managing symptoms of other bowel conditions outlined earlier may also question the timing and appropriateness of surgery. Where conditions can turn cancerous it is particularly important for the management of tumours at different stages to be discussed in a supportive and realistic manner so that any surgery subsequently performed is seen as a positive move to promote health rather than a failure.

GENETIC IMPLICATIONS FOR PATIENTS AND FAMILIES

The implications of diagnosis on genetically inherited conditions such as FAP and HNPCC for patients and their families are considerable. Ongoing monitoring, the possible or actual presence of other related conditions, and the possible or actual development of bowel cancer are more than enough for an individual to cope with. Additionally they may well be dealing with other family members in similar situations. It is important that the healthcare team, including staff in the related genetic departments, communicate and collaborate so that families and individuals gain appropriate long-term information and support (Neale & Phillips 2002).

SCREENING

Worldwide, cancers of the colon and rectum are the third most common cause of death in men and the fourth in women (Horton-Taylor 2001, p 57). From the survival figures cited in Table 3.1 it is apparent that treatment at an early stage substantially increases patients' survival. Growing knowledge of genetic conditions that can lead to cancer, and the mutations which cause them, is enhancing identification and monitoring of individuals and families who are at risk of developing them. However, cancer inherited via these families is only thought to be 5% of the overall colorectal cancer figures (Cole & Sleightholme 2001). Cole & Sleightholme also describe screening protocols being used with people who have colorectal cancer in their family but no recognisable gene disorder. These measures, while beneficial, only reach a small proportion of the population who may have bowel cancer.

In some countries colorectal cancer screening is already available for the general population. There are various reasons why this is thought desirable. Scholefield (2001) suggested that most colorectal cancers result from malignant changes in polyps (adenomas) that have developed in the lining of the bowel 10–15 years earlier. Only 10% of 1 cm adenomas become malignant after 10 years but the incidence of adenomatous polyps increases with age. He reviewed the various tests available, suggesting that screening of the general population for adenomas and colorectal cancer should target people aged 55–75. Horton-Taylor (2001, p 53) suggested that screening programmes for colorectal cancer now met the criteria for being plausible to implement. However, in the UK the next step was pilot studies to identify ways of extending screening to a wider population (Steele 2004). This has led to greater medical and political acceptance that the resources and programmes to implement a national bowel screening programme should be set up. However, for such a programme to be successful, the public must become aware that there is a risk of colorectal cancer arising without triggering major warning symptoms, and aware of and willing to undergo screening. Keighley et al (2004) report that levels of awareness need to be raised so that people realise the importance of screening and become willing to undergo it.

At present growing numbers of people who either have bowel cancer themselves, or know someone else who has it, are taking advantage of easier internet access to seek information about the disease and its treatment. During their searches they may learn that colorectal cancer screening is not universally available or, in their country, may only include a small number of the range of tests available elsewhere. They may need help to gain answers to questions and deal with a variety of issues. It is therefore important to regularly review and update information regarding screening availability and arrangements. This helps us both respond to questions and engage in debate about the best ways of achieving earlier diagnosis and treatment of colorectal cancer and related conditions. Nurses involved in stoma care and related fields are already well used to discussing bowel and urinary elimination, and how these systems function. As bowel screening programmes become more widely available so we can expand our practice to help the wider public to understand and gain access to them.

ADJUVANT CANCER THERAPY

The degree to which national health organisations and/or individual doctors recommend adjuvant chemotherapy and/or radiotherapy, and the availability of particular regimes, appears to vary for patients in different countries (Northover et al 2002). Chemotherapy variations can be in the drug(s) being used, dosage, mode and/or frequency of delivery. Radiotherapy variations can be in the length or dosage of treatment, and whether it is given pre- or postoperatively (Midgley & Kerr 2001, Young & Rea 2001).

This means patients and their families may have concerns or queries if they visit websites advocating different regimes to the treatment they are being offered. It is important that each patient's multidisciplinary team are agreed on the rationale for any adjuvant treatment and what its benefits, limitations and side effects are likely to be. These, in conjunction with patients' own queries, must be discussed appropriately with them. It is also important to be aware of reputable sources of information. For example, in the UK the National Institute for Clinical Excellence (NICE) issues guidelines for healthcare staff and patients on the use of chemotherapy in advanced colorectal cancer (e.g. NICE 2002).

Additional treatment may also become available because trials are taking place and patients are eligible to take part. It is therefore important to check the changing availability of trials as well as monitoring whether results are due to be, or have been, published. For example, healthcare staff and the public can access information on trials from Cancer Research UK.

In conclusion, many aspects of patients' situations and care may require consideration during the pre- and post-surgical period because they can affect their experience of treatment. Taking time to review factors such as those above, individually and with colleagues, can help us pinpoint additional knowledge to acquire and expand our perception of the breadth of care that patients may need.

References

Acheson A G, Scholefield J H 2002 What is new in colorectal cancer? Surgery 20(20):244–248

Association of Coloproctology of Great Britain and Ireland 2001 Guidelines for the management of colorectal cancer.

Association of Coloproctology of Great Britain and Ireland, London (www.acpgbi.org.uk, accessed 6.7.2004)

Bernick P E, Wong W D 2002 Ultrasonographic diagnosis of anorectal disease In: Zuidema G D, Yeo C J (eds)

Shackelford's surgery of the alimentary tract, volume IV: Colon. W B Saunders, Philadelphia, p 357–372

Black P K 2000 Holistic stoma care. Baillière Tindall and RCN, Edinburgh

Blackley P 1986 Female options – repercussions of construction of neo vagina. In: World Council of Enterostomal Therapists congress proceedings. Abbott International & Hollister, USA, p 51–53

Blackley P 2004 Practical stoma wound and continence management. 2nd edn. Research Publications Pty, Vermont, Victoria, Australia

Brown S R, Bishop D T 2000 Genetics of colorectal cancer. In: McArdle C S, Kerr D J, Boyle P (eds) Colorectal cancer. Isis Medical Media, Oxford, p 71–86

Cairns S, Scholefield J H 2002 Summary of recommendations for colorectal cancer screening. Gut (suppl V): V1–V28

Cancer Research UK 2003 Colorectal Cancer Fact Sheet. Office for National Statistics, London (www.cancerresearchuk.org/statistics)

Cohen A M 2002 Operations for colorectal cancer: low anterior resection In: Zuidema G D, Yeo C J (eds) Shackelford's surgery of the alimentary tract, volume IV: Colon. W B Saunders, Philadelphia, p 245–260

Cohen Z, Sabo G, McLeod R 2002 Inflammatory bowel disease In: Zuidema G D, Yeo C J (eds) Shackelford's surgery of the alimentary tract, volume IV: Colon. W B Saunders, Philadelphia, p 66–83

Cole T R P, Sleightholme H V 2001 The role of clinical genetics in management. In: Kerr D J, Young A M, Hobbs F D R (eds) ABC of colorectal cancer. BMJ Books, London, p 9–12

Dukes C 1937 The classification of cancer of the rectum. Journal of pathology 17:643–648

Enker W E, Martz J 2002 Abdominoperineal resection of the rectum for cancer. In: Zuidema G D, Yeo C J (eds) Shackelford's surgery of the alimentary tract, volume IV: Colon. W B Saunders, Philadelphia, p 261–268

Farthing M J G 1996 Medical management of Crohn's disease and ulcerative colitis. In: Myers C (ed) Stoma care nursing. Arnold, London, p 42–62

Finlay T 1997 Malignancies of the gastrointestinal tract. In: Bruce L, Finlay T M D (eds) Nursing in gastroenterology. Churchill Livingstone, New York, p 161–190

Forbes A 2002 Medical aspects of ulcerative colitis. In: Williams J (ed) The essentials of pouch care nursing. Whurr Publishers, London, p 1–26

Godber S L 2004 Palliation of colonic obstruction. Gastrointestinal nursing 2(3):33–39

Hardy R G, Meltzer S J, Jankowski J A 2001 Molecular basis for risk factors. In: Kerr D J, Young A M, Hobbs F D R (eds) ABC of colorectal cancer. BMJ Books, London, p 5–8

Horton-Taylor D 2001 Cancer and epidemiology. In: Corner J, Bailey C (eds) Cancer nursing: care in context. Blackwell Science, Oxford, p 46–60

Keighley M R B, Williams N S 1999 Surgery of the anus, rectum and colon. W B Saunders, London

Keighley M R, O'Morain C, Giacosa A 2004 Public awareness of risk factors and screening for colorectal cancer in Europe. European Journal of Cancer Prevention 13(4):257–262

Kerr D J, Young A M, Hobbs F D R (eds) 2001 ABC of colorectal cancer. BMJ Books, London

Knowles G 2002 The management of colorectal cancer. Nursing Standard 16(17):47–52

McCartney A J 1986 Pelvic exenteration for gynaecological cancer. In: World Council of Enterostomal Therapists congress proceedings. Abbott International and Hollister, IL, p 44–51

Midgley R S, Kerr D J 2001 Adjuvant therapy. In: Kerr D J, Young A M, Hobbs F D R (eds) ABC of colorectal cancer. BMJ Books, London, p 22–25

National Institute for Clinical Excellence 2002 Guidance on the use of irinotecan, oxaliplatin and raltitrexed for the treatment of advanced colorectal cancer. NICE, London

Neale K, Phillips R 2002 Familial adenomatous polyposis. In: Williams J (ed) The essentials of pouch care nursing. Whurr Publishers, London, p 27–42

NHSE (National Health Service Executive) 1997 Improving outcomes in colorectal cancer: the research evidence manual. NICE, London

NHSE (National Health Service Executive) 2004 Improving outcomes in colorectal cancer manual, 2nd edn NICE, London

Nicholls R J, Williams J 2002 The ileo-anal pouch. In: Williams J (ed) The essentials of pouch care nursing. Whurr Publishers, London, p 68–98

Northover J, Taylor C, Gold D, 2002 Carcinoma of the rectum. In: Williams J (ed) The essentials of pouch care nursing. Whurr Publishers, London, p 43–67

Pemberton J H (ed) 2002 Volume IV: Colon. In: Zuidema G D, Yeo C J (eds) Shackelford's surgery of the alimentary tract. W B Saunders, Philadelphia

Penna C, Parc R, 2002 Coloanal anastomosis. In: Zuidema G D, Yeo C J (eds) Shackelford's surgery of the alimentary tract, volume IV: Colon. W B Saunders, Philadelphia, p 269–276

Phillips R K S 2002 Rectal cancer. In: Phillips RKS (ed) Colorectal surgery 2nd edn. W B Saunders, London, p 89–123

Phillips R, Williams J, 2002 The colo-anal pouch and nursing care. In: Williams J (ed) The essentials of pouch care nursing. Whurr Publishers, London, p 117–127

Pringle W, Swan E 2001 Continuing care after discharge from hospital for stoma patients. British Journal of Nursing 10(19):1274–1288

Ruo L, Guillem J G 2002 Colorectal polyps, polyposis and hereditary nonpolyposis colorectal cancer. In: Zuidema G D, Yeo C J (eds) Shackelford's surgery of the alimentary tract, volume IV: Colon. W B Saunders, Philadelphia, p 157–179

Sagar P M, Pemberton J H 2002 Surgery for inflammatory bowel disease. In: Zuidema G D, Yeo C J (eds) Shackelford's surgery of the alimentary tract, volume IV: Colon. W B Saunders, Philadelphia, p 84–103

Salter M 1996 Sexuality and the stoma patient. In: Myers C (ed) Stoma care nursing. Arnold, London, p 203–219

Scholefield J H 2001 Screening. In: Kerr D J, Young A M, Hobbs F D R (eds) ABC of colorectal cancer. BMJ Books, London, p 13–15

Steele R J C 2001 Colonic cancer. In: Phillips R K S (ed) Colorectal surgery, 2nd edn. W B Saunders, London, p 53–88

Steele R J C 2004 Results of the first round of a demonstration pilot of screening for colorectal cancer in the United Kingdom. British Medical Journal 329(7458):133

Williams J, Nicholls R J 2002 Controversies and problem-solving with regard to ileo-anal pouches. In: Williams J (ed) The essentials of pouch care nursing. Whurr Publishers, London, p 143–164

Young A M, Rea D 2001 Treatment of advanced disease. In: Kerr D J, Young A M, Hobbs F D R (eds) ABC of colorectal cancer. BMJ Books, London, p 26–29

Young-Fadok T M 2002 Neoplasms of the anus. In: Zuidema G D, Yeo C J (eds) Shackelford's surgery of the alimentary tract, volume IV: Colon. W B Saunders, Philadelphia, p 373–382

Chapter 4

Practical management of bowel stomas

Barbara Borwell and Brigid Breckman

Although the conditions and operations that result in ileostomy and colostomy formation are often different, the main principles of practical stoma care are similar. When nurses and patients understand and apply these principles they acquire the ability and confidence to adapt their stoma care whenever changes are needed.

Research shows that learners who are new to a situation need some experience of it before they can apply principles of managing it (Benner 1984, Benner et al 1996, and outlined in Introduction). We can therefore best help novices in stoma care (whether patients, their relatives, or nurses) by first helping them learn stoma care as a series of steps or tasks. Once people have successfully learned these basic steps, they can then use that experience to understand and follow the underlying principles of stoma care. Our goal is to help patients use both the steps and principles of stoma care. This two-stage system has been used in this chapter to describe changing appliances so you can consider ways of including both in your own practice and when teaching others.

This chapter covers many of the principles that form the basis of care for all patients with bowel stomas, including those related to:

- siting of stomas
- management of loop ileostomies and colostomies
- choosing suitable appliances
- choosing suitable skin care aids
- changing an appliance
- disposal of used appliances
- storage of stomal equipment.

Specific elements of care that patients are likely to need because they have an end ileostomy or colostomy and the principles of care in the early postoperative period will be discussed in Chapter 5, as will principles for recognising when appliances should be changed. Principles for reordering stomal equipment are included in Chapter 8 as part of the wider discussion on preparing patients for discharge.

Stoma care should begin as soon as surgeons and patients know that surgery is likely and that this will, or may, include stoma formation as this is when patients begin to feel apprehensive about their future. Early referral to a stoma care nurse or other experienced colleague enables them to provide patients with realistic information about living with a stoma, and support to think about how this might become part of their lives. This helps patients reduce their anxiety and focus their attention on what they will still be able to do complete with stoma (i.e. most things).

If patients are not given such help during the time between when they realise they will, or may, have a stoma and when they are admitted for surgery their distress can increase considerably as they tend to spend the time worrying about what they will not be able to do. Information they do acquire (e.g. from people within their own social and work networks) may be out of date or not relevant to their condition and the type of surgery and stoma planned for them.

Stoma care involves systematic data collection and analysis of patients' needs in order to plan their care (Peters-Gawlik 1996). Care must be tailored to meet each individual's needs so they are enabled to manage their new style of bowel elimination, and reduce or resolve any problems in ways suited to their lifestyle.

PSYCHOLOGICAL CARE

Patients' attitudes towards their disease or condition which made surgery necessary may affect their adaptation to this new form of bowel elimination and changes to their normal body image (see Chs 19 and 20). Specific factors that might affect patients' reaction to, and acceptance of, their stoma should be identified in the preoperative assessment. These include their:

- quality of life and severity of symptoms experienced before surgery

- type of stoma to be created (e.g. temporary or permanent)
- prognosis, given their potentially curable or life-threatening disease
- age
- ethnic origin
- interpersonal relationships and their potential for physical and psychological support
- level of psychological preparation.

Ideally there should be time for at least two interviews between the patient, family and the stoma care nurse to take place before surgery. Time and privacy are essential so that all concerned can begin to build a relationship, and exchange relevant information. If possible nurses should visit patients at home, as this will help them feel more relaxed and likely to raise intimate concerns. Additionally, it enables nurses to gain useful information about patients' home environment, which will aid discharge planning. During these discussions it is important for the nurse to define her role within the healthcare team. This allows both patient and family to gain some understanding of how various team members will collectively promote continuity of care.

Although surgeons give each patient an explanation about their situation and proposed surgery, it may have only been partly understood or remembered. Gentle open questioning will encourage patients to tell the nurse what they have understood about their condition, planned operation, and stoma, and how they think their life might be affected by them. Knowledge of patients' past and current medical history, the proposed surgery, and whether the stoma is likely to be permanent or temporary should therefore be acquired before these preoperative discussions take place so that information can be repeated or expanded appropriately, and misunderstandings corrected. Most patients and their families welcome having an explanatory booklet about living with a stoma to refer to at leisure. We can use these to help patients understand information, for example by using the illustrations to show which areas of their bowel are affected or will be removed, as well as encouraging them to ask questions and clarify aspects of their particular situation. Most patients ask about the colour, size, look and position of the stoma and showing them slides or photographs can be helpful. Encouraging patients to look at and touch their oral mucosa can give them a sense of what their stoma will feel like. During their preoperative discussions most patients want to see and handle the type of pouch they are likely to wear. They should also be given the option of wearing an appliance preoperatively, which can increase their acceptance that equipment will be discreet and comfortable. Patients should be told that the appliance used in the initial postoperative period will probably differ from the type suitable for them in the long term.

Stoma surgery can affect patients' lives and sense of themselves in many ways. Nurses should encourage patients to explore their thoughts and feelings about living with a stoma, including how they think close relationships may be affected. Many of the approaches described in Chapter 7 can be used to aid such communication. Major pelvic surgery can impair sexual function (see Chs 3 and 5). The implications of their particular type of surgery should be carefully discussed with patients so that they can give informed consent to it. Discussion about sexual orientation and possible physical and psychological effects of their surgery is an important part of care. It needs to be skilfully and knowledgeably handled (Bancroft 1993, Huish et al 1998; see also the *patient scenarios* in Chapters 5 and 9).

Rehabilitation takes time, and regular monitoring of progress by the stoma care nurse, other relevant members of the healthcare team, and the patient will enable early identification of problems to take place, and help and support to be given. Referral to colleagues with specialised expertise should be made if this is needed by patients and their families; for example, if more advanced therapeutic interventions are required.

PHYSICAL CARE

Patients generally require the usual preparatory measures that people undergo prior to operation. Additional methods required because the patient's condition and surgery involves their bowel include:

- nutritional assessment and treatment to identify and minimise deficits
- preparation of the bowel itself.

Bowel that is as clean and empty as possible is more mobile and easier to handle surgically without spillage of intestinal contents, thus minimising the risk of postoperative sepsis. Preparation of the bowel for surgery depends on each patient's medical/physical condition and planned type of surgery, and a variety of oral and rectal preparations may be used (Keighley 1999). Patients also usually have their food restricted to a low residue diet and/or fluid diet to aid bowel emptying.

Undergoing bowel cleansing is difficult for most patients. Praise for their part in making their bowel as well prepared as possible may help them maintain self-esteem, as may tactful support and privacy at this time when they may feel particularly vulnerable.

SITING OF STOMAS

Preoperative siting is essential as a badly positioned stoma can make subsequent appliance management difficult and thus have severe repercussions on patients' lifestyles. Siting should take place at a time when patients are able to move around into different positions, and are alert enough to provide information about their needs and lifestyle. Ideally, it is therefore important to *avoid* times when patients' mobility or mental ability are reduced, or their attention is focused elsewhere (e.g. when bowel preparation or premedication has been given or patients are anaesthetised).

The quality of siting can have significant implications for patients' future stoma management and should therefore be carried out by an experienced stoma care or other senior nurse or surgeon (Blackley 2004, Readding 2003, Rutledge et al 2003). In situations where patients are undergoing emergency surgery and may not be fit enough to engage in all the usual elements of stoma siting it is often still preferable for an experienced nurse or doctor to mark the site they judge to be most suitable preoperatively. Muscle relaxants given during surgery can alter the abdomen quite considerably and make it even more difficult to choose an appropriate site (Davenport 2003).

The majority of permanent stomas are created below the patient's waistline and within the area of the rectus muscle to give support in the peristomal region and thus reduce the likelihood of later abdominal weakness and herniation. Traditionally, the correct position for these stomas has been held to be about one-third of the way along a line from the umbilicus to the anterior superior iliac spine, to provide a stoma that is visible to patients and adequately distanced from the main incision (Fig. 4.1). However, this may be unsuitable for people who are substantially overweight or whose height and/or waistline only gives them a small area in which to fit equipment.

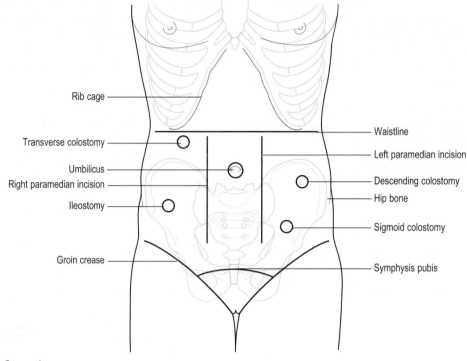

Figure 4.1 Stoma sites.

- An *ileostomy* is normally created on patients' *right* side.
- A *sigmoid or end colostomy* is normally created on patients' *left* side.
- A *transverse colostomy* is generally positioned in the *right upper abdomen*, midway between the costal margin and umbilicus and within the area of the rectus muscle. It is therefore more likely to be created on or near patients' waistlines. Whether intended as temporary or permanent stomas they require careful preoperative siting if major problems in appliance management are to be avoided.

The main goals which siting a stoma should achieve are that the chosen site will:

- be compatible with the planned surgery
- lie within an abdominal area which is of a size and shape that enables stomal equipment to adhere well to it
- allow the achievement of adequate appliance adherence, comfort and management when the patients are carrying out their normal lifestyle and activities.

Choosing a suitable stoma site

In order to achieve the above goals the siting process should include identifying:

- sites to avoid, generally and specifically (steps A and B)
- sites likely to be suitable for this person (steps C and D)
- a site acceptable to the individual patient (steps E and F).

Although the following six-step process may seem complex at first glance, it has been successfully used, and broken down into these small steps to teach colleagues, for many years (Breckman 1991).

Step A Identify where the type of stoma this patient is going to have is *usually* sited and consider whether this area of the patient's abdomen initially appears generally suitable. Does it enable the following areas to be *avoided*?

1. Rib cage
2. Waistline

3. Umbilicus
4. Left paramedian incision
5. Right paramedian incision
6. Hip bone
7. Symphysis pubis
8. Groin crease.

Step B Obtain the information you need to recognise sites that will be *unsuitable* because of the patient's body shape or lifestyle.

Identify sites to be avoided by asking the patient and yourself the following questions:

B1. Where is this patient's waistline?
B2. Where do clothes come on this patient's abdomen? (e.g. trousers, underpants, tights, suspender belts, roll-ons)
B3. Are there any scars from previous operations?
B4. Does this patient have any abdominal dips, gullies, creases or bulges when the patient is:
 – lying in bed
 – sitting in a low chair
 – standing
 – sitting in a low chair and leaning forward as if to put a cup on a low table. (This shows up problem areas which may also appear when the patient is sitting in the bucket-shaped seat of a car)
 – in any particular position used for work or hobbies (e.g. using particular equipment; digging the garden; playing golf).
B5. Does this patient travel by car? If so, where does the seat belt come on her abdomen when she is (a) a driver? (b) a passenger?
B6. Does this patient wear any supportive belt or other special fitments which might clash with possible stoma sites?
B7. Does this patient have pendulous breasts which could restrict her view of potential stoma sites?
B8. Does this patient's abdomen rest on her thighs when she sits down? (This can mean a bag placed too low on the abdomen gets squashed or cannot drain properly when the patient sits down.)
B9. If this patient has a partner who shares their bed, does the partner normally sleep on the same side of the patient as the stoma will probably be on? If this might cause difficulties could the patient and partner change sides in bed?

Step C Make a preliminary identification of sites that *might be suitable* for this patient's stoma. Then *check whether a site meets the criteria* of visibility, ad-

equate space for adherence of a bag, a reasonably flat surface for attachment of a bag, congruence with the patient's activities and lifestyle.

To do this ask the patient and yourself the following questions, and thus identify suitable sites if the answer is 'yes'.

C1. Is this site far enough away from the hips and rib cage to allow space for the bag adhesive/peristomal wafer to fit?
C2. Is this site far enough away from the probable incision site for this operation to allow sufficient space for bag application without impingement on the wound?
C3. Is this site free from abdominal dips, gullies, creases, bulges, scars, and the umbilicus when the patient is in the positions outlined in B4?
C4. Is this site high enough that the patient can see it clearly when standing? (Ask patients to point to the marked site with their glasses on if they will be worn when changing a bag. This points up problems with bifocals, or glasses that slip down their nose, altering visibility of the site.)
C5. If this patient will need to change her appliance sitting in a chair/wheelchair, can she see the stoma site in this sitting position? (This includes frail elderly people as well as those who have had a stroke, amputation or who normally use a wheelchair.)
C6. Will clothes impede drainage of the stoma bag or put pressure on the stoma itself in this position? (see B2)
C7. Is this site flat enough to be able to apply the type of equipment for this type of stoma?
C8. Does the patient understand why this site is suitable, and is she willing to accept it?

This is particularly important if patients have indicated they would prefer a different site that is anatomically unsuitable. Further explanation and discussion may be necessary to help them understand that the site which is chosen has implications for their future wellbeing because it will affect the ease or difficulty with which they can manage their stoma care and achieve good bag adherence.

Step D Ask the patient whether or not she would be willing to wear a bag before the operation, once the stoma site has been chosen and marked.

Benefits for patients in wearing a bag preoperatively:

• They can test the comfort of wearing a bag at that site.

- They can experience the feeling of wearing a bag with their normal clothing, and check their compatibility.
- They can see for themselves that their equipment will be unobtrusive under clothes.
- If they use a wheelchair they can check whether the abdominal movement which takes place when they move in and out of their wheelchair, and from bed to chair etc., causes problems with bag adherence at the chosen site.
- The site can be reconsidered if problems such as the bag adhesive or wafer lifting or creasing indicate that the original site is not really suitable.

Disadvantages for patients in wearing a bag preoperatively:

- Some patients find the experience emotionally disturbing, and it increases their anxiety.
- Some patients' normal method of coping with events is to wait until they happen, and then face that reality. Wearing a bag preoperatively may not be compatible with their preferred way of coping.
- A skin reaction to the trial appliance can affect the site and, if severe, can make it unusable at the time of operation.

It may be advisable for patients whose skins are sensitive to plasters, other adhesives, or who have a history of skin conditions (e.g. psoriasis) or burning easily in the sun, to avoid application of appliances to the stoma site preoperatively. They may benefit from patch testing of appliance adhesives and wafers on other parts of the body well away from the stoma site, to obtain information and reassurance about suitable equipment that will be available for their use after surgery.

Step E   Mark the stoma site and advise the patient to avoid washing it off. If appropriate, apply a suitable style of stoma bag (containing about 100 ml water) to the chosen site. Allow them to wear it for several hours, including overnight if they so wish.

The timing of this activity should allow sufficient leeway for reconsideration and testing of the site to be able to take place before the operation if necessary.

Step F   Evaluate the suitability of the site with the patient, and confirm or revise the site as necessary.

When siting stomas Black (2000, p 79–80) suggests the following:

- Special skin markers of the type used in dermatology and plastic surgery should be used. Biro pens and felt tip markers are unsuitable as they contain colophony, which may cause skin allergies.
- Stoma sites marked with a dermatological pen can be covered with a clear waterproof dressing, enabling the marker to be retained while patients bathe and when the dressing is removed. If biros or felt tip pens are used, their marks 'lift off' when the dressing is removed in theatre prior to skin prepping, leaving the site unidentifiable when the surgeon is later ready to create the stoma.
- Documentation in patients' notes should include:
  - where the stoma has been marked
  - any difficulties or special features identified when choosing the stoma site
  - whether the patient has understood the implications of the siting procedure and is in agreement with the site marked.
- Notes that do not contain this information can create difficulties if complaints or litigation about the site subsequently arise.

PATIENT SCENARIO 4.1: Khaliq Choudry is a 45-year-old Muslim who is a computer programmer. He does not think his activities at work will affect where his stoma could be sited. He is concerned as to how his religious activities might be affected by having a stoma. Mrs Reid encourages him to discuss these concerns so she can check whether they are the same as Muslims generally wish to address (see Ch. 19) and identify any additional concerns. The key points identified are:

- Mr Choudry wants to continue adopting the salaam position for prayer without worrying that his bag would lift and cause leakage.
- He does not think that whether his stoma is above or below his umbilicus will affect how he thinks of his stomal effluent or will manage his stoma care.
- Like most Muslims he generally uses his right hand for 'clean' tasks such as eating and greeting, and his left hand for 'unclean' tasks such as dealing with body waste. He thinks it would be acceptable to use his left hand for removing used equipment and cleaning around the stoma, and both hands for preparing and applying new equipment.
- He wants to use an appliance system that will enable him to be ritually clean for each of his five daily prayer sessions. Having been shown two-piece equipment and how the base can be left in situ whilst the bag is changed before each prayer session he expresses relief that this

system is available, and sufficiently discreet to avoid being noticed by other people.

Mrs Reid uses this information as well as that gained through the siting process described earlier. She asks him to adopt his usual position for prayer so she can make sure that the chosen site will remain flat and that the two-piece equipment will fit in with his body contours and not be put under strain in this position. These actions helped reduce the likelihood of problems arising from the stoma site and increased Mr Choudry's confidence that he could develop an acceptable way of managing his stoma.

Mrs Reid documents the key factors used in siting the stoma, and that Mr Choudry will need assistance to achieve appropriate cleansing prior to prayer.

MANAGEMENT OF LOOP ILEOSTOMIES AND COLOSTOMIES

Patients with loop stomas usually need general stoma care to be adapted because the circumstances under which these stomas are raised and their structure and function create some additional management requirements. The following features should be borne in mind when caring for these patients.

Their construction and purpose

A loop stoma is created by bringing a loop of bowel out of the abdomen and fashioning it so it has both a proximal (functioning) opening *and* a distal (defunctioning) opening exteriorised on the abdominal wall (Fig. 4.2). It is therefore generally larger than a single end stoma. Traditionally, loop stomas have been formed from transverse colon. Their size plus their site (usually the upper right quadrant and near the ribs) have made management difficult. More surgeons are now using ileum as this results in a smaller stoma, positioned in the usual ileostomy site, and thus easier management (Black 2000).

Creating a loop stoma is a relatively simple operative procedure, making it suitable for patients whose disease or condition, and/or general health, limit the extent and length of operation they can sustain but who require defunctioning of part of their bowel. Sometimes a loop stoma will be carried out in conjunction with resection of colon further

along the bowel pathway, or it may be created solely as a diversion. The main purpose of this type of stoma is to allow the bowel beyond it to rest/heal without effluent passing through it. The loop of bowel is often supported by a bridge or rod for 5–8 days following surgery. This creates a spur or ridge between the openings to prevent the loop from flattening or receding, which could enable faecal spillage from the proximal to the distal opening to occur. This rod is usually external and can thus be easily removed once the medical team think that the spur between the openings is well-established. An internal dissolvable Biethium plate is still sometimes used as an alternative loop support.

The choice of loop support system

The type and size of rod or bridge used to support and maintain the loop of bowel is important as it will influence:

- the style of appliance that can fit over it
- the ease with which the bag opening can fit around the stoma and thus protect the skin from effluent
- the ease with which skin protectives can be fitted snugly around the stoma
- patients' comfort
- the length of time equipment will adhere.

Generally the smaller rods and bridges now available provide sufficient support to maintain the loop whilst also being small enough to be compatible with effective application of stomal equipment. However, there can be problems, particularly if a transverse colostomy is created. If they are sited too near the rib cage, the rigid rod and rib cage collide when the patient sits or bends. Strain is put on the appliance, and the system is uncomfortable for patients.

The circumstances in which loop stomas are created

These fall into two main categories. Where a loop ileostomy is created as an integral part of planned surgery an appropriate site which can accommodate the stoma, rod and appliance should be marked. Examples include where colectomy or pouch formation is planned. Even though the loop stoma is larger than a single end stoma it will usually be relatively straightforward to manage.

The second category includes circumstances where loop stomas are created as temporary diversions

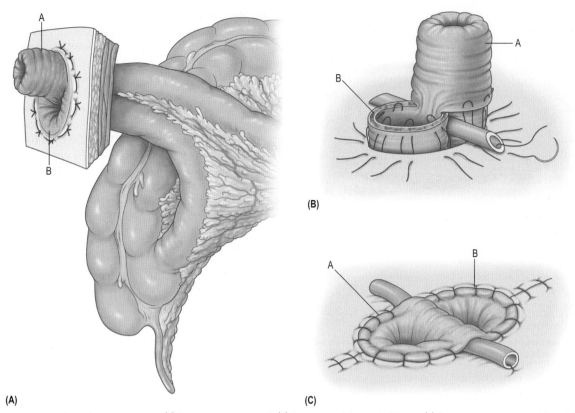

Figure 4.2 Temporary loop stomas. (a) Ileostomy without rod. (b) Ileostomy with supportive rod. (c) Transverse colostomy with rod. A, proximal opening; B, distal opening.

either during emergency surgery or in situations where the need for stomal diversion has not been identified or definitely decided upon before the operation takes place. The issue then arises as to whether preoperative stoma siting and provision of information about living with a stoma should take place. Some people suggest that if there is any uncertainty as to whether a stoma will be raised, potential sites should not be marked preoperatively as this might make patients anxious about living with a stoma they might never have. Similar reasons are also given for not engaging in preoperative discussion about stomas with patients in these situations. However, consideration also needs to be given to what may result if these patients do have a stoma raised without at least preoperative siting and hopefully some discussion, even if this has to be limited due to lack of time or patient frailty.

Loop stomas are often raised in patients whose condition makes shorter, simpler operations desirable so surgeons will naturally seek to create these stomas in positions where it is easy to exteriorise the bowel. In these circumstances transverse colostomies are sometimes created. When these sites are marked preoperatively it is usually possible to identify (right-sided) areas where it will be surgically easy to place the stoma *and* where there will be sufficient distance from the rib cage and waistline to accommodate the bulky stoma, support rod, and sizeable bag and skin protective adhesive area required. In other words, surgical and stomal management criteria can be met. In contrast, once patients are positioned on the operating table and their abdomen is relaxed under anaesthesia it can be much more difficult to identify appropriate sites. Loop colostomies that are not sited preoperatively are often brought out too near the rib cage to enable equipment to lie flat and adhere well. As effluent from transverse colostomies is normally semi-liquid any difficulties in obtaining a well-secured bag can result in substantial problems including leakage, skin damage and non-containment of odour.

Although many of these problems can be resolved with expert stoma care, the experience of having them at all, let alone frequently, can cause patients considerable psychological as well as physical distress. For example, faecal leakage can damage clothes, furniture, self-confidence, social interactions and relationships as well as peristomal skin. Such effects can be long-lasting and it is both inaccurate and inappropriate for healthcare staff to dismiss them as 'acceptable because patients only have these stomas temporarily'. Although many patients will have their loop stomas closed within 3–6 months others may have their stoma for much longer. Some patients may have to keep their loop stomas permanently if their condition prevents subsequent closure.

The effects of waking up postoperatively with an unexpected stoma must also not be minimised. Some patients do not trust assurances that their stoma will be temporary when given by staff who did not tell them they might need a stoma in the first place. The reduced trust can also increase the anxiety and distress felt by patients if management problems with their stoma do arise and staff should offer psychological support as well as physical care so rapport and confidence can be re-established.

Specific aspects of practical care

The main principles for choosing and using stoma bags and skin care aids should be followed in the care of loop stomas. There are also some additional aspects to consider:

Equipment should be of a size, shape and flexibility to accommodate the stoma and rod as well as effluent

Loop stomas are generally more oval in shape and quite bulky. During the first 5–10 days the stoma tends to be oedematous, and there may also be a support rod in situ. The upper portion of the chosen bag therefore needs to be of a shape that accommodates the stoma and rod easily. Drainable bags with a sizeable, oval, flexible faceplate are often suitable.

Stomas and equipment should be monitored carefully for compatibility as the stoma size can increase before subsequently decreasing in size, and prolapse of one or both loops can sometimes occur. Constriction of the stoma through too rigid or too tight equipment can also produce oedema.

Equipment should be suitable for accommodating sizeable amounts of effluent

Output, especially from transverse colostomies, may initially be substantial, semi-liquid and irregular, particularly if preoperative measures to empty the bowel were minimal. Forecasting how often bags will need emptying can be impossible. Emptying an overfull bag without spillage can be difficult and its weight can drag on, and reduce the bag–body adhesive seal. It is therefore advisable to check and empty patients' bags frequently, especially before moving them so that potential leakage sites are dealt with before seepage occurs as the patient changes position.

Patients can be concerned about the amount of faecal output and how they will deal with it themselves. They should be advised this will reduce to a more manageable amount and consistency as the bowel settles and they resume normal eating.

Skin care aids must be sufficiently substantial to protect the skin from effluent containing digestive elements (from ileostomies and transverse colostomies)

The amount and type of faeces being passed can affect both peristomal skin and any skin protectives being used within quite short periods of time so skin protection is essential. Appliances with pre-cut openings are generally less suitable as most loop stomas are not the same shape as the bag openings, and their use will leave some skin exposed to effluent. Generally, drainable appliances which incorporate a wafer which can be cut to fit around the stoma are most suitable as they provide maximum skin protection.

The rate of disintegration of protective wafers can vary considerably, depending on the amount and type of effluent, patients' body heat etc. Regular monitoring is advisable if adequate skin protection is to be maintained.

Preparation and positioning of skin care aids is important if maximum protection without stomal constriction is to be achieved

The tips described in Chapter 14 for creating a flat abdomen in fistula care are also useful when loop stomas are positioned near waist creases, rib cage curves etc. They can be used in addition to the following basic process which enables well-fitting equipment to be applied.

- Select suitable equipment which either has an integral wafer or includes a separate wafer to use in conjunction with the drainable bag.
- Make a paper template of the stoma and then use it to cut out the wafer/flange, ensuring a snug fit is obtained.

- If the stoma is oedematous, make radial slits in the wafer hole to allow it to expand slightly if oedema increases.
- If using a separate protective wafer, this can be fitted before applying the bag or they can be combined first, leaving the backing paper on the wafer while attaching the bag to its outer side. The combined approach is useful if the stoma is active.
- Slit the backing paper of the wafer/flange in two to four places but leave it in situ.
- Having cleansed the stoma and surrounding area, position the equipment, tucking the rod inside the bag. (This is much easier to do if the backing paper is still in place, preventing the wafer from sticking to you or the rod!) Now remove the backing paper in sections, sealing the lowest part of the equipment first and working up to the highest point on the patient's body. This ensures any wrinkles are above the stoma, minimising leakage risk.

Faeces and mucus can be passed from both the proximal and distal stomal openings and via the rectum

It is usually helpful to tell patients quite early on postoperatively that this may happen, coupled with a basic description of their type of diversion, so that they are not alarmed or fear that something has gone wrong if this does later take place. Although staff may easily accept this is a normal occurrence, patients can find it difficult. Help with personal hygiene and a tactful supportive approach can enable patients to retain their sense of personal dignity and reduce anxiety.

Many patients will spend time at home enabling their bowel to settle down/heal to a degree that will allow bowel continuity to be restored. This means they will need to be taught all the usual aspects of stoma care if they are to manage this period, including their stoma care, confidently and with adequate ability. It is important not to assume patients will have understood and accepted that this will be necessary, particularly if their operation was an emergency and they had little opportunity to absorb such information, even if it was given. It is advisable to clarify with the surgical team at an early stage postoperatively whether they plan to send patients home with their temporary stoma. This gives patients time to understand the importance of giving their bowel adequate rest, and the

contribution that they will make to their ultimate wellbeing by accepting time at home with a temporary stoma. This will help them be more positive and active when learning stoma care. However, some patients may believe that if they exhibit adequate stoma care abilities, their surgeon will not close their stoma. This possibility should be borne in mind if the patient refuses to learn self-care or appears to find it extra difficult to remember and carry out. In such circumstances a counselling approach can be used to encourage the patient to talk about their situation as *they* experience it, as this will enable any further information and help to be responsive to their individual concerns and needs.

Closure of loop stomas

Patients are usually told that their bowel will need to be assessed as ready for closure before that operation can take place. They often optimistically assume the tests to assess bowel condition are mere formalities and that closure will automatically and speedily take place after the tests. These assumptions can lead to much distress if patients have to undergo a longer period for healing and further reassessments before a decision to close the stoma can be made. It can be more helpful to describe stoma closure to patients as a series of stages, each of which requires successful completion in order for them to progress to the next one.

Stage 1: examination of the section of bowel from the distal loop to the rectum

The purpose is to assess the degree to which healing of any anastomosis and restoration of normal bowel appearance and function has taken place, and whether this is sufficient to cope with faecal flow once the stoma has been closed. It entails:

- washouts of the defunctioned section of bowel via the distal loop so that mucus, old faeces etc. can be evacuated rectally, leaving the bowel sufficiently empty for its condition to be assessed
- administration of barium enema and X-rays to portray the state of the distal bowel and anastomosis with subsequent assessment of their condition and readiness for bowel continuity to be restored
- distal loop washout to be given to remove residual barium so it does not solidify and become retained in the bowel.

Stage 2: preparation of the patient's bowel for stoma closure

The purpose is to ensure that both proximal (functioning) and distal (defunctioning) sections of bowel are sufficiently empty to enable the surgeon to re-anastomose the bowel. It entails:

- patient admission to hospital, usually 24 hours prior to surgery
- the patient going on a low-residue diet for 24 hours prior to hospital admission, and oral fluids only from the time of admission until the commencement of the period of nil by mouth prior to surgery
- administration of antibiotics and aperients by mouth to prepare the *proximal* bowel
- *distal* loop washouts the day before operation with warm water to prepare the bowel section between the distal loop and rectum for operation.

It is important to remember that most oral aperients will only aid emptying of the functioning proximal bowel, although aperients that stimulate bowel wall contraction may have some effect on the distal bowel too (see Ch. 17). Washouts can take time so the patient must be kept warm and as comfortable as possible, seated on a toilet or commode with enough privacy to help them relax and allow the water to pass through their distal bowel and be expelled rectally. The position of the distal loop will depend on whether a loop ileostomy or colostomy has been raised (Fig. 4.2). Normally effluent can be noted passing from the proximal opening, making identification of the other loop as the distal one straightforward. This should be verified by gentle insertion of a gloved finger into the opening to check that the internal direction of the bowel is congruent with the defunctioning ileal or colonic distal bowel. An irrigation set, as described in Chapter 15, can be used for these washouts. The cone rests snugly in the stomal opening so water passes into the stoma easily and with minimal spillage, helping to maintain the patient's dignity. Washouts should be gentle, to avoid putting pressure on the anastomosis.

Stage 3: surgical closure of the bowel

This involves re-anastomosis of the proximal and distal stomal openings.

Stage 4: normal postoperative care

This will include monitoring of bowel function, resumption of oral fluids and normal diet, and establishment that normal faecal passage is taking place without problems before the patient goes home.

TYPES OF APPLIANCE

The majority of appliances used in the UK are disposable and made of light, easy to handle, odour-proof plastic which may be transparent, opaque or patterned. Modern adhesives are usually made of hypoallergenic substances to minimise any skin irritation. Some patients prefer reusable appliances, or their circumstances may make these the most appropriate choice. For example, patients may live in countries where they have to buy their stomal equipment, or where maintaining reliable supplies of equipment is difficult. Where these circumstances could arise it is important that their implications are tactfully discussed with patients, and the possibility of choosing reusable equipment is considered.

Appliances are generally divided into drainable and closed/non-drainable categories. Each of these may consist of a one- or two-piece system.

Drainable appliances

These have an outlet to enable effluent to be emptied in between bag changes (Fig. 4.3). Many appliances have integral systems for closing the outlet securely. Where separate clips are provided there may be fewer clips than bags in a box. It is prudent to retain the clip when bags are changed. This style of appliance is generally used where patients' faeces is of a sufficiently soft or fluid consistency to be easily drained out of it. This means drainable bags are most likely to be used when:

- the stoma is situated in the ileum, ascending, or transverse colon and thus effluent is diverted from the body before colonic reabsorption of fluid can occur
- patients' food intake is curtailed or of a more fluid consistency, resulting in a more fluid faecal output, including in the early postoperative period.

The nature of this more fluid effluent means that fairly substantial skin protection will be needed. Therefore the adhesive or flange provided on drainable bags is usually of a style that will provide such skin protection for the 3–4 days they will be worn.

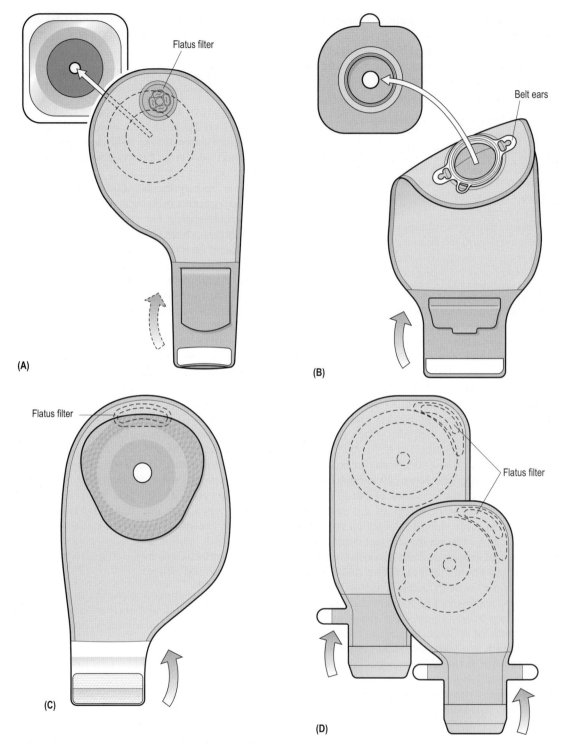

Figure 4.3 Drainable appliances with cut to fit adhesives. (a) Flexible base with an adhesive bag with an integral outlet closure and integral flatus filter. (b) Two-piece with separate clip-on bag which has integral 'ears' for belt. (c) One-piece with flexible flange. (d) One-piece standard and mini sized bags.

One-piece systems

The adhesive area for attachment onto the skin is an integral part of the appliance. It may incorporate a skin protective wafer for additional protection around the stoma. This wafer may have a microporous type adhesive surround to provide a more extensive yet flexible adhesive area. Some one-piece bags may need to be worn with a belt to provide support and security. The complete appliance will be changed every 3–4 days, depending on individual circumstances (see Chapter 5).

Two-piece systems

These consist of a flange or base and the attachable bag. One type incorporates a welded plastic ring onto which the bag is clipped, while another has a reinforced area onto which the bag is stuck. With both types the material of which the flange/ base is made can remain in place for several days. The bags may be replaced in between without disturbing the base. Bags may be available in standard and shorter (mini) lengths. The adhesive flange may be made entirely from a combination of sodium carboxymethylcellulose, gelatin, pectin, and polyisobutyline made up as a protective wafer, or may have an inner ring of protective wafer bonded onto an outer, more flexible adhesive collar.

Closed appliances

These bags are non-drainable and therefore are usually more suitable for patients with the fairly solid faeces that occur when fluid has been reabsorbed from the remaining colon before it leaves the body via a descending or sigmoid colostomy (Fig. 4.4). Effluent is less abrasive to the skin by the time it reaches these types of stoma. Thus the skin protection provided in this type of equipment may be less substantial than that of drainable equipment.

One-piece systems

The closed ended bag has an integral adhesive area for attachment to the skin. When used the complete bag is removed and replaced with a clean one. Several types are available in either transparent or opaque odour-resistant plastic. Most styles incorporate an activated charcoal filter for the expulsion of flatus without odour.

Two-piece systems

The base or flange, made of hypoallergenic substances, allows bags to be replaced several times before the base needs to be changed, using similar attachment processes to those described above for drainable equipment. Various transparent and opaque designs of bag are available, depending on the style of product chosen.

Other types of appliance

Some appliances are stylistically similar to those described above in that they are drainable or closed, one- or two-piece. However, they are often primarily identified in accordance with the features described below.

Reusable or non-disposable systems

These appliances are generally made of butyl or similar material and can be used for about 3 months before being replaced. Most are two-piece, and the circular opening of the bag is stretched to hook over the lip of the flange and then fit snugly around the flange neck. A double-sided plaster is used: one side is applied to the base of the flange, the other side to the body. This system can be used with peristomal wafers if additional skin protection is required. Bags can be changed daily, leaving the base for several days, if patients have enough strength and motility in their fingers to fix the bags over the flange. When the whole system is changed the double-sided plaster (plus wafer if used) is discarded. The remaining equipment is washed thoroughly with warm soapy water, rinsed and hung up to dry and air. The inside of bags should then be lightly powdered to prevent the sides sticking together before storage ready for reuse.

Toilet disposable appliances

There are two types that may be described as disposable. Firstly, there are closed one-piece bags made from plastic film attached onto a protective adhesive and which have a combined charcoal filter. They are only suitable when colostomy effluent is solid as they are manufactured to disintegrate in the fluid of the toilet pan. Their *advantage* is ease of disposal. *Disadvantages* include being unsuitable for bathing, water sports, liquid effluent. They are not suitable for all toilet systems.

Secondly, there are appliances that have an outer and inner bag. Once the appliance has been used it can be pulled apart. The inner section containing faeces is removed and disposed of in the toilet. The outer section is placed with the usual home or hospital rubbish for disposal.

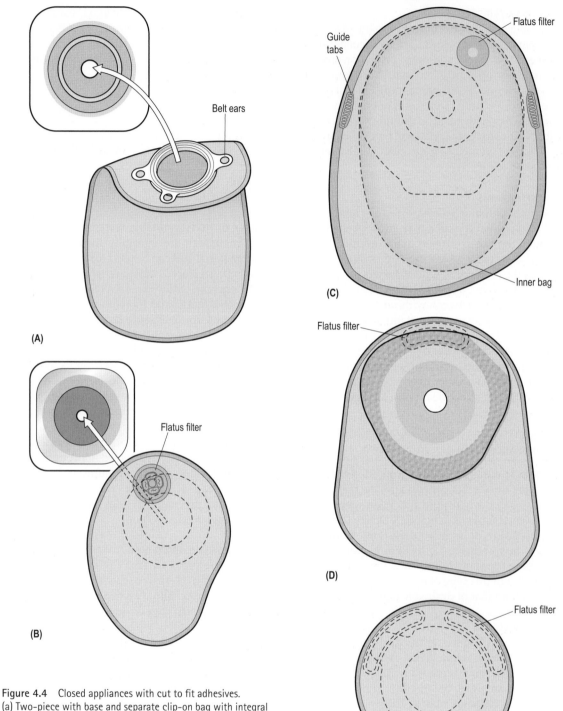

Figure 4.4 Closed appliances with cut to fit adhesives.
(a) Two-piece with base and separate clip-on bag with integral belt 'ears'. (b) Two-piece with flexible base and an adhesive bag with flatus filter. (c) One-piece with inner bag that is disposable in toilet. (d) One-piece with flexible flange and flatus filter. (e) Stoma cap with flatus filter.

Convex systems

Flanges with a convex curve push back the abdomen immediately around a stoma. They make it protrude from skin level into the appliance, enabling effluent to be deposited into the bag instead of pooling or leaking at skin level. They are available in one- and two-piece appliances. It is important that convex systems are fitted and monitored by a stoma care nurse. Although they are particularly helpful when managing retracted or badly sited stomas (see Ch. 21), problems can arise from their use. These include:

- bruising or discolouration around the stoma
- stoma prolapse.

Further research into convex system usage is being conducted.

Colostomy plugs

These are alternative one- or two-piece systems. Faecal evacuation is managed by plugging the end colostomy except when it is expected to act. Patients must have enough colon functioning to make their faeces sufficiently solid to prevent leakage around the plug.

Plug systems are somewhat T- or mushroom-shaped in overall appearance. The pliable stalk or plug is inserted into the stoma. The material, which has kept the plug compressed, then disintegrates through contact with bowel mucosa. The plug expands to prevent faeces leaving the stoma until it is removed. Plugs are single use only, and contain a filter to allow deodorised passage of flatus.

One-piece: the plug is attached to an adhesive faceplate which adheres to the peristomal skin.

Two-piece: a separate faceplate is applied to the peristomal skin. The plug is passed through the faceplate opening for stomal insertion and removal. When plugs are removed an appliance can be attached to the faceplate to collect faeces. Faceplates are changed two to three times a week (Black 2000).

A stoma care nurse should assess patients' suitability for plug usage and monitor their subsequent management of any system with which they have been fitted. Factors to consider include:

- *Stomal diameter and condition.* Stomas that are larger than 45 cm diameter, protruding, or prolapsed are unsuitable.
- *The likely thickness of the abdominal wall* and whether any available plug length is suitable.

- *The patient's usual faecal consistency* and whether it is sufficiently solid to prevent leakage around the plug.
- *The patient's ability to manage the system.* This includes their potential adeptness to manage the system and manage evacuation following plug removal, and the levels of confidence and comfort they could gain from its use.

Blackley (2004, p 189–190) suggests patients should be advised:

- to build up their plug wear times gradually from 1–2 hours daily to a maximum of 12 hours
- that wear times and comfort vary, and can depend on factors such as diet, faecal consistency, and flatus volumes
- that plugs left in situ for too long may allow leakage of faeces or mucus, or plug extrusion
- that sufficient time for faecal evacuation must be left between plug insertions.

MATCHING PATIENTS AND APPLIANCES

The range of appliances available can be confusing for both nurse and patient seeking to choose a suitable appliance. The point at which stomal diversion occurs in the bowel pathway should first be ascertained. This is because the type of effluent produced will largely be determined by the amount of bowel left in situ above that division (see Fig. 3.2). Previous resection of bowel above the stoma site is also likely to affect bowel function. Once this information is known it should be used as part of a systematic approach in order to highlight potential problem areas that need to be taken into account, and thus guide choices (Borwell 1994). The following areas should be considered:

Type of effluent to be contained: is the faecal consistency likely to be fairly solid or more fluid, given the amount of bowel still in situ above the stomal diversion, and the digestive functions that this patient is still likely to have in action? What capacity will the bag need to have (see earlier, plus Chs 2, 3).

Drainable appliances will be needed in the immediate postoperative period for all types of stoma, fistulas, wound drainage, where the effluent is soft to fluid consistency. They should be transparent to aid monitoring of the stoma and effluent.

Long term, patients with ileostomies, caecostomies, ascending and transverse colostomies will need drainable appliances. Patients with sigmoid or descending colostomies can use a closed bag. Some patients whose transverse colostomy passes faeces with a soft to solid consistency can also use a closed bag if they do not need to change it more than twice a day and skin protection can be maintained.

Physique: what is this person's body structure: are they short, tall, slim, obese?

The flange and the bag should be of a size and shape that will lie flat and fit snugly into the patient's body contours. Some peristomal areas will require a flexible flange whilst others will need a firmer base (see also Ch. 21).

Potential for skin problems: does this patient have a history of skin disease, or sensitivity to plasters/plastic, which might mean the material in some appliances makes them unsuitable to use?

Flange adhesives may need to be patch tested in order to obtain this information. Patients who sweat a lot may need to wear bags with an integral fabric backing, or use an appliance cover.

Physical ability and dexterity: is there any impairment of visual or manual dexterity?

Background knowledge of patients' usual levels of independence can help identify what skills they are capable of attaining, whether they need an appliance with particular features and, if they may need assistance with their stoma care, who might be able to provide it.

Mental ability, age and intelligence: is the retention of knowledge and acquisition of new skills likely to be difficult for this patient?

Some (but not all) elderly people may find physical and mental frailty affects their abilities for self-care, which can lead to frustration and even despair. Choosing a simple appliance which can be fitted with the minimum number of steps may be helpful.

Patient's personal choice: does this person have particular factors that they want their equipment to provide or avoid, perhaps influenced by their social background? (see Patient scenario 4.1).

The information gained from considering these factors can then be used to identify which style of appliance is potentially suitable. One-piece systems are:

- easy to handle
- suitable for the elderly or those with physical or mental impairment
- cosmetically light, flexible, discreet.

Two-piece systems are suitable where:

- trauma to sensitive skin from bag changes needs to be minimised
- the patient wants to be able to use bags of different lengths easily when engaging in different activities.

SKIN CARE

The goal of skin care is to maintain peristomal skin in good condition. Aids used to achieve this goal should be chosen according to:

- the function that is needed in the particular situation
- the capacity of the aid to fulfil that function and be easily used by the patient.

Skin protection provides a barrier or film against effluent or potential skin trauma from adhesives, and may be used as a prophylactic measure.

Skin restoration is necessary when the epidermis of the skin has been exposed to trauma and requires repair. An agent with therapeutic and protective qualities is needed to enable healing and subsequent protection to take place.

Types of skin care aids

Skin protective (peristomal) wafers are available in squares or rings in a range of sizes. They will adhere to moist weeping areas and are useful to heal or protect skin from effluent or adhesives.

Wafers are cut to fit snugly over the relevant area and can be left in situ for several days providing there is no effluent seepage underneath them. A paper template of the area to be covered is usually made as a pattern for cutting the actual wafer accurately, as they are expensive and this reduces wastage.

Rings or washers can be fitted to provide a snug seal immediately around a stoma or wound drain, and are an integral part of many appliances.

Protective powders are often made of similar ingredients to wafers and act as therapeutic agents, which will adhere to moist raw areas. The powder forms a layer that offers protection from adhesives and effluent. This is a less substantial barrier than that provided by wafers or rings, but is more flexible than they are.

Pastes can be used as a filler, to level out irregular contours, or to provide an additional seal immediately around a stoma or fistula (see Ch. 14). Once applied, paste can be flattened with a moistened finger or spatula. Some pastes contain alcohol.

These should not be used on excoriated areas as they can be painful (Black 2000).

Barrier creams protect skin by forming a film. They are not recommended for broken weeping skin, as they do not give sufficient protection to promote healing. Creams should be used sparingly, massaged into the skin, and excess removed with a tissue so the skin surface is in a condition to allow appliance adhesion.

Skin gels, lotions and wipes can be used on intact skin to produce an elastic film which helps protect the skin from stomal effluent and trauma when appliances are removed. They should be applied sparingly and allowed to dry before stomal equipment is applied. Some products contain alcohol to aid fast drying. These should not be used on broken or sensitive skin. Products without alcohol, such as Cavilon, can be used to aid skin care around stomas, wounds and fistulas where sore skin is present.

Medical adhesive sprays/wipes and removers aid appliance adhesion and offer skin protection. Most patients find the impregnated adhesive/removal wipes easier to use, especially when away from home. Aerosol adhesives should be carefully applied to the bag flange/base, which will then be applied to the skin, and not applied to the skin itself. This helps ensure the spray is only applied to the relevant area of skin. However, some people have found these sprays inhibit adhesion when used with hydrocolloid flanges. Proprietary adhesive removers should be used where residue occurs, to minimise trauma to the skin.

Cleansing lotions and wipes can be used for cleansing peristomal skin, particularly when it is sore or sensitive. Non-oily impregnated wipes are useful for travellers or when toilet facilities are inadequate.

MATCHING PATIENTS AND SKIN CARE AIDS

The sophisticated adhesives on modern appliances have reduced the incidence of skin trauma and sensitivity reactions. This fact, coupled with financial constraints, can mean questions are asked as to whether skin care aids are necessary. Assessment of the prophylactic and restorative requirements of each patient should be made. The aspects to consider cited by Stewart (1984) remain relevant today.

Condition of the skin immediately around the stoma and within the appliance field as a whole   This enables actual or emerging problems to be identified and decisions made as to whether a protective aid is required (e.g. barrier cream for slightly dry or reddened skin) or whether a restorative/substantially protective aid is required (e.g. a wafer to protect all the red and sore-looking skin beneath the bag flange).

Whether the skin is likely to be sensitive and thus susceptible to problems   People with fair skin or who burn easily in the sun generally need prophylactic protection as well as people who have a history of skin problems such as psoriasis or eczema. This is usually achieved through choosing a style of bag whose flange incorporates a wafer, or using an additional form of skin protective routinely.

The type of stoma or fistula and the nature of effluent   Potential damage from effluent must be considered. For example, ileal effluent is rich in enzymes which can excoriate the epidermis, and create problems of pain and difficulty in appliance adhesion with physical and emotional consequences for patients. Substantial protective skin care will normally be included as routine prophylactic care. The cost of providing this is much less (in monetary and human distress terms) than withholding such protection.

Ability of patients to handle various skin care aids   This includes considering the effects of factors like the patient's dexterity, eye-sight and mental ability to recall how to use aids.

ACCESSORIES

Generally stoma care is best kept as simple as possible. Many patients achieve efficient and self-confident self-care with minimal or no use of accessories.

Belts

These are usually adjustable. The range of sizes varies between manufacturers. Patients may find some belts are easier to attach and detach than others. It is important that patients are taught how to fit and wear belts. They should be worn at stoma level, not at waist level. The latter can create an upward drag on appliances which reduces rather than aids adherence. Belts may be used to:

- hold a non-adhesive appliance in place
- provide additional security (e.g. during sporting activities, at work, at night)

- provide extra support if there are particular demands on the appliance which could reduce its adherence (e.g. from the weight of a prolapse; if substantial amounts of effluent are being passed)
- help a flush stoma to stand out more from the surrounding abdomen, so effluent falls into the bag rather than pooling or leaking at skin level.

Corsets

Some patients require additional back or abdominal support. They may adapt their usual support corsetry to accommodate their stomal equipment. However, certain types of corset are available on prescription in the UK. These are individually made by specialist companies to accommodate stomal equipment and patients' support requirements. If patients have not worn these specialist support garments before, it is prudent to have only one fitted and made initially. The patient then assesses the corset's comfort and usefulness before more are ordered.

Bag covers

These are available in both disposable and poly cotton reusable forms from various manufacturers. Some patients make their own, for example to match their wedding dress or underwear. The purpose of bag covers is to:

- reduce sweating and/or skin problems by preventing contact between the appliance and patients' skin
- help patients promote the kind of self-image they find acceptable.

The covers should resemble the shape of the bag and be easy to apply and remove. Covers for use with drainable bags should include an opening which will enable bags to be emptied without removal of the cover.

Many stoma bags are now made with a 'comfort' backing to reduce sweating and skin problems. Some patients prefer these products as they tend to be less bulky than using a bag and cover. However, the 'comfort backing' can cause skin problems for some patients.

Odour-reducing agents

These are available in a variety of formats and generally have some effect in combating or reducing odour.

Flatus filters

These activated carbon patches are an integral part of some bags or are available as separate patches for patients to apply to their bags themselves. Their purpose is to reduce faecal odour as flatus is slowly filtered through them as it leaves the bag. It is important that patients understand that it will take time for their wind to leave the bag and that if they stick extra holes in the filter or press on the bag to force flatus through more quickly, efficient deodorisation will not take place. Patients with impaired vision or limited manual dexterity may have difficulty using the separate filters and prefer integral ones.

Deodorising drops, gels and powders

These can be used sparingly in the bottom of appliances (e.g. 2 drops or 6 puffs of powder) in order to contain or reduce faecal odour. Patients tend to be particularly concerned about odour in the early postoperative period. The presence of a couple of deodorant drops in the container into which faecal contents or a used appliance are to be placed can help patients feel less embarrassed and confident that any odour is being minimised. Patients with malodorous wounds may also use these deodorising products on their dressings to minimise odour.

Household derivatives

Some people prefer to place substances such as natural yoghurt, charcoal tablets or aspirin tablets in their appliance to reduce odour. Care must be taken that aspirin tablets do not come in direct contact with the actual stoma as this could cause mucosal damage.

MATCHING ACCESSORIES AND PATIENTS

A series of questions can be used to consider each accessory and whether it would be suitable for individual patients. Clarity about the help an accessory is meant to provide will enable patient and staff to subsequently monitor whether it is achieving the desired outcome at an acceptable level. Useful questions include:

- Is there a potential or actual difficulty or problem that use of this accessory would prevent, reduce or relieve?
- Is using this accessory the best way for this patient to manage their potential or actual difficulty?
- Would use of this accessory substantially enhance

this patient's comfort, self-confidence, and/or wellbeing? How would it achieve this?

- Does the level of benefit this patient should gain from use of this accessory warrant its provision on a temporary or ongoing basis?

CHANGING STOMAL EQUIPMENT

The principles of changing stomal equipment are basically the same whether the patient is in hospital or at home. These principles should be used to inform and create the steps of the procedure through which an appliance is changed (Trainor et al 2003). Generally when nurses and patients are first learning to change stomal equipment it is taught as a series of steps, as shown in Box 4.1. However, once the basic procedure is understood it is then helpful for patients to also learn the main underlying principles so that they can adapt the steps of their bag change successfully in different situations.

We are following this two-stage approach here by firstly outlining the procedure or series of steps which nurses generally use when changing an appliance. We then discuss the underlying principles, and ways of helping patients adapt their care procedure to fit in with their home and other situations where they might change their equipment.

Patients tire easily and any appliance changes in the early postoperative period are generally done with the patient lying on their bed. This enables them to feel comfortable and in a good position to pay attention to what the nurse is explaining and doing. It is important that patients, their families, and staff all understand that concentration and retention of information is usually temporarily reduced following major surgery and anaesthesia, and accept that information will often need to be given several times.

Basic equipment for an appliance change

1. New appliance of correct size and type (+ spare clip if required for drainable bag)
2. Skin care and other accessories as required (e.g. skin gel, deodoriser, adhesive tape)
3. Soft paper tissues
4. Strengthened wipes
5. Stoma measuring guide
6. Scissors
7. Bowl of warm water
8. Mild soap
9. Jug for contents of appliance
10. Plastic disposal bag
11. Disposable gloves
12. Hand mirror
13. Protective sheet (e.g. absorbent, plastic backed for bed and patient's clothes)
14. Pen (if wafer template to be prepared).

In hospital most of these items can be stored in a box at the patient's bedside. As equipment needs may alter, for example as the stoma shrinks, it is best only to leave equipment for a couple of changes in the box, and restock immediately after use so patient and staff know it is always adequately stocked. This also encourages patients to automatically restock their box once they return home.

Basic routine for changing an appliance – by the nurse

The main steps for nurses to follow when changing an appliance are given in Box 4.1. Preoperatively patients should have been given a description of the pinky-red colour which their stoma is likely to be. This should be repeated again *before* removal of the bag at the first equipment change. When patients understand that this colour is healthy because it is caused by the plentiful supply of blood to normal bowel to promote effective function it helps them find the colour more acceptable.

Nurses can do much to help patients acquire and follow both procedural steps and underlying principles by describing and demonstrating them while attending to patients in the early postoperative period. This 'talking the patient through' what we are doing helps them link what to do with how and why right from the very start.

For example, while carrying out steps 8 and 9 (Box 4.1): 'I always check that this slight reddening of the skin which comes when the bag is first removed is fading by the time I apply the new bag. That helps me know that it is just the usual flushing and not a sign that your skin might be reacting to the adhesive, which it could be if the skin stayed pinked up.'

Patients are now discharged very soon after surgery and this limits the time available in which to help them acquire sufficient knowledge and skills to adequately manage self-care at home. They need to have regained sufficient mental and physical energy to 'take in' information and use it to successfully carry out elements of stoma care. Starting self-care too early may mean patients fail to retain knowledge and skills and this can reduce their self-

Box 4.1   Steps for changing stomal equipment

1. Inform patient of proposed activity.
2. Ensure privacy.
3. Collect all necessary equipment and place it where it is easy to reach.
4. Explain the procedure simply.
5. Place protective sheeting to cover bedding and patient's clothing. Ensure they are lying comfortably and able to watch the procedure, and that their abdomen is flat enough to aid bag application.
6. Put on disposable gloves, reminding patient they will not need to use gloves.
7. If the bag is drainable put 1–2 drops of deodorant into the jug ready to reduce odour and then empty bag contents into jug before removing the bag.
8. Remove appliance. Peel adhesive or base off the skin with one hand while easing the abdominal skin away with the other hand. Help patient relax by talking to them while removing the bag. Point out normal reddening/erythema and quick fading to patient.
9. Remove excess faeces or mucus from the stoma with a dry tissue. Observe patient's non–verbal reaction.
10. Examine the skin and stoma for soreness, ulceration, colour or other unusual signs of damage/reaction. If the skin is unblemished and stoma is a healthy red colour, proceed.
11. Wash the skin and stoma gently until clean. Remind patient that cotton wool should not generally be used. (Strands of wool remaining on skin can reduce bag adhesion.)
12. Dry the stoma and skin gently but thoroughly.
13. Measure the stoma using a guide so that the relevant size of bag gasket or opening can be selected. Remind patient that stomas usually shrink after surgery so monitoring is needed in the first few months to identify size changes.
14. Prepare clean appliance plus skin care aids and accessories if needed.
15. Apply any skin care aid necessary so it protects the area to be covered by the appliance adhesive.
16. Apply clean appliance and any accessories if used. Check whole system is adhering well and that outlet on (drainable) bags is securely closed.
17. Make patient comfortable. Ask how they are feeling, and monitor their readiness to ask questions or discuss the change process at this time.
18. Dispose of soiled tissues and used equipment. Rinse the bag in the sluice or toilet; wrap it in a disposal bag and place in appropriate bin.
19. Discard gloves and wash your hands. If patient has taken part in change process give them the wherewithal to wash their hands too.
20. Restock patient's box as necessary.
21. Record observations on patient's stoma and skin conditions; potential or actual problems and actions proposed or taken to manage them. Indicate patient's response, stage in learning, proposed next learning activity.

confidence and make them more anxious as to whether they will be able to manage well at home. However, patients do need to have completed enough changes of their equipment to be able to carry out all of the steps in the correct order while recalling what to do and why in order to retain these abilities once they go home. Getting the balance right between giving a patient enough time to recover but also leaving enough time in which they can complete sufficient practice changes before discharge to gain basic expertise and confidence is not always easy.

The most effective way of monitoring whether a patient's progress in learning to manage their stoma care is sufficient is to consider whether the goals are being achieved in terms of *their experience*. The issue is not just whether we have told them the information, or shown them the procedure (although these are important nursing goals for us to achieve). What we need to monitor, with the patient, is whether *they* have:

- understood and retained sufficient information to adequately manage their stoma care when they go home
- acquired adequate basic skills in all the steps required to manage their stoma care.

Patients may well be sufficiently recovered from their surgery to be deemed medically fit for discharge before they have acquired adequate self-care abilities. It is important that all members of the healthcare team have a shared concept of the minimum standard of self-care that must be reached, and the knowledge and skills that must be gained sufficiently to reach that basic standard, before discharge home is allowed.

The learning programme for each patient is usually planned by the stoma care nurse or an experienced ward nurse in consultation with the patient and it should actively promote acquisition of the relevant knowledge and skills (see Ch. 8, including Patient scenario 8.2). Nurses who are teaching and supervising patients' self-care must give descriptive and constructive feedback to them so they know what they are doing correctly, where they need to do something differently or more adeptly, and what it is they should seek to do or remember (see Patient scenario 7.2 in Ch. 7). Likewise nurses must record the patient's progress in specific and descriptive terms so that any nurse can identify from them which elements of self-care the patient has learned or has yet to acquire when they come to supervise and help a patient do a practice change, and whether there are problems that require further monitoring and attention. Such detailed recording enables staff to be helpful and consistent in their teaching and provides the essential information on which realistic planning of discharge can be based and agreed upon by all concerned.

USING THE PRINCIPLES OF STOMA CARE TO INFORM AND ADAPT SELF-CARE

Having begun to learn the steps of a bag change, patients can then be helped to use these experiences to make sense of and follow the underlying principles of care.

We can ask them, in the light of their experience so far, to identify how they might use each principle (or group of principles) to adapt the self-care being learned in the hospital context so it is easily managed at home and in other contexts. This approach helps patients actively apply what they are learning. It also enables nurses and patients to identify where gaps in knowledge and skills exist and need rectifying. It is a form of *coaching* which sends explicit messages to patients that they can and should take charge of their stoma and its management, and find ways of fitting it into their normal lifestyle (see Patient scenario 4.2 and the scenarios in Ch. 5).

The principles can be grouped so patients understand their links and implications, or they can be taught one at a time when an opportunity arises. The *main principles* related to appliance management, with some possible groupings, are listed below.

1. *Assume the stoma might be active while equipment is being changed, and follow a self-care system that ensures stomal action causes minimal disruption and difficulty in completing the change procedure.*
   (a) Protect floor and clothing from possible stomal action.
   (b) Collect all necessary equipment before beginning the change process and position it so it is easy to reach and use.
2. *During the first few weeks postoperatively the stoma size and shape, and the appliance and skin care used, may change. Therefore during this time preparation of new equipment is done as steps 13 and 14 (Box 4.1). Once the stoma size, appliance type and skin protective needs have become established (i.e. basically consistent at each equipment change) then preparation of new equipment should be done before removing used equipment.*
3. *Basic rules of cleanliness and prevention of infection for self and others should be followed.*
   (a) Wash hands before and after completion of the appliance change.
   (b) Products that would normally be disposed of in the toilet, (faeces, toilet paper) should be discarded there, including rinsing out the bag if possible (see disposal, later). Other products that could block the toilet, which includes most stoma bags, paper towels etc., should be wrapped up securely before being added to the usual waste bag/bin/disposal system.
   (c) The stoma and peristomal skin should be cleansed before application of new equipment.
4. *Effluent normally drains downwards from the highest point towards lower points.*
   (a) Remove used equipment from the top or highest point downwards, so the maximum amount of effluent can be caught in the bag.
   (b) Apply new equipment so the lower half is first secured and then the upper half; this enables stomal effluent passed during this procedure to be contained in the new bag.
   (c) Securing the lower half of the flange/adhesive first and working from below upwards means that if any creases occur they are likely to be in the upper section above

the stoma, and effluent is thus less likely to track along them.

5. *The amount of energy available to use for appliance changes is likely to be limited during the first weeks of recovery, and at times when additional activities are being resumed or taken on and themselves depleting energy levels.*

   (a) Keep a container permanently stocked with the equipment to do two to three bag changes so time and energy does not have to be used gathering these when a change is needed. Store in a cool dry place near where the change procedure will be carried out.

   (b) If possible, change equipment at a time of day when energy levels are normally higher (e.g. after a night's rest rather than at the end of the day).

   (c) If flanges or peristomal wafers have to be cut out, prepare these at a different time to when the bag is being changed thus shortening and simplifying the change procedure. (NB: due to the likelihood of stoma shrinkage in the first month only prepare one or two items in advance.)

   (d) If tiredness is likely to impair self-care abilities then enlist the help of family or friends for specific activities, such as to prepare or restock equipment so energy can be conserved for the main process of actually changing the equipment.

   (e) If easily tired *sit* to prepare new equipment, remove used appliance and clean around stoma and peristomal skin and only *stand* to flatten or straighten abdomen for application of new equipment.

6. *Equipment adheres best when the abdomen is as flat as possible and bulges and creases are minimised. Generally this occurs when someone is standing to apply new equipment. A high stool, bed etc. can be used to lean against if extra support is needed.*

7. *A balance should be sought between (i) getting the fit of an appliance or wafer snug enough around the stoma to prevent effluent lying in contact with, and damaging, the skin and (ii) preventing damage to the stoma which can arise from too tight a fit or poor centring of equipment over the stoma.*

   (a) Generally bag and flange openings should be about 3 mm larger than the base of the stoma. Peristomal wafers are softer and can be cut to fit around the stoma base, using a piece of paper to make a template of the relevant size before cutting the wafer. NB:

date templates and indicate top and bottom so current and old templates can be differentiated, particularly during the first few weeks when the size required often alters.

8. *Monitoring the colour and condition of the stoma and peristomal skin should be an integral part of stoma care.*

   (a) Patients need to be able to recognise normal phenomenon as well as cues which signal problems. This entails pointing out elements such as:

   the bright red normal stoma colour

   minimal spotting of blood on a tissue that has been used to cleanse the stoma, which is a common and normal phenomenon

   peristaltic movement/wiggling of the stoma

   normal skin condition, including the temporary flushing/erythema which occurs on bag removal as well as abnormal conditions (e.g. too dry/soggy; reaction to appliance adhesive or wafer)

   equipment that is well sized and centred

   equipment that is adhering well and that which is beginning to lift and/or require changing (see Ch. 5).

   (b) Damage or other alterations to the stoma and surrounding skin do not have to be painful to require attention: soreness is often only a feature when skin damage has become quite substantial. Sometimes soreness is experienced without visible signs of damage to skin or stoma. Generally, advice should be sought promptly from the stoma care nurse or experienced hospital/district nurse if the patient is concerned that a problem might be present. This enables assessment and help to be given in ways that help patients recognise the presence or absence of a problem and any treatment that may be required. Problems and their management are discussed in Chapter 21.

9. *Appliances that are leaking or lifting away from the body should be changed promptly so that leakage and damage to skin (and clothes, furniture etc.) are prevented or minimised.*

10. *It is advisable to carry a 'change kit' so that equipment can be easily replaced whenever and wherever necessary.*

    Equipment that is well adhered to the body prevents effluent from skin contact and damage. Once this seal is broken faeces can become trapped between the appliance and the body and thus damage the skin. It is important that equipment is changed (rather than just patched up) as soon as possible after it starts to lift so that the skin can be cleansed and adequate protection reinstated through new equipment being applied. Ways of recognising when equipment should be changed are discussed in Chapter 5.

Patients should be encouraged to carry the wherewithal to change their equipment (see Patient scenario 4.2, below) and to regularly use that equipment and replace it with fresh stock so the quality of products in the change kit is maintained. Care should be taken that change kits are stored in reasonable conditions avoiding excess heat or squashing.

11. *Stomal equipment should be stored in cool dry conditions which enable the quality of the adhesives on bags and skin protective products, and the shape of skin protectives, to be maintained.*

These can be affected in conditions that are too warm (e.g. near a radiator or in direct sunlight) or too moist (e.g. in a bathroom that gets steamy). Patients should be given this information and encouraged to use it to identify suitable places for storing equipment in their home. Such discussion before discharge enables tactful guidance to be given if their initial choice is unsuitable. The chosen storage place also needs to be easily accessible to patients as their energy levels will be low when first discharged and can be drained if extra efforts are needed to get to their stored equipment.

Generally it is helpful to suggest to patients that *adaptation* of the system of self-care in hospital to fit in with their lifestyle circumstances is normal and easy when the principles are followed. Like any skill this is learnable, and staff who spend some time identifying several ways in which they can introduce patients to the underlying principles of care and encourage them to use them will enhance patients' ability to rehabilitate. This is often a two-stage process. Firstly, principles can be pointed out, using phrases such as:

The main aim here is to … (add relevant principle).

When you adapt this way of looking after your stoma to fit in with your home/work/holiday circumstances it will still be important to … (add relevant principle).

Secondly, after indicating a principle (or group of principles), statements and questions can be used

which invite patients to consider how they could *apply* the principle(s), such as:

I remember you told me you like going camping … how might you go about changing your bag when you have your next camping holiday?

Encouraging patients to apply principles to their own circumstances (rather than overly advising or instructing them) helps them increase their flexible use of them. As they plan resumption of normal activities this boosts their confidence as well as their levels of information, and misunderstandings can be identified and corrected.

PATIENT SCENARIO 4.2 Mrs Reid is discussing with John and Mary Fletcher how he can adapt the stoma care procedure he is learning in hospital so it fits in with conditions at home and when he returns to work as a self-employed decorator. Mary had brought in the two clothes pegs and about 2 feet of string as requested and Mrs Reid had shown them both how John could loop the string around the back of his neck and use the clothes pegs (attached to each end of the string) to keep his shirt etc. pegged well back from his stoma. John felt confident that this would help him see his colostomy easily and prevent clothes from getting soiled if his stoma worked during a change.

Mary had already watched John's equipment being changed and he was now able to prepare his new equipment, remove the used appliance and clean the peristomal area. Mrs Reid encouraged them to use the knowledge gained from these experiences to come up with ideas as to how and where he would store and change equipment at home. Mary was relieved when John said he would use newspaper to protect the bathroom floor as she had been worrying about where they could store the large protective pads she had seen used in hospital. After discarding the airing cupboard (too hot) and the bathroom (too steamy), they decided that new equipment, including John's 'change box', could be stored in their wardrobe, which is cool and dry and near the bathroom where he will do his bag changes.

A lively debate takes place over how John could change his equipment when he is working in a customer's home. At first John thought this would be an impossibility because of needing to clean around the stoma. Mrs Reid asked them what could be used instead of soap and water in these circumstances (encouraging them to find another way of fulfilling principle 3 above). Mary suggested baby wipes or moist toilet tissues and these are agreed to be an acceptable alternative (as long as they are non-oily) for use when John does not have easy access to his usual cleansing system. Both John and Mary are beginning to use principles to shape his future care.

DISPOSAL

Used stomal equipment must be disposed of in a manner that minimises any risk of infection to people coming in contact with it. This includes patients, carers, and employees involved in waste disposal.

Most patients discard used equipment via the waste disposal system in operation wherever they change their appliances. Since these systems may not include incineration, and most stoma bags are not biodegradable, it is possible that appliances will still be intact at the end of the waste disposal process. Effluent remaining in them could become a source of contamination both during and after completion of the waste disposal process (Black 2000). These factors must be borne in mind when disposal of used equipment is discussed.

Disposal in hospital – by nurses

1. Disposable gloves should be worn for emptying and changing stomal equipment, complying with healthcare policy on handling any patient's body fluids or waste products.
2. All materials used for cleansing the peristomal area, and those soiled by stomal effluent (e.g. pads used to protect clothing) should be collected in a disposal bag and subsequently deposited in the appropriate (coloured) disposal sack for that ward or department after completion of the change procedure.
3. The used appliance should be placed in a separate bag or container on removal so that, once the change procedure has been completed, it is easily available for rinsing through before being wrapped up and bagged and then placed in the appropriate waste disposal sack.
4. Hands should be washed both before gloves are put on at the start of the change procedure and as the final step following disposal of used equipment and cleansing materials.

5. Clean disposal bags should be routinely re-stocked in patients' boxes in addition to new appliances, skin care and cleansing aids.

Disposal – by patients

Many patients are concerned about disposing of used equipment (Kelly & Henry 1992). Individual needs can be addressed when decisions as to how patients will manage disposal are shaped by:

- legal requirements regarding health and safety
- criteria which a disposal system should meet in order for that person to experience it as acceptable and achievable in most contexts
- disposal options available in their locality
- the practical steps that they are willing and able to take when disposing of used equipment.

Preparing patients to manage disposal effectively in different contexts can be covered in four stages, each with its own guiding principles.

(1) Identification of an appropriate disposal system

- *Non-biodegradable equipment should not be disposed of in a toilet as it can cause blockage.*
- *The level of risk thought likely from a particular patient's stomal effluent and equipment should be identified.*

Classification of the equipment for disposal purposes should be made in accordance with legal requirements and the level of risk posed by the used equipment.

In the UK waste that is deemed likely to be infected or hazardous to patients, carers, and employees involved in waste disposal will be classed as 'clinical waste'. Where waste is deemed non-infectious it falls outside the category of clinical waste. It is then classified as 'household waste' and can be disposed of via the patient's normal system of waste collection (HSC Health Services Advisory Committee 1999). Equipment from stoma patients can usually be classified as low risk, household waste.

- *Any differences in advice likely to be given by different professionals whose remit includes waste disposal should be identified and resolved.*

Advice is likely to depend on whether the adviser classes stomal equipment as clinical or household waste, and how they interpret legislation. Swan (2001) found that, in some UK localities, environmental health officers (EHOs) and nurses were giving different advice on disposal. Nurses' advice was based on equipment being classed and disposed of as household waste. EHOs who classified stomal equipment as clinical waste were advising patients to use special collection services. This appeared to arise from their interpretation of the Environmental Protection Act (1990), which makes those who produce, carry, keep and dispose of controlled waste (including clinical waste) liable to ensure safe disposal under criminal law. Factors that influenced how EHOs classified used stomal equipment included whether patients lived in rural or urban communities, whether waste was finally incinerated or not, the quantity of waste being produced and whether the costs incurred collecting small amounts of waste by special services were justifiable. Conflicting advice causes confusion and reduces recipients' confidence in their ability to dispose of equipment safely and acceptably.

- *Criteria that a disposal system should meet must be discussed with patients early enough to enable an appropriate system to be chosen, demonstrated and practised before discharge.*

It is generally helpful to include information about how to minimise the risk of infection in our discussion with patients about the goals they want to achieve when disposing of equipment (and thus the criteria that their system must meet).

This allows us to pay attention to two additional key factors as well as their goals and infection risks:

(a) Rehabilitation includes patients' acquisition of the ability to change equipment in most circumstances. Constraints on disposing of equipment in household waste systems can affect people's ability to go to work, socialise and travel.

(b) Waste collection via special services can be observed by neighbours. Some patients report feeling stigmatised using this system, and having difficulty maintaining their privacy and dealing with neighbours' questions.

Discussions should enable patients to identify:

- situations in which they might change their equipment
- what a safe, discreet, practical disposal system would entail in order to make it acceptable to them
- how this system could be adapted in different contexts while maintaining adequate standards of health and cleanliness

- whether they want to use a special collection service if this is available.

When we help patients think about disposal in practical terms, relating it to their everyday lives, it enables them to envisage resumption of work and social activities. Informing them of suitable strategies which other people use in similar situations to those they describe increases their expectations that they will also manage to change and dispose of equipment successfully.

(2) Demonstration of chosen procedure

- *Demonstration of how, specifically, to empty, rinse out, and wrap up used stomal equipment should generally be carried out in a normal sized toilet.*

This helps patients accept the procedure is possible to complete in most toilets. Carrying out a full demonstration enables us to convey, verbally and non-verbally, that the disposal system is acceptable from health and social perspectives. It also enables us to 'talk through' how the various steps meet the chosen disposal criteria/goals, and remind patients of any different steps they will need to do in other contexts.

The following procedure meets many patients' criteria for cleanliness, reduction of odour, usability in most circumstances and social acceptability:

1. Materials used for cleansing the peristomal area and those soiled by stomal effluent (e.g. newspaper used to protect the floor) are collected in newspaper or a plastic bag.
2. The used appliance is emptied, rinsed in the toilet (either by the flush of water or using a jug) and then also placed in the newspaper or plastic bag.
3. The newspaper/plastic bag is then sealed and placed in the correct hospital disposal bag (whilst reminding patients they will use a household rubbish bag or dustbin).
4. Routine hand washing before and after appliance changes and disposal takes place. Patients should be reminded that they do not need to wear gloves to handle their own body waste when changing and disposing of equipment.

Key criteria to be met in order to minimise infection risks are that waste shall be properly wrapped and free from excess fluid (Swan 2001). Patients who are able and willing to rinse out their bags after emptying them can be encouraged to do so. This reduces any worries they may have about odour, health risks, or embarrassment from exposure of their equipment if rubbish bags get torn. It is important to provide guidance on the level of cleanliness that it is reasonable to obtain from rinsing used bags, as some patients end up scrubbing their bags because they think (wrongly) that total effluent removal is required.

(3) Supervised practice by patient

- *Patients should be supervised completing the disposal procedure before discharge from hospital.*

This enables any difficulties to be identified and resolved, and any (incorrect) beliefs that effluent coming from a stoma is somehow more infectious than that discharged from a rectum can often be picked up and dispelled at this stage. Support and feedback should be used to help patients develop competence and confidence in completing this task.

(4) Evaluation

- *Patients and staff should evaluate whether the disposal method achieves the criteria identified for it to meet prior to discharge and during follow-up appointments.*

Some patients have more difficulty emptying or rinsing out their equipment than had been envisaged (Swan 2001). As they rehabilitate, some patients may need to discuss management of disposal in additional circumstances, such as in new work or social situations. It is therefore advisable to encourage patients to review their criteria for disposal and whether they are being achieved or need adaptation as an integral part of their follow-up.

Alternative disposal systems for home use

In the UK some healthcare providers who operate a soiled dressings collection service also enable patients to have their used stomal equipment collected. However, many patients dislike having a collection van arriving at their home and view it as stigmatising or a potential trigger for questions by neighbours.

Some organisations provide clinical waste disposal units for patients with a regular collection and replacement system. The cost of this service may have to be met by patients although, if specific circumstances warrant it, costs may be met by health or social services. Although some patients find this system beneficial, many dislike storing used equipment or having a special unit taking up space in their home, and perhaps triggering questions from visitors.

Disposal away from home

Stomal equipment can be changed and disposed of in virtually any circumstances where elimination might have taken place before the patient had surgery. It is important to clarify which aspects of stoma care *patients* believe they can do, and are willing to do, outside their home as otherwise they may curtail their activities and lifestyle. For example, some patients refrain from eating if they are planning on being out of their home (e.g. shopping or socialising) in an attempt to stop the stoma working and necessitating a visit to a public toilet.

Patients should be encouraged to adopt a system of changing and disposing of appliances which they can use easily outside the home. Helping them understand the rationale for their home disposal system, and identify criteria that disposal away from home should achieve, will aid identification of an acceptable alternative system which they can use confidently. Many patients' goals are twofold: firstly, they want to avoid drawing attention to their new elimination system either through the presence of odour and/or through the presence of a used appliance; secondly, they want to deal with used equipment in a competent and socially acceptable way.

It is essential that patients know they must not dispose of their appliance in the toilet (unless that appliance is specially constructed for this form of disposal). Dealing with waste pipes blocked by stoma bags can be unpleasant, and embarrassing for the culprit! The same rinse and wrap system described earlier can be used to prepare equipment for disposal. Most women's public toilets and those for disabled people have sanitary bins into which this cleansed stomal equipment can be placed. Men may have to use other disposal bins accessible to them, and should be informed that it is socially appropriate to so dispose of their rinsed and wrapped equipment.

BATHING

People with stomas can bath normally, with or without an appliance in situ. Many stomas (particularly colostomies) settle into a fairly predictable pattern of action as normal eating and other activities are resumed. This enables most people to bath when their stomas are less likely to act. They should be informed that stomal action during bathing is not harmful (although it may be inconvenient), and that water will not enter their stoma if they are enjoying a good soak without their appliance. Well-secured modern stomal equipment will not be affected by water and dries quickly, so bathing, swimming and water sports of any type may be enjoyed.

CLOTHING

Many people feel that their clothes are an expression of who they are and enjoy wearing clothes chosen to fit in with both their sense of themselves and their lifestyle. Concern that their usual clothes will not accommodate stomal equipment discreetly is common and may be expressed as hints that a change of wardrobe and/or the wearing of baggy clothes are being assumed to be a necessary part of their future life. Identification of the type of clothes patients normally wear should be an integral part of preoperative siting as this will aid choice of a site that is as compatible as possible with their usual clothes.

Certain styles of clothing may be impractical, such as overly tight clothing in the early days following surgery, or tight hipster jeans. In the male with a transverse colostomy or with a stoma sited on their waistline, problems with trousers can arise if they are tightly fitted or supported with a belt. In such instances braces may be advisable and, in the longer term, trousers purchased with extra fullness around the waistline or with a deeper waist may be more satisfactory.

Women who normally wear pantie-girdles, roll-ons etc. may adapt them to accommodate stomal equipment themselves if they are handy with a needle, or use made-to-measure ones made by one of the commercial companies. Some commercial firms produce swimwear with an inner lining to disguise an appliance when the costume is wet, and boxer style swim trunks for men are also available. However, many patients find swimwear within the normal range carried in stores if they are encouraged to shop around and find a style that accommodates their appliance comfortably with a pattern and fabric that camouflages the equipment outline.

DIET

Patients are understandably apprehensive about the effects that food and drink may have on their stomal action and this is discussed in Chapter 16. Generally patients should be encouraged to re-introduce their normal foods into their meals gradually so their shortened bowel becomes used to them. Experimentation with the amount and frequency with which preferred foods are taken can often result in foods that were initially thought to cause problems being incorporated into normal meals later.

CONCLUSION

These principles of stoma care will generally serve patients well and help them incorporate their stoma into their normal lifestyle with increasing levels of knowledge and competence. Additional aspects of living with an ileostomy or colostomy are discussed in Chapter 5. However, all these practical aspects of care need to be provided in ways that aid patients' psychological as well as physical rehabilitation. The patient scenarios throughout this book aim to give you a sense of what such care can be like in action, and ideas for further developing your own practice.

References

Bancroft J 1993 Human sexuality and its problems, 2nd edn. Churchill Livingstone, London

Benner P 1984 From novice to expert. Addison-Wesley, Menlo Park, CA

Benner P, Tanner C A, Chesla C A 1996 Expertise in nursing practice. Springer, New York

Black P K 2000 Holistic stoma care. Baillière Tindall and RCN, Edinburgh

Blackley P 2004 Practical stoma wound and continence management, 2nd edn. Research Publications Pty, Vermont, Victoria, Australia

Borwell B 1994 Colostomies and their management. Nursing Standard 8(45):49–56

Breckman B 1991 Communicating stoma care. Unpublished teaching manual, BA (Hons) submission, University of East London

Davenport R 2003 Choosing the site for a stoma. In: Elcoat C Stoma care nursing, 2nd edn. Hollister, Wokingham, Berks

Environmental Protection Act 1990 Waste management – the duty of care code of practice. HMSO, London

HSC Health Service Advisory Committee 1999 Safe disposal of clinical waste. HSE Books, Sudbury, Suffolk

Huish M, Kumar D, Stones C 1998 Stoma surgery and sexual problems in ostomates. Sexual and Marital Therapy 13(3):311–328

Keighley M R B 1999 Mechanical bowel preparation. In: Keighley M R B, Williams N S Surgery of the anus, rectum and colon, 2nd edn. W B Saunders, London, p 73–95

Kelly M, Henry T 1992 A thirst for practical knowledge. Professional Nurse 7(6):350–356

Peters-Gawlik M 1996 Planning of care as an aid to rehabilitation. Eurostoma 15, Summer: 10–11

Readding L A 2003 Stoma siting: what the community nurse needs to know. British Journal of Community Nursing 8(11):502–511

Rutledge M, Thompson M J, Boyd-Carson W 2003 Effective stoma siting. Nursing Standard 18(12):43–44

Stewart L 1984 Stoma care: preoperative preparation of the patient. Nursing 2(30):886–887

Swan E 2001 Waste disposal for the ostomate in the community. Nursing Times 97(40):51–52

Trainor B, Thompson M J, Boyd-Carson W, Boyd K 2003 Changing an appliance. Nursing Standard 18(13):41–42

Chapter 5

Specific aspects of care for patients with ileostomies and colostomies

Barbara Borwell and Brigid Breckman

Most aspects of practical stoma care which are similar whether someone has an ileostomy or a colostomy are discussed in Chapter 4. However, there are also differences in the information and care that patients with ileostomies and colostomies require. This chapter enables you to clarify and compare some differences, which can be the result of:

- the type and extent of operation (outlined in Chs 3 and 10)
- the physiological functions that are retained or lost due to the position of the diversion in the gastrointestinal pathway.

Aspects of care discussed in this chapter include the following:

1. principles for monitoring ileostomies and colostomies in the early postoperative period
2. care of people with an ileostomy, including:
   - types of effluent and 'control' of stomal action
   - when to change equipment
3. care of people with a colostomy, including:
   - types of effluent and 'control' of stomal action
   - management of flatus
   - when to change equipment
4. responding to sexual concerns, including:
   - ways of reviewing physical effects of surgery on sexual function
   - ways of helping patients with sexual concerns and problems
   - contraception and pregnancy
5. urinary problems that may arise following bowel stoma surgery.

As you will see, the section on helping patients with sexual issues is more detailed than some other sections. This does not imply that people who have a stoma are primarily concerned with sexual issues, nor that all patients will want to discuss the sexual implications of their surgery in detail. The material on sexuality-related care provided in this chapter and others has been included in response to the difficulties expressed by many colleagues in both gaining adequate knowledge of the likely effects of particular operations and in knowing how to help patients and their partners discuss and deal with sexuality-related issues. This information can increase the helpfulness and ease with which you can engage in this aspect of care, and recognise when referral of patients for more specialised help is advisable.

PRINCIPLES OF STOMAL MONITORING AND CARE IN THE EARLY POSTOPERATIVE PERIOD

These *principles* are similar in many respects for both ileostomies and colostomies although what is normally observed with each stoma type may partially differ.

1. *The **colour of the stoma** should be routinely observed when patients are receiving general care so that cues signalling possible impairment to the blood supply can be noted and reported promptly to medical staff.*

Bowel (including stomas) normally has a plentiful blood supply which gives its red colour, similar to the lining of the mouth. The colour and evaluation of it as denoting adequacy or otherwise of blood supply should be recorded on completion of surgery so subsequent monitors have a baseline with which to compare what they observe. Changes to a more dusky or a more pallid colour *should be reported* to the medical team, likewise any major size changes. Transparent appliances are therefore used postoperatively to enable adequate observation to take place.

2. *Stomas should be monitored for **alterations in size and the presence of oedema** as these may lead to an alteration in the size and shape of the hole in the appliance and skin care aid being necessary to protect the skin and avoid stoma blood supply impairment.*

The gasket or opening of an appliance should normally be about 3 mm larger than the stoma itself so it does not cause friction or constraint, both of which can affect the blood supply. This is also a close enough fit to protect the peristomal skin from effluent, encouraging it to fall into the bag. However, any stoma may become oedematous, enlarging before subsequent shrinkage, necessitating an increase or decrease in the size of the bag and/or skin protective opening.

Ileostomies and colostomies usually differ in appearance. As the digestive elements of ileostomy effluent are more likely to damage peristomal skin most ileostomies are formed as spouts of about 2.5 cm length so effluent passes through them falling into the bag rather than collecting at skin level. End colostomies tend to be created flatter as effluent is less abrasive on the skin, but transverse colostomies can be oedematous and produce some skin-damaging effluent.

3. *Stomal effluent should be measured and recorded (including presence or absence of flatus) postoperatively, and a brief description of faecal consistency given, as part of the monitoring of patients' overall intake and output.*

The amount and consistency of faeces passed from an ileostomy or colostomy will vary depending on the position of the stoma in the bowel pathway and the condition and circumstances through which the patient has come to surgery. Accurate recording of faecal output is important as this enables progress of the patient's bowel towards appropriate functioning to be monitored and any problems to be recognised and dealt with promptly.

4. *Appliances need to be of a style and size to accommodate flatus and fluid effluent and enable these to be emptied out without removing the bag.*

An odour-proof drainable bag should be used, positioned to allow ease of emptying, for both ileostomies and colostomies. A flatus filter is initially not used; thus when flatus is passed from the stoma for the first time it remains visibly trapped in the bag to be noted before release.

Patients' abdomens are tender following surgery and this, coupled with the need to avoid damaging the peristomal skin, means that well-adhered appliances should be left in situ and emptied of effluent/flatus via the outlet rather than changed unnecessarily.

5. *Appliances should be checked and emptied sufficiently often to prevent over-filling and leakage.*

Leakage from stomal equipment causes much distress to patients, diminishing their confidence in both the equipment and the possibility of a leak-free future life. Generally the volume of effluent should not exceed half an appliance capacity and it is prudent to check and empty bags regularly and before changing a patient's position. If an appliance is more than half full it leaves insufficient room for flatus (which also takes up space) to be accommodated without pressure on the bag seams, the seal between flange and bag in two-piece equipment, and the seal between the bag adhesive and the patient's body. The weight of an overfull bag also drags on the body-bag adhesion seal, thereby reducing its efficiency as well as being uncomfortable for patients.

6. *Skin products should be appropriately used as soon as the stoma has been created to prevent the occurrence of skin damage.*

This includes recognising factors liable to give rise to problems (e.g. patient's skin type; abrasiveness of effluent likely to be passed; level of skin problems known to occur with the type of bag adhesive being used) and then incorporating suitably substantial skin protectives in the equipment being used (see Ch. 4 and below).

Patients and staff should also use certain *principles* to identify when stomal equipment needs changing because problems, or the potential for problems, are present. *Equipment should be changed when:*

(a) *Leakage of faeces occurs.* Even slight leakage can indicate faeces are likely to be lying on the skin underneath the bag adhesive, creating skin damage.
(b) *Burning or tingling sensations are experienced beneath the appliance.* These symptoms can be due to the skin reacting to the equipment. Alternatively, some faeces may have become trapped beneath where the seal of body and bag immediately around the stoma has been broken.
(c) *Discolouration of the equipment's adhesive area is present.* This signals faecal spillage has occurred and the potential for leakage and skin damage is high.
(d) *Softening or discolouration of the skin protective wafer is present.* Whether the wafer is an integral part of the bag or used in addition to it this indicates the wafer is breaking down with subsequent loss of skin protection and possible

faecal damage to the skin (see Patient scenario 5.1, below).
(e) *Odour is experienced coming from an odour-proof bag.* This can indicate the appliance is beginning to lift away from the body, so changing the equipment may be advisable. It is worth checking first that the end of an outlet on drainable bags (i.e. below the clip) has been adequately cleansed as faeces left there can create odour.

SPECIFIC ASPECTS OF CARE FOR PATIENTS WITH AN ILEOSTOMY

TYPE OF EFFLUENT

The position of an ileostomy in the digestive pathway results in effluent that contains digestive elements being diverted from the body, carrying with it the potential for peristomal skin damage (see Chs 2 and 3 and Fig. 5.1). Thus management of ileostomy output needs to be considered in terms of its likely constituents, volume and consistency, all of which affect the kinds of skin care and appliance that can be used. A drainable appliance combining substantial skin protection is normally worn (see Ch. 4).

Ileostomy output in the early postoperative period differs in both amount and consistency from that found once patients are eating and drinking normally. Initial output is generally watery and low in volume. This gradually increases and thickens until a volume of 400–500 ml of faeces of toothpaste or porridge-like consistency is being passed (Blackley 2004). However, Nicholls (1996, p 118) reports that large volumes (several litres) of effluent may be passed in the early postoperative period and sodium replacement will be necessary in such cases. Accurate measurement and recording of all fluid intake and output is therefore vital if metabolic problems are to be promptly detected in this early period.

'CONTROL' OF ILEOSTOMY ACTION

The position in the ileum where the stoma diverts effluent largely determines which physiological processes will affect composition, consistency, and frequency of elimination. These factors, coupled with the absence of sphincter muscles, mean ileostomy action cannot be 'controlled'. This aspect of living with their stoma must be stressed to patients right from the start. It is essential they accept this fact as metabolic disturbances can occur if patients seek to limit stomal action by substantially restricting their fluid or dietary intake (Fumi et al 1996). Restriction of fluids does not affect the volume of ileostomy effluent but can give rise to long-term urinary and renal problems. Patients should be encouraged to discuss their preoperative diet and ways in which this can now be adapted to be nutritionally balanced and thicken stomal effluent (see Ch. 16; Black 2000).

Dietary intake does affect ileostomy effluent and some patients have reported that occasionally they restrict their diet to avoid social embarrassment. Generally it is more helpful for patients to gain the ability and confidence to empty and change equipment in a wide variety of situations as most people need to empty their bags three to four times daily. An ileostomy will usually be active about half an hour after a meal, with output being greatest 3–4 hours after a main meal. Patients should be invited to discuss ways of fitting stomal management into their normal lifestyle so they avoid restricting their lives. Drugs are not usually required in the long-term control of ileostomy volume.

WHEN TO CHANGE EQUIPMENT

Usually a one-piece appliance can remain in position for 3–4 days and two-piece equipment may last longer. Manufacturers recommend complete equipment renewal at least every 7 days. However, other factors can influence the length of time equipment will last and it is more important for equipment to prevent skin damage and leakage than it is to stay in situ for a set number of days.

In the short time between surgery and discharge home the main goal is for patients to gain adequate self-care abilities. Decisions on changing equipment are usually based on achieving the best balance between giving patients sufficient change practice to gain skills whilst leaving equipment in place for enough time to avoid skin damage through too frequent removal. These frequent changes may mean patients do not readily have the opportunity to experience what equipment is like when it needs changing either because it is coming to the end of its functional life or because there are cues signalling that problems are arising. It is therefore important to teach patients the principles through which they can recognise when to change their equipment, as listed earlier in this chapter.

> **PATIENT SCENARIO 5.1**   Student Nurse Green and Staff Nurse Hill are looking after Ruth Goldsmith on her third postoperative day. While Nurse Hill is showing Ruth and Nurse Green how to empty Ruth's ileostomy bag she notices the flange's protective wafer is softening and changing colour, indicating skin protection is diminishing and the equipment needs changing. Before changing the bag she takes this opportunity to point out these cues to Ruth and Nurse Green, so that in future they will be able to recognise such cues while equipment is in situ. Once Ruth's equipment has been changed Nurse Hill shows them both the used bag flange. As they look at the undersurface (i.e. the side that had been applied to the body) they can now see more clearly where the wafer was melting away and thus no longer providing adequate skin protection. Now that they can look at the upper (outer) side more closely they can see the difference between the firm outer area of the flange and the melting paler inner area.

SPECIFIC ASPECTS OF CARE FOR PATIENTS WITH A COLOSTOMY

TYPE OF EFFLUENT

As faeces passes along the colon, fluid is reabsorbed for use within the body and the remaining faeces becomes more solid (see Ch. 2). Mucus is also secreted and this aids passage of faeces along the colon and creation of an alkaline bowel content. The type of effluent passed from a colostomy will therefore largely depend on the amount of colon which remains in situ to fulfil normal colonic function before the faecal flow is diverted via the stoma. This needs to be borne in mind when discussing appliances, skin care aids, and frequency of stomal action with patients (see also Ch. 4). The more common positions for colostomies are shown in Figure 5.1.

The type of faeces resulting from these stoma positions are generally as follows:

- *caecostomy*: effluent is liquid, may sometimes contain digestive enzymes, has a rather pungent odour, and is frequently passed

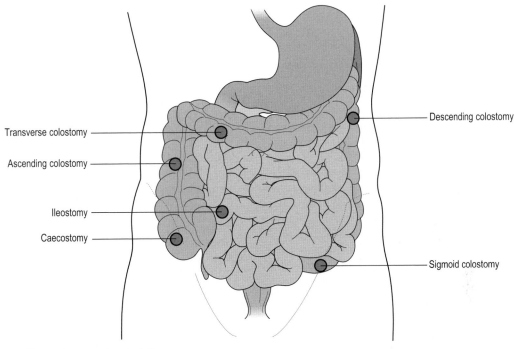

Figure 5.1   Types of stoma and typical sites.

- *ascending colostomy*: effluent is semi-liquid, may intermittently contain digestive enzymes, and is frequently passed
- *transverse colostomy* (usually right upper abdominal position): effluent varies between semi-liquid to soft unformed stool which may contain some digestive enzymes
- *descending colostomy*: effluent varies between a soft to a more formed stool
- *sigmoid colostomy*: a formed stool without digestive enzymes is normally passed.

'CONTROL' OF COLOSTOMY ACTION

Lack of an anal sphincter means patients cannot control when and where they defecate in the way they did before surgery. Many patients use the irrigation method to regulate colostomy action (see Ch. 15). Others may use the colostomy plug to help control the times when the stoma is free to evacuate (see Ch. 4). Some patients may use diet and/or medication to promote more consistent or manageable forms of colostomy action (see Chs 16 and 17). Whilst the restriction of certain foods can reduce odour and flatus, it is generally misleading to assure non-irrigating patients that they will be able

to 'regulate' their bowel to produce a daily stomal action at a time that is totally predictable and arranged by them. It is possible that action from sigmoid colostomies may settle into a pattern derived from the reaction of the bowel to food intake. However, the frequency and consistency of output from ascending and transverse colostomies make regulation particularly difficult. It is much more helpful to encourage patients to view their growing ability to manage their stomal equipment in the various situations arising from their lifestyle as their new form of bowel control.

MANAGEMENT OF FLATUS

Preston (1994) reports that individuals pass between 300 and 1000 ml flatus daily, expelling it between 10 and 14 times a day! Patients' absence of sphincters to aid control of when and where they pass flatus can create problems, particularly when it is being expelled from the colon and its faecal odour is more recognisable. Understandably, flatus is reported more frequently, and designated as problematic, by more people with a colostomy than an ileostomy (Wade 1989).

Generally patients with a colostomy want to know:

- which foods and fluids produce flatus *and* which ones create more odour
- how to manage the noticeable bulge created by flatus in their bag
- how to remove flatus from equipment without creating embarrassment or difficulties from its odour or faecal spillage.

Some people find as they resume normal eating and activities that flatus reduces but others report it as an ongoing occurrence (Pringle & Swan 2001). Certain foods and drinks do seem to cause flatus more often and patients can be advised of these (see Ch. 16, Meadows 1997, Preston 1994). However, eating is part of many enjoyable social activities and if people adopt a very curtailed diet they may also withdraw from social occasions where they think they might have to eat flatus-producing foods. It is therefore important to use dietary information and patient handouts such as those in Chapter 16 to help them.

Flatus can also build up from swallowed air (Preston 1994). Blackley (2004, p 179) lists activities that can contribute to flatulence as: rushed eating, chewing gum, smoking, missing meals, eating and drinking at the same time. It may therefore be helpful to discuss with patients whether any of these activities could be contributing to their problems.

The options for managing flatus with the different styles of equipment described below also have their limitations.

Use of a closed appliance with a flatus filter

The majority of closed appliances have a smaller capacity than drainable bags in which to accommodate flatus with or without faeces. Most bags incorporate filters to deodorise flatus as it passes through them and out of the bag. Although the quality of filters has improved, successful deodorisation often depends on flatus passing at quite a slow rate through the filter. Some patients find the time it takes to reduce the size of their bulging bags via filters unacceptable because they have to handle worries (or events) arising from an obviously bulging appliance or one where the bag-body seal, or the bag itself, bursts. The time taken to dispel flatus and bulge can seem endless to patients, particularly in the early days when their confidence and ability to handle explanations may be low. However, many patients find this type of appliance acceptable, even though they might prefer the flatus to be released from their bag more speedily. Occasionally the filter can be too

effective, creating a negative pressure in the bag which results in *pancaking* (where faeces collect around the stoma instead of dropping down into the bag). This faecal collection has to be accommodated somewhere as it grows larger and tends to force its way between the bag and body, enabling odour and faeces to escape as that seal is broken. Blackley (2004, p 190) suggests that faeces can be encouraged to slip down into the bottom of pouches by:

- puffing talcum powder into the pouch
- inserting a piece of facial tissue into the pouch
- painting the inside of the pouch where it touches the stoma with cooking or baby oil.

Some patients may complain of odour escaping via the filter. A change of appliance (and filter type), or use of an attachable filter instead, may resolve the difficulty if it only occurs with the particular make of filter and is not being caused by an ineffective bag–body seal.

Use of a drainable one–piece appliance

Many drainable bags now have filters but patients report varying levels of satisfaction with the way these control odour and release of flatus. Some people prefer to release flatus via the bag outlet. Care needs to be taken so faecal spillage is avoided as flatus is being released, and patients normally require some privacy when using this method. Although flatus can be released easily and speedily, removal of the more solid faeces through the bag outlet can be difficult. Thus patients may have to accept decreased ease of faecal removal in order to gain increased ease of flatus removal. Drainable appliances are more costly than closed ones. If patients change drainable bags with the same frequency that they would do with closed bags (in order to dispose of faecal content) this can have considerable cost implications over time.

Use of a two–piece appliance

This type of appliance can be 'burped' by briefly uncoupling the bag from the base in order to release flatus and then reconnecting them. If this method is adopted, patients should be given details of the various deodorising products available on prescription so they can minimise the amount of odour released with their flatus from the bag (see Ch. 4; Preston 1994). It enables speedy reduction of bulging equipment to be achieved but does require patients to be adept at reconnecting their equipment.

Use of continent colostomy plug

Both one- and two-piece plugs have filters to deodorise flatus. In a recent small study patients reported they did not think plug usage reduced flatus, but they liked experiencing less noise and no bulge from flatus collecting in a bag. There did not appear to be a build-up of flatus to be released on plug removal. Patients experiencing problems with flatus or insufficiently solid faeces for plug usage kept a diary for at least one week to identify when flatus and/or faecal action was most prevalent. Use of loperamide once or twice daily at such times was reported as helpful (Bobb & Liles 2003).

None of these systems provide ideal solutions but patients can be encouraged to decide which option will best help them manage their flatus in their particular situation.

WHEN TO CHANGE EQUIPMENT

The principles of stomal monitoring and care, and the reasons for changing stomal equipment outlined earlier in this chapter, are relevant for colostomy as well as ileostomy care. However, the consistency of faecal output from colostomies changes as normal meals are resumed and fluid reabsorption from the colon becomes re-established. The style of equipment used and frequency of changing it may have to be revised when these changes occur.

In the immediate postoperative period a one- or two-piece transparent non-sterile drainable appliance should be used so that the stoma and effluent can be easily observed and managed without frequent removal. More substantial skin protection is advisable for ascending and transverse colostomies where effluent may be more abrasive to the skin. The frequency of appliance change in the initial postoperative period will be partly determined by when the stoma begins to act. This varies depending on the condition that necessitated surgery. For example, a transverse colostomy performed to decompress a bowel in acute intestinal obstruction will act almost immediately. In contrast, patients who have had elective surgery following effective preoperative bowel preparation may find their (sigmoid) colostomy takes a few days to act. Depending on the amount and effects of stomal action in this early postoperative phase a one-piece appliance may stay in position for 3–4 days. If two-piece equipment is used the base can remain in situ for several days while the bag is changed more often if necessary.

Most patients with *sigmoid colostomies* will be able to use a closed appliance once their faeces has sufficiently solidified. The decision for patients to change from drainable to closed appliances needs to be primarily based on whether the type of faeces they are passing meets certain *criteria*:

- the *amount* of faeces being passed can easily be contained in the capacity offered by the closed appliance without making it necessary to change the bag more than twice daily
- the *consistency* of faeces is sufficiently solid to be contained by the degree of adhesiveness and size of the adhesive area provided by the closed bag's seal/flange.

Both criteria need to be met in order to avoid leakage or skin damage. This can be caused if closed equipment is being changed too frequently and/or is not effectively containing effluent. It can be tempting to change from drainable to closed appliances too early because of their simplicity of use and neater size, which many patients prefer. However, if the above criteria are not met the resultant problems can markedly affect patients' confidence in both the new closed equipment and their ability to use it successfully.

Patients who wish to use continent colostomy plugs should be advised to wait until their faecal consistency is sufficiently solid to prevent leakage, and of an amount to be containable for the time each plug is in situ.

Patients and staff must be made aware that it is these criteria which must be met, and why. We must also discuss with patients who they should contact, and how, to get help in choosing appropriate equipment and learning how to use new items once they meet the above criteria for changing to closed bags or plugs. Usually such help will be provided by their stoma care nurse (especially for initial plug fitting) or an experienced outpatient or community nurse.

Although faeces from *transverse colostomies* usually changes from fluid to semi-liquid as normal meals are resumed, effluent does not generally thicken and reduce in amount sufficiently to enable closed one-piece equipment to be worn. Some patients do use closed two-piece equipment but this is only advisable if the frequency with which the base has to be changed is sufficiently low to maintain good skin protection. It is therefore unwise to assure patients with transverse colostomies that they will be able to use closed equipment.

RESPONDING TO SEXUAL CONCERNS

GENERAL POINTS AND WAYS OF HELPING

Several aspects of sexuality-related care are similar whether patients have an ileostomy or a colostomy. These will be discussed next before the sections more specifically related to patients with ileostomies and colostomies.

Sexuality and sexual expression are still topics that many people (including healthcare staff and patients) have difficulty thinking about, let alone discussing in explicit and detailed ways. However, the majority of people who have stoma surgery do have concerns which can be described as 'sexual' whether these are about their changed body image, possible or actual changes in how they can engage in physical sexual activities, or (most commonly) a combination of both. They therefore need access to staff who can help them resolve concerns and rehabilitate as fully as possible in these areas.

Much of the anxiety that nurses express about providing sexuality-related care is triggered by the inaccurate belief that if we embark on sexual discussions we then have to provide all the information and help ourselves (Penman 1998). This is no more true than for any other aspect of living with a stoma, where we may equally find we can provide some help and then liaise with colleagues when more help is needed. Indeed it is a key area where liaison with the surgical team is important in order to establish the likelihood of impairment in view of the actual operation they have performed, and whether the expertise of specialist colleagues could benefit individual patients.

Since patients gain most of their stoma care and information from nurses they are also likely to seek their help with sexuality-related issues. Many nurses build up their ability to respond to such requests for help through a series of steps through which they gain knowledge, skills and confidence. These *steps* include:

- *Revising and extending knowledge of normal sexual function.* This is described by a number of authors (e.g. Herbert 1996, Fillingham 2004).
- *Gaining knowledge of how different operations that include stoma formation may affect sexual function* (e.g. using the material and references in Chs 3, 6, 10, and this chapter).
- *Learning to translate such knowledge into appropriate levels of information for patients* (who may require anything from minimal to detailed explanations about their surgery and its implications for sexual function).
- *Practising ways of giving relevant information until it can be given skilfully.* Essentially, we need to be able to give relevant information in ways that are helpful to the particular patient, with or without a partner, and of whatever sexual orientation. Like any skill, confident imparting of information and helping recipients use it takes practice and that also helps reduce any embarrassment felt when imparting sensitive and intimate material (Borwell 1997). These explanations can be practised with a colleague, having first briefed them on the kind of constructive feedback you want (e.g. on the clarity of your explanation; comfort or discomfort that you exhibit whilst explaining etc.). This will help you gain skills and confidence in providing accurate and easily understood information, which you can subsequently use when discussing these areas with patients and their partners.
- *Learning to use a range of approaches with which to help patients discuss and deal with sexuality-related concerns.* This includes the communication skills described in Chapter 7, approaches described later in this chapter on responding to patients' sexual concerns, and the approaches for helping with loss and change described in Chapters 20 and 22.

There are certain *principles* that it is essential for all staff who might be asked about the effects of 'stoma surgery' on sexual function to understand:

- The procedure of creating a bowel stoma without a more extensive operation (i.e. solely to create a diversion) does not usually damage the nerves associated with physiological sexual function. Therefore the diversionary procedure does not in itself generally create permanent physiological sexual impairment.
- The potential for pelvic nerve damage (the main cause of long-term physiological sexual impairment) depends on the surgical field involved in the different operations as it is the proximity of the surgery to the relevant sympathetic or parasympathetic nerve pathways that creates the potential for damage.
- Temporary physical effects on sexual function may well be experienced as tissues in the field of operation recover (e.g. from any bruising and swelling from being handled) and healing from stomal, abdominal and/or perineal surgery occurs.

- It is unhelpful, when talking about patients' operations, to talk about it in terms of the type of stoma raised, such as 'your ileostomy operation'. Unfortunately this can lead all concerned to assume that any subsequent sexual impairment arises as a result of the procedure of stoma creation and (as you can see from the above principles) this is not the case. This is compounded when research into sexual function reports impairment described by 'ileostomists' and 'colostomists' without stating (or even ascertaining) the nature and extent of those patients' total operation. These practices have led to some patients being given inaccurate information about the effects of their surgery just because they have a diversionary stoma, and have caused much distress.
- The presence of a stoma impinges on people's sense of themselves as a sexual being, and the assumptions and beliefs derived from that experience can affect both their physiological and psychological sexual functioning.
- Patients' response to their changed body image will often be related to their attitude, self-esteem and experiences before surgery. Their perception of their desirability, ability to function, and their relationship with an established or potential partner is likely to affect physiological functioning, just as the physical effects of their surgery are likely to affect their psychological experiences.

Concerns often raised by patients reflect the wider areas of expressing sexuality through their body image and loving interactions as well as issues around what is physiologically achievable (Salter 2002, Huish et al 1998). It is therefore important to have some wider understanding of body image changes which they may experience. These are discussed in Chapter 20, coupled with some ways of helping people with such experiences. Common concerns include:

- how the surgical procedure might have physically affected their sexual abilities
- whether having sex can be detrimental to recovery and/or harm the stoma
- whether the perineal and/or abdominal wounds will cause pain or discomfort during sexual activities, or alter the satisfaction experienced by the patient or their partner
- when sexual activities can be resumed postoperatively
- how to prevent problems with stomal equipment during sexual activity

- the degree to which they appear and/or feel desirable to themselves and/or to actual or potential partners
- how and when to tell potential lovers that they have a stoma.

Many of the skills described in Chapter 7 can be used to help patients clarify their sexual concerns so that the amount of information they need and the type of help that will be most beneficial to them can be identified (see, *for example*, Mrs Reid's initial response to Gary Cook in Patient scenario 7.1). Sensitive clarification of the issues with which patients are concerned, and identification of sources of help available, are both responses that patients value highly. They convey clear messages that the patient's concern warrants attention even though these approaches may not be sufficient help in themselves to resolve concerns. In Patient scenario 9.2 in Chapter 9, you will see that Nurse Linden explicitly told John Fletcher that it is fine with her that he has told her of his sexual problems, so that he would not misinterpret her additional information (about who else could help) as an indication that he should not have raised these issues.

Some patients may wish to discuss sexual concerns in conjunction with their partner whereas others may prefer to talk to the nurse without their partner. The absence of an identified partner should not lead staff to assume one does not or will not exist, or that the patient who has no apparent partner will not have concerns to be addressed. Although the following tips related to sexual activity can be given during an explicit discussion about sexual concerns most of them can actually be incorporated into the information being given generally on living with a stoma. It is well worth developing ways of doing this as it will enable you to use such tips to discreetly signal to patients (with or without partners) that sexual activities are possible, and that it is permissible for concerns to be discussed either at that time or later.

Some people suggest that being 'ready' for sexual activity includes preparatory tasks such as emptying their appliance and ensuring it is well adhered to their body. Some people avoid foods known to give them excess flatus beforehand as they feel embarrassed if their stoma is noisily passing wind or faeces during love-making, particularly in the early days of readjustment. A change of position from, for example, sitting to lying down may also lead to bowel activity and the couple may incorporate a little time for this to settle down into their routine (Salter 1996, p 209).

Many patients have concerns about their stomal equipment. Some people like to wear a belt to give added security when they are more mobile generally, and this can also be used during sexual activities. Others may wish to tuck the whole bag into a wide belt or cummerbund. Attractive belts can be made using the upper half of underpants or panties: cutting off the crotch area and making a hem on the new lower edge through which elastic can be threaded. Some women find crotchless panties or a pretty waist slip aesthetically pleasing and a boost to feeling feminine. Some people think their appliances look more attractive if they use a bag cover, whether supplied by an appliance company or one of their own design. A cover can also reduce the possibility of the bag sticking to either its owner or their partner in inopportune ways if sleeping together or if love-making makes them a bit sweaty. When discussing bag covers generally (see Ch. 4) giving the example of a young woman who made her own lace bag covers to match her wedding dress has proved to be a really successful invitation to patients, prompting many of them to start discussing sexuality-related concerns and review their beliefs about the desirability of people who have stomas.

General discussion on the need to allow healing of all surgical areas before full lifestyle activities are resumed can also be used to help patients apply this idea to sexual activities. For example, a diagram that includes the sexual organs and perineal area can be used to show women the field of surgery where healing will be taking place, so the close relationship between the line of bowel dissection and the posterior vaginal wall can be seen. Most patients have little difficulty understanding that they will not feel comfortable allowing children or pets to bounce up and down on their abdomen in the early postoperative period. The inadvisability of a partner's penis thrusting too hard against the posterior vaginal wall (which may well have less elasticity to accommodate it comfortably) can be given as a similar example of why healing time must be given before full lifestyle activities are resumed. Assurances should be given that, although penetrative sex should wait until healing has occurred, sharing a bed and engaging in cuddles and close body contact can be resumed as soon as the couple wish to do so.

The timing of sexual information and the level of detail that particular patients might want should be carefully assessed with them. For example, they can be told that more detailed information about positions etc. can be given if they indicate they want it, either at the time of the conversation or in the future and with or without a partner. Likewise it may be helpful for patients to know that it is often only several months into their physical and psychological recovery that many patients indicate they now want information about alternative ways of sexual expression and/or assurances that (for example) sexual satisfaction from oral and manual sex, or the use of sex aids, are acceptable alternatives.

While some nurses develop the ability to provide relevant information others may not accept that providing detailed sexual information is part of their role. It is helpful if patients are clearly told these are reasonable enquiries for them to make, coupled (if necessary) with the information that the nurse receiving this enquiry is not in a position to provide the level or scope of information that might be of most benefit to them. Leaflets and help are available from the ostomy organisations and others (see Ch. 24) and nurses can also take steps to help patients gain specialist referral. The increasing number of sexual videos and books for heterosexuals, gay men, and lesbians which are now available in ordinary shops may also be useful as their level of detail is sufficiently explicit to help people who want to extend their sexual repertoire to gain ideas for doing so.

People who are building up a new relationship may seek advice as to how to talk to their potential sexual partner. Salter (1996, p 214) suggests it is important to avoid putting off telling a potential partner about the stoma as it is likely to result in the stoma being discovered by accident. She suggests that by the third or fourth date people usually know if the relationship is going to deepen and that this may well be a good time to explain. Generally it is more helpful to encourage individuals to develop an explanation with which they feel comfortable than to advise them what specifically they should say and/or do. Inviting them to identify *what* information would help their partner understand, and *how* they might provide such information is useful. It gives them some practise in discussing the issue, and enables gaps or misunderstandings in their knowledge to be recognised and addressed. Awareness that they needed help to handle explanations can also help patients understand that inept, disappointing or rejecting reactions from a potential partner arise from that person's lack of knowledge and/or appropriate skills and beliefs with which to respond. They do not constitute evidence of 'facts' about the acceptability or desirability of people with a stoma.

The following section focuses on patients whose 'conventional' surgery includes an ileostomy. There is a subsequent section on patients with colostomies. Additional information regarding patients with bowel pouches can be found in Chapter 10. The effects and treatments related to urinary surgery (including penile implants) are discussed in Chapter 6.

SEXUAL CONCERNS AND FUNCTIONING OF PEOPLE WITH ILEOSTOMIES

Physical effects of surgery on male sexual function

Men whose surgery only involves creation of an ileostomy are unlikely to have physical sexual impairment as the operative field should be sufficiently distant from the presacral nerves to avoid damage.

Where surgery is for non-malignant conditions, a close rectal dissection can be performed for men undergoing panproctocolectomy or restorative proctocolectomy, thus avoiding sexual nerve damage. Patients with dysplasia should not have a close rectal dissection. However, Nicholls & Williams (2002, p 79) suggest that most surgeons will dissect the rectum with its mesorectum in a manner that preserves the presacral nerves (required for ejaculation) and the autonomic nerve plexus in the lower part of the pelvis on the lateral wall (required for erection).

Some patients do report difficulties maintaining an erection in the first few months postoperatively while healing is still taking place (Salter 2002).

People who include anal sex in their activities should be encouraged to refrain from this after pelvic pouch construction as it may damage the sphincter muscles and can lead to incontinence and leakage (Borwell 1997). Use of their stoma for sex should also be discouraged (Black 1992).

Physical effects of surgery on female sexual function

Women are also unlikely to have physical sexual impairment if they have ileostomy formation only.

Similar attention to nerve-sparing to that described above for men should also be employed during panproctocolectomy and restorative proctocolectomy for women. However, the proximity of the surgical field to women's vagina and perineum can create subsequent difficulties if scar tissue makes the posterior vaginal wall and/or perineum more rigid. Healing may take several months and is often influenced by patients' preoperative condition. For example, people with Crohn's disease may have abscesses or fistulas resulting in infection and/or general debility affecting the rate of healing. Adequate time for healing must be given before penetrative sex takes place. It is important that both patient and partner understand that, if intercourse takes place too early and pain (dyspareunia) is experienced, anxiety that this will recur can make it difficult for the woman to relax and become sufficiently aroused and lubricated for satisfactory vaginal penetration on subsequent occasions.

Salter (2002, p 193) states that vaginal discharge and dyspareunia are well-known problems following panproctocolectomy. She suggests that this is due to anatomical changes if the vagina and uterus fall back and adhere to the sacrum. In contrast, such problems may be uncommon in pouch patients when the pouch replaces the rectum by being positioned between the sacrum and internal genitals. If secretions pool in the vagina due to its changed position, their intermittent discharge can be successfully managed through regular vaginal douching (Blackley 2004).

Many patients whose surgery includes ileostomy formation have their operation after living with chronic, debilitating conditions for a substantial time. These circumstances may have affected their interest and ability to engage in sexual activities. Questions about how their operation will affect them sexually may be minimal preoperatively. As their general health and wellbeing improve postoperatively so their interest in sexual expression may also increase and patients, with or without a partner, may seek more detailed information and advice from healthcare staff.

Where absence of the rectum following surgery results in alterations to the position of a woman's vagina, the angle at which her partner inserts his penis may also need to change for intercourse to be satisfactory. Diagrams can be used to help couples understand this information and the suggestion that some people find varying their position from the missionary (man on top) one to a side to side or woman on top position is more comfortable (because the penile angle becomes more in line with the altered vaginal position). Extra lubrication may also be helpful. Some people use saliva or water-based (KY) jelly whilst others take advantage of the various lubricants available from sex shops, mail order or the internet.

As indicated earlier, it is important to develop sensitive and flexible ways of imparting this kind of information so *what* we say, *how*, and *when* is appropriate for patients and partners. You may also wish to use some of the approaches described in the colostomy section, below, more widely than just in response to patients with a colostomy.

Contraception

Specialist advice may be necessary for premenopausal women following ileostomy creation because of anatomical and physiological changes (Black 2000). Major pelvic surgery can alter women's pelvic anatomy sufficiently to make insertion of a vaginal cap difficult. Intrauterine devices (IUD) are generally contraindicated as they can also become difficult to insert following some operations and, in cases where ileostomists have a history of pelvic infection, an IUD could provide a locus for infection.

Williams & Nicholls (2002, p 163) state that most contraceptive pills are absorbed within the duodenum so patients with an ileostomy or ileo-anal pouch should be able to absorb them. However, they also recommend that both partners should use some form of contraception.

Pregnancy

Patients may be advised to wait a year after stoma surgery to allow scar tissue to heal. A 2-year wait may be advised for patients who need to recover from the effects of inflammatory bowel disease (Black 2000). Many women with an ileostomy do have a successful pregnancy delivered by the vaginal route. Kirsty, now in her thirties, has had three successful pregnancies which included twin boys and all three were uncomplicated vaginal deliveries. Antenatal care required in the early months is likely to be the same as for all women. As the pregnancy progresses, closer medical monitoring may be necessary and the care required is likely to be influenced by the effects of a woman's original condition and surgery (Blackley 2004). Taylor (2003, p 187) suggests that in pregnancy:

- vaginal delivery is usually possible for patients who have had ulcerative colitis, but forceps delivery may be required

- women with Crohn's disease may be delivered by Caesarean section if it is thought an episiotomy might not heal well and/or fistula formation could occur
- intestinal obstruction may occur if changes in the peritoneum result in adhesions becoming taut around the intestine.

The possibility that signs of intestinal obstruction could be masked by, or interpreted as, signs of early labour should be borne in mind.

Practical aspects of stoma management may need to be modified as the abdomen increases in size and seeing the stoma becomes more difficult. Use of a mirror or enlisting help from a partner may be necessary. Reassessment of equipment may also be needed if the type being used is not sufficiently flexible to mould around the changing body contours, or if prolapse occurs. Medication should be reviewed both to ensure it is compatible with pregnancy and to ascertain whether it will affect stomal output (Blackley 2004, p 223–224).

SEXUAL CONCERNS AND FUNCTIONING OF PEOPLE WITH COLOSTOMIES

Many of the underlying issues and concerns discussed earlier ('General points and ways of helping') also occur when patients have colostomies. However, people undergoing surgery including colostomy formation tend to be in the middle to elderly age group and so have to deal with the additional problem of ageist beliefs that unfortunately still seem to be widespread. For example, assumptions that such 'older' patients will not (or should not) have much concern over any sexual impairment arising from their surgery can lead to information about possible impairment not being given preoperatively. Likewise access postoperatively to information and help may not be provided if patients feel unable to indicate that it is, or could be, needed. It is usually helpful to tell patients that people of any age and background can have concerns about how such surgery might affect them as a man or woman, and that this is a normal topic which many patients and staff discuss both before and after surgery. However, it is also important not to impose overly detailed explanations about possible sexual impairment and alternative sexual practices on patients who might not want them at that particular time, or indeed at any time. Some (but not all) older people may have other conditions that are affecting their sexual activities, such as arthritis, general physical or mental debility, which may also need to be considered when information and advice is offered (Huish et al 1998).

Identifying the potential for impairment

The effects of operations including colostomy formation are often less straightforward to identify than is the case with ileostomies. Additionally, changes in operative techniques are altering the likelihood of impairment. This means that automatically attributing specific impairments to particular operations is often inappropriate. It is more useful to review the extent of operations, and the implications of the surgical field and techniques used, in order to deduce whether sexual impairment is likely. For example, surgery that solely entails creation of a colostomy is unlikely to result in permanent sexual impairment in men or women as the field of operation can usually be kept clear of the nerves that could cause it. Now consider the other operations which include colostomy formation that are described in Chapter 3 (anterior resection; abdomino-perineal excision of rectum; pelvic exenteration). The goal in each of these major operations is often removal of cancer with surrounding tissue clearance. However, the extent of the surgical field (and therefore the potential for sexual impairment) differs in each operation.

With each operation we must therefore systematically consider:

- the extent of the field of operation and whether any sexual organs will be removed or directly operated upon
- the proximity of the surgical field to the sympathetic and parasympathetic nerves which enable/affect sexual function
- the degree to which blood vessels which supply the sexual organs may be damaged or bruised and thus affect sexual function
- the likely extent and effects of soft tissue damage and bruising
- any alterations in sexual organs and the surrounding areas due to the operation and/or subsequent scarring of tissue
- whether sperm banking should be offered preoperatively (Salter 1996 p 210).

In addition, the condition of patients' wounds, and the level of healing that has occurred, must be considered postoperatively as these can affect the levels of comfort, or discomfort, patients experience when engaging in sexual activities.

We can also use the above list as a framework for discussions with surgical colleagues about particular operations for specific patients, to clarify possible or actual effects and implications. Such discussions enable team members to offer compatible explanations and helpful support to patients and their partners.

The references cited in Chapter 3 for anterior resection and abdomino-perineal excision of rectum clearly describe refined surgical techniques through which colorectal surgeons can remove cancers more effectively whilst preserving the nerves required for sexual function. Development of such approaches, and increased training of surgeons in their use, should be reducing the number of patients experiencing permanent sexual problems. However, identifying what percentage of patients are having sexual problems from the different operations, and why, remains difficult. Much research from earlier years was reporting results from earlier techniques of anterior resection, and the wider excision and blunt dissection then used for abdomino-perineal excision of rectum. More research about the effects of current operations is needed. Many patients, understandably, want to know whether any sexual impairment will be temporary or permanent, what such impairment might entail, and whether it can be effectively treated. The *timing* of when they want such information can differ, but the majority like to have a sense that such information will be available to them if or when they want it, and will be knowledgeably and sensitively provided.

More work is being done on the factors that influence surgical outcomes such as cancer recurrence, but McArdle (2001) describes how difficult it is to pinpoint the elements that promote or interfere with successful outcomes. Increasing use of audit may lead to greater clarity about the results that particular surgeons normally have with patients undergoing particular operations for specific cancer stages.

If staff do not inform patients that problems can arise and then they do occur, this can create substantial distress and distrust of healthcare staff in patients. It can affect their relationship both with staff involved in their current care and with those who provide future care, and has been known to decrease patients' subsequent willingness to believe information and accept treatment.

Physical function can be affected by psychological factors such as anxiety. Therefore patients, their partners, and their healthcare team must find helpful ways of managing sexual concerns and problems now. That is not just a matter of imparting any relevant information available: our attitude and skills must enable us to provide it, or refer patients to more experienced colleagues, in an informed and helpful manner. Striking a balance between ensuring patients have sufficient information about the possible effects of their planned operation to enable them to give informed consent to it *and* avoiding creation of such anxiety in them that their sexual function is impaired through the resultant psychological experience is not easy. Staff should consider whether their levels of knowledge and skills are sufficient to achieve this balance before providing detailed information. The two *patient scenarios* later in this chapter indicate ways of giving helpful responses while the provider keeps in mind the boundaries of her competence.

Some information linking tissue damage to particular dysfunction is available.

- Damage to the presacral sympathetic nerves that supply the bladder and sexual organs will result in the inability to ejaculate, although men will still be able to achieve an erection. Ejaculation may be retrograde into the bladder if the inner bladder sphincter can no longer close.
- Damage to the sacral parasympathetic supply in the nervi erigentes can cause problems in penile erection and ejaculation (Northover et al 2002, p 54).
- Damage to the parasympathetic nerves which control blood flow to the penis can occur (Keighley 2002, p 320).

Problems can also arise from indirect damage where bruising and swelling of tissues around nerves and blood vessels involved in sexual function temporarily cause impairment, and from direct damage of blood vessels supplying the penis. For example, there is evidence that impotence can occur following radical cystectomy when damage to the blood vessels supplying the penis causes veno-occlusive dysfunction and cavernosal artery insufficiency, reducing the penile engorgement that normally occurs in erection and thus affecting men's ability to gain and maintain an erection (De Luca et al 1996). If similar blood vessel damage occurred, for example during abdomino-perineal excision, this could affect the penile vascular supply and thus men's erectile function.

More is also becoming known about the series of chemical reactions that take place during sexual stimulation in order to initially produce vasodila-tion to aid erection and subsequently inhibit it. For example, the commercial drive to create pharmaceutical substances such as sildenafil (Viagra) to treat sexual dysfunction has also led to increased research into the physiological processes that occur in sexual activity. Interference with these chemical reactions can also affect erection (see Ch. 6; Webb & Holmes 1999). The need to ascertain the effects of drugs on people's sexual function is focusing attention on how such information can be elicited in adequate detail. Likewise increasing information gained from psychosexual counselling research and practice is also aiding understanding of how such personal information can be elicited and responded to most helpfully. Questionnaires are being developed to aid elicitation of sexual information (e.g. Huish et al 1998, Rosen et al 1997). Hopefully these activities will create a more specific knowledge base which could be of real use with stoma patients.

Increasing public and professional knowledge of the existence of treatment for sexual dysfunction is creating changes in attitude towards sexual assessment and treatment. For example, public debate as to whether oral medication for erectile dysfunction should be provided inside or outside mainstream health care carries an inbuilt assumption that such treatment is acceptable for people to obtain. Likewise public discussion as to whether particular treatment is sufficiently reliable in reducing or resolving sexual dysfunction has enabled detailed and explicit discussion and assessment to become accepted as necessary for professionals and patients to engage in as a prelude to identifying appropriate treatments.

Once explicit description of sexual function, and the questions used to elicit it, are designated normal and necessary assessment activities it becomes more acceptable for professionals to learn how to fulfil such assessments skilfully, and for patients and professionals to focus on sexual function in sufficient detail. Information as to what sexual functions appear to be present and absent aids identification of what tissue damage has occurred, and what treatment options may therefore be available to correct or minimise problems.

More ways of helping

Given the diversity of possible physical and psychological causes of sexual dysfunction it is obvious that full and careful assessment of patients will be needed if problems persist. This may be undertaken by the team involved in patients' original surgery or through referral to a specialist. However, patients' initial questions and concerns are most likely to be raised with stoma care nurses and other members of the healthcare team who they view as sufficiently knowledgeable and approachable to be likely sources of help. The support and help we provide (or ask others to provide) can be considered in four areas.

Preoperative management of sexual information and concerns

It is essential for the healthcare team to work collaboratively to minimise provision of any conflicting information. Where there is a possibility of some sexual impairment this should generally be stated so that patients can give informed consent to surgery. The amount of detailed information that is given should be primarily shaped by the level of detail individual patients wish to receive at this time. Most patients are able to indicate this level when asked to do so. Many patients, faced with major surgery for cancer, are more concerned preoperatively about whether their surgery will be curative, and how they will fit their stoma and its management into their lives. However, the way in which sexuality-related issues are handled by staff should send clear messages to patients and their partners that subsequent concerns and needs for more information and treatment will be responded to sensitively and helpfully (see Patient scenario 1.1 in Ch. 1).

Pacing resumption of sexual activities

All the information given earlier in this chapter for helping people with ileostomies regain sufficient general health, energy, and healed body tissues will also benefit people with colostomies. Similarly, preparation of stomal equipment so it is secure and unobtrusive should be discussed. It can also be helpful to encourage patients and their partners to actively consider how they can create an ambience conducive to relaxed participation in sexual activities, and rediscover previously used strategies for fostering sexual pleasure and closeness.

Management of uncertainty over time

Some patients report they have some erectile ability but that it is less firm or lasts for less time than was the case preoperatively, and thus still causes difficulties (e.g. in penetration). Others who initially experience sexual impairment subsequently report that this has reduced or resolved, usually within the first 2 years following surgery. This means that doctors may be reluctant to assume impairment is permanent and initiate substantial assessment and treatment within this period of time. Patients may experience both the uncertainty and the inaction to resolve their problems as difficult, and may require help to manage this situation resourcefully. Most of the help we can give during this time will not resolve their uncertainty over the levels of impairment with which they could be left but will aid rehabilitation in many aspects of their lives. This in turn can reduce patients' overall sense of difficulty and increase their sense of wellbeing as a whole.

Firstly, difficulties are often experienced as less overwhelming if people feel understood and that their difficulties are acknowledged. Providing patients with time and attention to express their problems and feelings can help them feel valued and less alone in handling them. The skills described in Chapter 7 can be used to convey respect, concern and empathy as well as to help patients clarify their experience and needs. Giving such support also helps us pick up anything that a patient may be doing to help himself handle his situation but which actually could be making it worse, such as drinking too much alcohol (which can depress sexual capability) in order to reduce his anxiety over possible sexual inability before love-making.

Secondly, patients may feel less distressed and powerless if they can 'do something' to actively promote their physical and psychological recuperation. Help here can include encouraging patients to plan and fulfil realistic programmes for regaining physical fitness, resuming work, hobbies, and social activities etc., all of which can enhance people's sense of confidence and self-worth.

Thirdly, patients who undergo such major surgery usually experience loss due to the various changes in the way their body looks and functions. Helping patients work through their responses to many of these changes can enable them to develop a new sense of who they are becoming and increasing acceptance of how they now function generally (see Chs 20 and 22). Although who they are as sexual beings may yet to be resolved it can feel less burdensome as confidence increases in other aspects of themselves.

Helping patients prepare for sexual assessment and treatment

Assessment is likely to be fuller and more useful if patients can provide detailed description of the sexual function which they do and do not experience. Firstly, this requires them to notice and remember what happens during sexual activity (e.g. with a partner; when masturbating). However, some people find paying attention to what is or is not happening raises anxiety and reduces the level of function they attain when they are not trying to act and to monitor at the same time. It is therefore beneficial to help them find ways of monitoring their sexual function sufficiently to gain the information needed for assessment without acquiring a habit of constantly assessing their performance.

Secondly, patients need to be able to talk about their concerns and describe their sexual experience with the nurse, doctor or therapist who is assessing them. Patients can have difficulty finding the words to describe their experience and/or understanding the terminology used by their assessors. Embarrassment over revealing such intimate details is likely to be compounded if patients do not understand the jargon used in assessors' questions. Patients can be prepared for assessment by telling them what kind of information they will probably be asked for, and what they can do to be ready to give the answers. Such guidance enables them to decide whether they want to have such an assessment and, if so, what they will do to prepare for it. This kind of information-giving needs to be used as part of a counselling approach that focuses on patients' experiences and needs (see Chs 19 and 20) rather than staff seeking to fit the patient into their pattern of preparation.

The *patient scenarios* with John Fletcher in Chapters 1 and 9, coupled with this next one, indicate how this four-stage process can be used. From reading these scenarios and the following one you can see that in each instance the rapport built up between patient and staff enable him to lead into sexual issues when he is ready to do so. Their responses have helped him become confident that they will want to help him.

PATIENT SCENARIO 5.2   It is now a year since John Fletcher had his abdomino-perineal excision of rectum. He feels well generally and pleased to have resumed his normal work and social activities. He has come to see Mrs Reid, the stoma care nurse, to find out how he can get more help with his ongoing sexual difficulties. He reports that he went to his GP to ask if these new sex tablets he has heard about could help, and had been told to

discuss it with his surgical team. When he did so he was advised to give his body more time to settle down. John says he is fed up with not getting specific answers to his problem and that he wants some action. He wants to know what to do when he goes to his forthcoming medical outpatient appointment. Mrs Reid acknowledges the frustration he is expressing, and how difficult it is for him to wait patiently for his body to recover. She explains that his doctor will need to know in detail what does and does not happen sexually in order to identify what specific help is required. She explains that if someone gets some erection but it isn't hard enough to be useful, then their treatment is likely to be different from the treatment which may be given if a man stays flat as a pancake or doesn't get any hardening of his penis. John grins slightly nervously but does not say anything. On noticing this Mrs Reid goes on to tell him that sometimes men have difficulties if they try to resume sex too soon after surgery, and then either anxiety prevents them from seeking to have sex subsequently, or it interferes with their ability if they do try. She remembers that John has expressed concern about possible sexual impairment on a number of occasions (e.g. see Patient scenario 1.1 in Ch. 1) and thinks it would be helpful to clarify the basis of those concerns. She also wants to check whether John wants an assessment now he has more of an idea of what it would entail. She therefore asks him if he would be willing to give his doctor this information if he himself knew it. John says yes, even if it was embarrassing he would do so now he understands providing such information would help him move towards getting a solution.

Mrs Reid now asks John if it would be helpful if they identified what information he already knew and what information he had yet to find out about himself, so he could prepare for his medical appointment. She uses this approach to give John the opportunity to experience talking more specifically about his sexual situation, and thus engage in some rehearsal for his actual medical assessment. Mrs Reid has completed fairly substantial counselling training in addition to her nursing courses but she makes it clear to John that she is not a psychosexual therapist. She can use her skills to help him prepare well for his medical assessment, and has found that this kind of rehearsal does help patients and their doctors discuss intimate concerns more readily, which is a good start to identifying the treatment that will best help them.

John is now sufficiently relaxed to agree to this suggestion. She uses broad statements to indicate aspects of his sexual experience his doctor is likely to ask about, coupled with open questions to help him reflect on his situation.

For example: she tells John that the doctor is likely to ask him if he has noticed any hardening or erection of his penis since his operation. She then asks him when did he get an erection before his illness and operation? This encourages John to remember he sometimes used to wake in the morning with an erection, as well as getting one when making love with Mary. Mrs Reid now asks him whether (if he wanted to at the time) he thinks it might be an idea to pay attention to what happens nowadays in any situations where previously he might have got an erection, so that he would have such information available when he had his assessment? She is careful not to imply what he should or should not be experiencing or doing, but her question gives him an option to consider. She also uses reflecting and summarising to check her understanding of what John tells her, using his words and phrases so as to avoid putting words into his mouth or changing the meaning of what he is saying. This approach enables her to pick up some of John's beliefs about sex as well as enabling both of them to gain a more specific understanding of John's current situation. This includes the following:

- John does feel sexual desire but is quite anxious about initiating love-making with Mary in case he can't translate desire into adequate sex.
- He equates successful sex with penile penetration as he thinks this is what satisfies Mary as well as himself.
- He can get a partial erection sometimes but this is not very hard and goes down quickly when he tries to use it for penetration.
- John has rarely masturbated since surgery because he was worried he might be doing something damaging as he did not ejaculate when he climaxed. He does get some erection and a sense of climax.
- He normally takes the on top missionary position when making love. He and Mary 'don't go in for fancy sex' and he knows little about what else he could do to make their love-making satisfying.

- Some of the times John has tried to make love with Mary were either at the end of a full day's work or after he has had several beers to relax him.

John is now in a much better position to provide specific information to his doctor. However, Mrs Reid gives him additional information to help him now. She tells him some men do not ejaculate externally following his kind of operation and he will not damage himself if he has a climax without ejaculation. She also points out gently that he may be contributing to his difficulties if he embarks on sex when he is physically or mentally overtired or has had too much alcohol. Mrs Reid tells John that some men retain the ability to experience orgasm even if they do not get an erection, and that it is important for John and Mary to know of this possibility. She links this to the suggestion that John and Mary go back to earlier days when they may have paid more attention to helping each other feel sexy and aroused, and spend more time and attention now on enjoying the early stages of love-making too. John thinks they could do this, and also that it would be a good idea to try masturbating again (so he gets a better idea of how much erection he can get and how long it lasts) before his medical appointment.

Mrs Reid recognises that John and Mary could benefit from learning ways of extending their sexual repertoire because this could increase their levels of satisfaction without being dependent on full intercourse. She realises that the presence of some erectile ability indicates that certain nerve, vascular, and chemical activities can occur and therefore medication to enhance the period of penile tumescence might well enable John to get a more usable erection. However, she thinks John should have a full assessment and examination before useful techniques and treatments are discussed in detail. She therefore just establishes with John that he feels he can now prepare himself more confidently to talk to the doctor and will tell Mary what he has learned from this discussion.

John is pleased when Mrs Reid suggests she could talk to the surgical team to ensure a senior doctor gives him sufficient time at his forthcoming appointment to discuss assessment and treatment. She is aware that John and Mary are likely to need more time and explicit help than she can provide if they do wish to extend their ways of making love. She wants to ensure that the possibility of referral to a trained sexual counsellor is included in the options considered by John, Mary, and the healthcare team. This would broaden the style of help given to include psychological as well as physical assessment and treatment, and could be supportive for both of them. As John leaves he says he is more hopeful now that he will get more help, and that already he feels better in himself.

In the above *scenario* the patient asked directly about medication for erectile dysfunction. Nurses and doctors will increasingly need to be able to respond to questions about the usefulness of such drugs for stoma patients in an informed and sensitive manner. Currently, both medical and public attention is being paid to a class of drugs known as phosphodiesterase type 5 (PDE5) inhibitors. Their reactions have been outlined by various authors (e.g. Israel 1998, Webb & Holmes 1999), and can be summarised as follows:

- In order for phosphodiesterase type 5 (PDE5) inhibitors such as sildenafil (Viagra) to be effective sexual stimulation is required so that penile nerve endings and endothelial cells release nitric oxide.
- Nitric oxide activates the enzyme guanylate cyclase, which results in the production of cyclic guanosine monophosphate (cGMP); this is a vasodilator that relaxes smooth muscle in the corpus cavernosum, enhancing blood flow to the penis and leading to an erection.
- Cyclic GMP is degraded by phosphodiesterase 5, so when a PDE5 inhibitor is taken this slows down the rate of degradation of cyclic GMP and thus its tumescent effects on the penis are prolonged for longer.

It is important for patients to understand that taking PDE5 inhibitors will not in itself cause them to have erections. Firstly, they will need to engage in sexual stimulation to trigger the above cycle of events. Secondly, these are only likely to result in improved erections if their relevant nerve and vascular pathways are sufficiently intact to enable tumescence to occur and be prolonged. Medical assessment prior to the use of PDE5 inhibitors is also important, as there are conditions that contraindicate their use, such as severe cardiovascular disorders, or when patients are taking medication containing nitrates (Blackley 2004).

At this stage there is insufficient published research into the use of these products with patients whose surgery included stoma formation. However, if there is sufficient detail as to what sexual processes a man has or has not retained, then it may be possible for research into PDE5 inhibitor efficacy with other patients to be used to decide whether it could be appropriate to prescribe them for that individual. For example, Zippe et al (1998) found that 12 out of 15 patients, who had erectile dysfunction following radical prostatectomy where bilateral nerve-sparing procedures had been used, reported they gained sufficient penile erection for vaginal penetration after taking sildenafil (Viagra) whereas none of the 10 patients who had undergone a non-nerve-sparing prostatectomy procedure responded to it. Derry et al (1999) studied men with erectile dysfunction caused by spinal cord injury between levels T6 and L5 who were able to achieve at least a partial reflexogenic erectile response to penile vibratory stimulation. Nine out of twelve patients improved the quality of their erections after taking sildenafil and reported improved satisfaction with their sex lives.

The action of these drugs and other aids which may be of use to some men are also discussed in Chapter 6 and by Webb & Holmes (1999). Sexual function and satisfaction is a complex area involving both physical and psychological factors. It is essential that elements of the background information included here are selected carefully for both relevance to individual patients' situations and appropriateness of the timing for discussing them with any particular person. In addition, staff must consider whether they have got the level of communication skills required to engage sensitively in such discussions, or whether patients would be better helped through referral to a specialist.

Historically much of the discussion and research about sexual impairment following surgery involving stoma creation has focused largely on male dysfunction. Indeed Coates (1986, p 83–85) suggests that insufficient attention is paid to the effects that pelvic nerve damage may have on women's sexual experience given the physiological similarities between the clitoris and penis. However, as women in many cultures are increasing their willingness to discuss their sexual needs and experiences, and perceive sexual satisfaction for themselves as well as their partners is important, so members of the healthcare team are more likely to be asked for information and help.

Theoretically the surgical approaches outlined in Chapter 3 should be resulting in women having fewer problems following either anterior resection or abdomino-perineal excision of rectum. However, problems can still arise. Firstly, removal of the rectum in either operation can lead to the vagina falling back towards the sacrum unless prevented (e.g. by a colo-anal pouch following anterior resection). Secretions can pool in the repositioned vagina, creating malodorous discharge. Vaginal douching can help women deal with this situation. The angle used for entry by a partner may also need to change, as described earlier and in Patient scenario 5.3, below.

Secondly, the proximity of the vagina and the perineal wound can mean that difficulties are caused by scarring and rigidity in the perineum, or soreness and discomfort until perineal healing is well established.

Thirdly, damage to nerves and blood vessels can decrease the amount of vaginal lubrication and the speed of lubrication which women may experience during love-making compared to their preoperative experience.

In addition, part of the vagina may be removed during *abdomino-perineal excision of the rectum*. This may occur either because a wider excision is still viewed as the correct approach in that centre, or because there already is tumour spread by the time women come for treatment. In these circumstances the vagina will be shortened, and some loss of elasticity is likely along the remaining posterior vaginal wall due to the scarring of tissue in close proximity to it where the rectum was removed. This often leaves less room to accommodate a partner in it.

These various changes can lead to dyspareunia (painful intercourse) if patients and their partners are not helped to understand them and adapt their love-making accordingly (Topping 1990, Schulte 1994). It is important to help women avoid such difficulties as once a woman experiences pain during sexual activity it can lead to anxiety and tension on subsequent occasions which in turn can make vaginal relaxation and lubrication more difficult to achieve.

Women can benefit from knowledgeable, skilled help in the same four areas discussed earlier for men having this operation. For example, women should also be informed preoperatively that their surgery could affect sexual function if they are to give informed consent to it. Discussion about pacing resumption of intercourse can help patients and their partners take account of how perineal healing is progressing and whether it is sufficient to allow pain-free love-making. Women can be helped to use knowledge of normal sexual function to monitor any changes that occur following surgery. This information can help patients and their partners work out ways of adapting their love-making to accommodate such changes. It can also be used to help women get the best help from sexual assessment and treatment.

PATIENT SCENARIO 5.3   Mrs Reid is talking to Jean Baker, a 48-year-old woman who had abdomino-perineal excision of her rectum for cancer 9 months previously. She is managing her colostomy well and has resumed most aspects of her normal working and social life. Jean and her partner Jo had reported some problems with sex at a previous appointment. At that assessment her surgeon was pleased with the way her body had healed and could find no physical cause for their difficulties. Mrs Reid had also spent some time then with Jean and Jo discussing the possibility that Jean may now take longer to respond to foreplay and achieve enough lubrication. They had agreed to give more time and attention to preliminary sexual activities and to try using KY jelly to give additional lubrication. Mrs Reid had also discussed ways in which Jean might help herself feel more feminine and desirable, such as using pretty bag covers or wearing a half-slip while making love to discreetly mask her bag. Although for some patients this is sufficient to enable them to deal with difficulties, Mrs Reid had sensed at that time that more substantial help might be needed. She had tentatively raised the possibility that Jean and Jo might benefit from seeing a psychosexual therapist who had training in both physical and psychological approaches, and they had gone home to think it over.

At this visit Mrs Reid learns that Jean has had some really helpful sessions with a psychosexual therapist recommended by her GP. Mrs Reid expresses her pleasure at this news, and asks Jean if she would be willing to tell her how the sessions have helped. Jean says she got both practical and emotional help. Firstly, the therapist helped both Jean and Jo use finger examination to discover the angle of Jean's vagina. They were then helped to discover how to position themselves so that Jo could enter Jean more easily in line with her current vaginal position. After a little practice they can now use a side to side position or Jo can use rear entry if Jean is supported by pillows. Jean says it felt a bit strange at first but now they are taking up these positions more naturally during love-making. Jean said the therapist had shown them diagrams to help them understand why these positions were likely to be more suitable, and that had helped them relax and feel more confident.

Jean also said the therapist had given them some exercises to help them discover what gave them most sexual pleasure and arousal, with instructions to tell each other at the time what they found enjoyable. This had helped them both gain confidence and skill so they were now getting and giving more pleasure from non-penetrative sex. Jean felt these practical measures were also building her self-esteem and sense of herself as a good lover. However, she had also benefited from the time spent with the therapist exploring her experience of having cancer, needing such body-changing surgery, and having to live with a permanent colostomy. She said she had not realised how much anger and grief she had been holding on to, and that she had needed to deal with her emotional state and lack of self-acceptance as well as the physical sexual discomfort she had been experiencing. As Jean thanks Mrs Reid for her interest and support she mentions that it was her suggestion that specialist help was available, and often useful in their kind of situation, which had given them the courage to seek it out. Mrs Reid has also benefited from Jean's description of the specific help she gained as this information is giving her ideas as to how she could further develop her own practice.

Notice in the above *scenario* that Mrs Reid had used the expertise she does have to start Jean and Jo along the road to getting the level of help they subsequently turned out to need. Her initial help was important as it enabled them to discover sexual issues were an acceptable topic to raise, would be taken seriously, and that they did have the capability to discuss them and try out some of the strategies suggested. This gave them sufficient confidence to consider her next suggestion (i.e. what was important was that they got sufficient help to meet their needs, and that it was acceptable for them to

consider other sources of help besides herself) and act on it. The feedback Jean gave her shows that the value of this kind of preparation and support was recognised. It is typical of that expressed by many patients receiving this kind of initial help.

Careful consideration must be given to the needs of patients undergoing *pelvic exenteration* (see Ch. 3). The overall physical effects of removal of all the pelvic organs are considerable. Patients may report feeling drained of physical and emotional energy for months. Incorporating management of a colostomy and urostomy into their life is more daunting and time-consuming than coping with one stoma. Coming to terms with having such extensive cancer that it necessitates this radical surgery is also difficult.

Patients must recover well physically from their exenteration before further treatment is considered. Therefore there can be sizeable delays before patients reach a position where they can establish what alterations in their body image and function they will ultimately have to accommodate. For example, men may later be offered penile implants, or other help normally offered to men having cystectomy (see Ch. 6). Women may undergo construction of an artificial vagina (Blackley 1986, McCartney 1986).

The approaches described earlier to help patients manage uncertainty and raise their confidence and self-esteem through general rehabilitation are also useful for these patients. Specialist help may be needed by some individuals.

Contraception

Abdomino-perineal excision of rectum does not always make men sterile. Contraceptive precautions to avoid pregnancy should therefore be continued. Taylor (2003, p 188) reported that some men who have undergone rectal excision find using a sheath unacceptable as it reduces sensation which may already be impaired due to nerve damage during surgery. However, since the advent of AIDS and HIV the importance of practising safer sex must also be considered.

Many women undergoing radical rectal surgery for cancer are postmenopausal, but premenopausal women will need to use contraceptive measures if they wish to avoid pregnancy. This should be discussed with their surgeon, so that the nature and extent of their surgery can be taken into consideration. The proximity of the surgical field to the vagina, and any alterations to the vagina from scarring or repositioning, may mean women are advised not to use an intrauterine device. The contraceptive pill can be used (unless medically contraindicated) as the absence of the resected colon will not reduce its absorption and effectiveness.

Pregnancy

The presence of a colostomy is not in itself a contraindication for women becoming pregnant. Women should discuss the extent of their particular operation with their surgeon before beginning a pregnancy so that their decision to conceive can take account of any possible problems that could arise. For example, vaginal shortening and/or vaginal or perineal scarring could affect whether vaginal delivery can be achieved. Many patients have had successful pregnancies: what is important is to help patients and their partners clarify what is possible and desirable in their particular circumstances.

Alterations in bowel function as well as stoma position can occur. Monitoring of these as pregnancy advances will enable problems to be identified, and revisions of stomal equipment and management to be made where necessary (Blackley 2004, p 223–224).

URINARY PROBLEMS

Patients should be asked about their urinary function as an integral part of postoperative monitoring. Hopefully, current nerve-sparing operations will reduce the numbers of patients having problems. However, damage to the sympathetic nerves in the hypogastric plexus can cause problems in bladder emptying (Northover et al 2002, p 54). Enquiries should be made sensitively. Patients have already undergone surgery that has created major alterations in their body image and bowel function. Understandably, some patients may have difficulty in acknowledging they could, or do, now have urinary problems.

Patients who report urinary problems are often told that it will take some months for bruised or oedematous tissues within the area of operation to regain their normal size and function. Urinary problems often resolve as tissues recover. An initial strategy of 'wait and see' before embarking on more medical interventions is reasonable. However, patients have to deal with their problems during this period and should be given help to do so. The

team should discuss who will provide such help and what it should entail so that individual patients' requirements are addressed.

It is not always possible to identify which patients will continue to have problems. Pringle & Swan (2001) reported that 11.5% of patients in their study had urinary incontinence one year after their bowel surgery. It is therefore important that patients develop management strategies that can be used long term without creating further problems. Some patients try to minimise problems by curtailing their fluid intake and social activities. These strategies should be discouraged as they can turn into lifestyle patterns which affect urinary function and their level of rehabilitation. Instead we can help patients to plan ways of achieving an adequate fluid intake and understand that this aids the overall function of their urinary system (e.g. patient handouts in Appendix 16.1).

Referral to a continence adviser is sometimes not suggested until problems are deemed to be 'permanent'. However, they can also suggest ways in which patients could manage temporary difficulties, giving them more confidence and ability to engage in their normal activities and thus continue to rehabilitate. Discussing patients' situations informally with a continence adviser can be useful. It enables us to clarify whether we can use their advice to help particular patients or whether a direct referral would be more appropriate.

Some patients find it difficult to cope with the sense of uncertainty which may arise from waiting to see whether urinary problems resolve. We can use the approaches to help patients handle uncertainty over time which were described earlier ('Management of uncertainty over time')

Problems may persist if there has been nerve damage, or if the bladder flops back (due to absence of the rectum) when urethral kinking may also occur. In these circumstances urine may be less easily eliminated: residual urine can collect and become infected. Patients may therefore require referral to a urologist and continence adviser for investigations (e.g. cystogram, ultrasound) and treatment (e.g. learning self-catheterisation).

CONCLUSION

Most qualified nurses who have some experience of stoma care, and easy access to support from colleagues with more extensive expertise, can provide much of the practical care described in this chapter. In contrast, the information and approaches for handling sexual concerns require staff to have much more advanced knowledge and skills.

A useful intermediate stage is acquiring a broader understanding of the issues involved in providing sexuality-related information and care. This enables us to respond to patients' preliminary expressions of a need for help in more sensitive, informed ways *and* be more aware of the kind of expertise we are looking for in colleagues to whom we might refer them. It is impossible to forecast when individual patients will raise these kinds of concerns but they often put out subtle 'feelers' or comments to see if it is acceptable to voice concerns at different times as they go through surgery and rehabilitation. The information and help described here is also relevant when helping patients prepare for discharge (Ch. 8) and when supporting their ongoing rehabilitation (Ch. 9).

References

Black P 1992 Body image after enterostomal surgery. MSc Thesis, RCN Steinberg Collection, London

Black P K 2000 Holistic stoma care. Baillière Tindall & RCN, Edinburgh

Blackley P 1986 Female options – repercussions of construction of neo vagina. In: World Council of Enterostomal Therapists congress proceedings. Abbott International & Hollister, USA, p 51–53

Blackley P 2004 Practical stoma wound and continence management, 2nd edn. Research Publications Pty, Vermont, Victoria, Australia

Bobb K A, Liles L 2003 A question of choice. Presentation at Living with a Stoma research conference, 30 September, Knebworth Park, Hertfordshire

Borwell B 1997 Developing sexual helping skills. Medical Projects International, Maidenhead

Coates R 1986 Urological/sexual problems. In: World Council of Enterostomal Therapists congress proceedings. Abbott International and Hollister, USA, p 83–85

De Luca V, Pescatori E S, Taher B et al 1996 Damage to the erectile function following radical pelvic surgery: prevalence of veno-occlusive dysfunction. European Urology 29(1):36–40

Derry F A, Dinsmore W W, Fraser M et al 1999 Efficacy and safety of oral sildenafil (Viagra) in men with erectile dysfunction caused by spinal cord injury. Neurology 51(6):1629–1633

Fillingham S 2004 Penile disorders. In: Fillingham S, Douglas J Urological nursing, 3rd edn. Churchill Livingstone, Edinburgh, p 224–227

Fumi L, Berntsson R N, Aberg K, Hulten L 1996 Water and electrolyte losses in ileostomy patients: evaluation of a new oral rehydration solution. In: World Council of Enterostomal Therapists congress proceedings. Hollister, Libertyville, IL, p 105–107

Herbert R A 1996 Reproduction. In: Hinchliff S M, Montague S E, Watson R Physiology for nursing practice, 2nd edn. Baillière Tindall, London, p 679–734

Huish M, Kumar D, Stones C 1998. Stoma surgery and sexual problems in ostomates. Sexual and Marital Therapy 13(3):311–328

Israel M 1998 Viagra: the first oral treatment for impotence. Pharmaceutical Journal 26(1):164–165

Keighley M R B 2002 Ostomy management. In: Zuidema G D, Yeo C J (eds) Shackelford's surgery of the alimentary tract; volume IV: colon. W B Saunders, Philadelphia, p 305–331

McArdle C 2001 Primary treatment-does the surgeon matter? In: Kerr D J, Young A M, Hobbs F D R (eds) ABC of colorectal cancer. BMJ Books, London, p 19–21

McCartney A J 1986 Pelvic exenteration for gynaecological cancer. In: World Council of Enterostomal Therapists congress proceedings. Abbott International and Hollister, USA, p 44–51

Meadows C 1997 Stoma and fistula care. In: Bruce L, Finlay T M D (eds) Nursing in gastroenterology. Churchill Livingstone, New York

Nicholls R J 1996 Surgical procedures. In: Myers C (ed) Stoma care nursing. Arnold, London, p 90–122

Nicholls R J, Williams J 2002 The ileo-anal pouch. In: Williams J (ed) The essentials of pouch care nursing. Whurr Publishers, London, p 68–98

Northover J, Taylor C, Gold D 2002 Carcinoma of the rectum. In: Williams J (ed) The essentials of pouch care nursing. Whurr Publishers, London, p 43–67

Penman J 1998 Action research in the care of patients with sexual anxieties. Nursing Standard 13(13–15):47–50

Preston J 1994 A perspective on the physical and psychological implications of odour for the ostomist. In: World Council of Enterostomal Therapists congress proceedings. Hollister, Libertyville, IL, p 245–247

Pringle W, Swan E 2001 Continuing care after discharge from hospital for stoma patients. British Journal of Nursing 10(19):1274–1288

Rosen R C, Riley A, Wagner G et al 1997 The international index of erectile dysfunction (IIEF): a multidimensional scale for assessment of erectile dysfunction. Urology 49(6):822–830

Salter M 1996 Sexuality and the stoma patient. In: Myers C (ed) Stoma care nursing. Arnold, London, p 203–219

Salter M 2002 Sexual aspects of internal pouch surgery. In: Williams J (ed) The essentials of pouch care nursing. Whurr Publishers, London, p 180–198

Schulte A 1994 Disturbances of sexual function after rectal amputation, and possible therapeutic measures. In: World Council of Enterostomal Therapists congress proceedings. Hollister, Libertyville, IL, p 172–174

Taylor P 2003 Other considerations in stoma care In: Elcoat C Stoma care nursing, 2nd edn. Hollister, Wokingham, UK

Topping A 1990 Sexual activity and the stoma patient. Nursing Standard 4(41):24–26

Wade B 1989 A stoma is for life. Royal College of Nursing, London

Webb V, Holmes A 1999 Assessment and management of erectile dysfunction. Nursing Times 95(2):48–49

Williams J, Nicholls R J 2002 Controversies and problem-solving with regard to ileo-anal pouches. In: Williams J (ed) The essentials of pouch care nursing. Whurr Publishers, London, p 143–164

Zippe C D, Kedia K, Nelson D R, Agarwal A 1998 Treatment of erectile dysfunction after radical prostatectomy with sildenafil citrate (Viagra). Urology 52(6):963–966

Chapter 6

Care of patients with urinary stomas

Sharon Fillingham

Despite the development of a variety of new reconstructive procedures the majority of adults undergoing urinary diversion will require the formation of a traditional incontinent stoma. Internal (continent) urinary pouches are less widely available and require specialist surgeons' expertise/experience. The selection criteria are usually more rigid and multiple admissions are often necessary.

INDICATIONS FOR URINARY DIVERSION

CANCER

Bladder cancer is the most common reason for undergoing urinary diversion. Surgery can involve radical pelvic clearance which is undertaken both as a curative and as a palliative procedure (Blackley 2004).

UNMANAGEABLE INCONTINENCE

Some patients with severe incontinence, neuropathic bladder or interstitial cystitis may choose urostomy surgery in preference to other alternatives now available (see Ch. 12) or may not meet the selection criteria for such systems. However, children with congenital abnormalities such as spina bifida and bladder exstrophy now rarely have stoma formation suggested as the best system for managing their urinary problems, although occasionally it is necessary to convert their original continent diversion to a stoma in later life.

URINARY FISTULA

Trauma causing urinary fistulas may necessitate a temporary urostomy to allow healing to occur, or a permanent urostomy to be formed where damage is beyond repair.

TYPES OF URINARY DIVERSION

ILEAL CONDUIT

This is the most common form of urinary diversion, and was described by Bricker in 1950. A 15–25 cm section of terminal ileum with a good blood supply is isolated from the rest of the bowel in order to create a conduit or tube through which urine can leave the body. The remaining ends of ileum are reanastomosed in order to restore gastrointestinal continuity. Care is taken to preserve the conduit's future blood supply as well as that of the rest of the bowel.

The proximal end of the isolated bowel segment is closed and the ureters, once resected from the bladder, are implanted and sutured into the isolated loop. The style of anastomoses used varies in accordance with the surgeon's preference, e.g. Wallace I (Wallace 1970; Fig. 6.1). The distal end is brought out through a premarked site on the abdominal wall and then everted to form a spout (Brooke 1952). Ideally the spout should be 1.5–2.5 cm long so it projects sufficiently to enable urine to flow into the appliance rather than pool around the stoma.

Ureters are only about 6 mm in diameter so the patency of their anastomoses to the conduit is temporarily protected by using fine bore catheters, or ureteric stents. These are passed along the ureters (from above where they are implanted into the conduit), through the uretero-ileal anastomosis, and along the conduit to exit via the stomal opening.

COLONIC CONDUIT

Conduit creation from either transverse or sigmoid colon is now rare. Unlike ileal conduits they are usually sited on the left side of the abdomen and are generally much larger in circumference. Mucus formation is greater and stomal colour is darker in the sigmoid colon where blood perfusion is poorer.

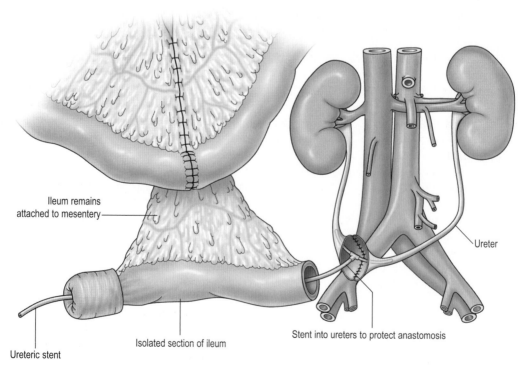

Ileum remains attached to mesentery

Ureteric stent

Isolated section of ileum

Ureter

Stent into ureters to protect anastomosis

Figure 6.1   Formation of an ileal conduit.

CONVERSION OF CONTINENT DIVERSION TO CONVENTIONAL UROSTOMY

In recent years some patients have undergone conversion of the continent pouch to an 'incontinent urostomy'. Reasons for this are multifaceted and the surgical decision is never taken lightly either by surgeons or by patients. Often the surgeon's first action is to use the existing 'continent pouch' (see Ch. 12) and bring it to the surface as an 'incontinent stoma'. The advantage of this is that the procedure itself is simpler but the disadvantage is that the resulting stoma formed is often flush to the skin, which can make maintenance of intact skin and a leak-proof seal more difficult to achieve.

CUTANEOUS URETEROSTOMIES

In this procedure one or both ureters are brought to the surface of the skin rather than implanting them into a conduit. They may be single, bilateral or double-barrelled stomas, but are rarely created now (Fillingham & Fell 2004). They can be a useful temporary or palliative measure, for example if there are difficulties maintaining patients' homeostasis in emergency situations or if patients' general condition precludes more extensive surgery.

Benefits of ureterostomy diversion are that there is no excessive mucus production or electrolyte absorption as can occur in bowel conduits. Unfortunately there are often difficulties with ureterostomies because their flushness to the skin creates difficulties in maintaining a leak-proof appliance and also because these small, often slightly retracted stomas are prone to stenosis.

OTHER UROSTOMIES

Patients may present (usually in the outpatient department) with established urostomies which have been formed using other methods. These include cutaneous vesicostomy, cutaneous pyeloplasty, jejunal ureterostomy (Fillingham & Fell 2004). These are now uncommon, and are also generally managed by an external drainable urinary device.

PREOPERATIVE CARE

General information and care needed to help all patients prepare for, and rehabilitate after, stoma surgery is primarily discussed in Chapters 1, 3–5, 19 and 20. Additionally, many practical aspects of bowel stoma care covered in Chapters 4 and 5 are also relevant in urostomy care. All these chapters should be used in conjunction with this one to plan, provide and evaluate care. Specific aspects of care required because the diversion is a urinary one are covered in this chapter.

Formation of a urostomy is considered major surgery and the general preoperative care and investigations will reflect this. In particular, urinary diversion as part of radical cystourethroprostatectomy (removal of bladder, prostate and urethra) is an extensive and often debilitating procedure. It is therefore essential to (a) identify whether patients are fit for surgery and (b) prepare them both physiologically and psychologically.

Assessment of the whole urinary system and its level of functioning includes:

- baseline measurements of urea and electrolytes through haematological investigations
- urinary sample examination for evidence of malignancy (cytology) and infection (culture and sensitivity)
- radiological examination through ultrasound of the kidneys and bladder; intravenous urogram; and computerised tomography (CT scan)
- glomerular filtration to assess creatinine clearance and renal function.

BOWEL PREPARATION

Gastrointestinal clearance is necessary to minimise problems when resecting the bowel segment for conduit formation and reanastomosing the remaining bowel. Preparation varies according to local policy but usually involves the ingestion of several doses of an effective purgative laxative, e.g. sodium picosulfate. Care must be taken to maintain hydration prior to surgery and intravenous fluids are sometimes necessary.

SKIN PATCH TESTING

Patients who have skin problems or a sensitive skin which might react to stomal equipment should be patch tested before surgery (see Ch. 4). Urine will drain as soon as the stoma is formed and therefore it is essential for theatre staff to know which appliance(s) will provide skin protection and adhesion without allergic reaction and blistering so these can be immediately fitted.

SITING A UROSTOMY

All patients should see a stoma care nurse prior to surgery. Urostomy formation is usually an elective procedure, thus allowing adequate time for planned siting.

A site chosen should be within the rectus abdominis muscle as the stoma is secured to the rectus sheath to minimise the possibility of retraction due to peristaltic movement. Ideally ileal conduits are sited on the right side below the level of the umbilicus. It is essential that an area of at least 5 cm² is available that is free of scar tissue and uneven contours to provide an adequate surface area for appliance adhesion.

Consideration is given to left-sided siting if this surface area cannot be achieved on the right side of the abdomen. Some patients engage in activities that could affect or be affected by a right-sided stoma (e.g. if a golf swing knocks against an appliance there is the potential to dislodge it). It can also be useful to enquire whether a night drainage system connected to the stoma bag might be affected because of the position in a double bed in which the patient has to sleep (e.g. partner has to sleep on patient's right to shield their right arthritic shoulder). This question often prompts patients to divulge concerns about their acceptability as a sexual partner, so it can be a useful lead into further discussion. Stoma siting is discussed in detail in Chapter 4.

POSTOPERATIVE CARE

The general postoperative care of patients who have undergone formation of a urostomy is consistent with other stomal surgery (see Chs 4 and 5). Specific care is centred around urine colour, volume and mode of output.

Colour

Initially moderate haematuria is expected. Urine should gradually become clearer. Heavy or persistent haematuria may indicate bleeding from any point within the urinary system and should be reported and investigated.

Volume

Unlike gastrointestinal stomas the output from a urinary stoma is immediate. This should not fall below 30 ml per hour but will obviously depend on the overall fluid balance.

Mode of output and ureteric stents

The ureteric stents (see earlier) maintain the patency of the new system until primary healing has taken place. Stents should be checked regularly in the early postoperative period. Clear appliances should be chosen to allow both the stoma and stents to be viewed easily (see below). It is important to observe drainage is occurring from both stents (and thus both left and right urinary pathways). Most surgeons identify the left from the right stent in some manner, e.g. by cutting one end straight, the other obliquely. Occasionally, if urinary drainage is absent from either stent, flushing may be necessary. This should be undertaken very gently using approximately 1 ml of saline to dislodge any mucus deposits blocking the stent. This is an aseptic procedure and should only be carried out after consultation with the surgeon or stoma care nurse. The procedure will vary depending on the type of stent used.

Stent removal varies from 7 to 10 days (longer if previous radiotherapy has taken place). Pressure should not be exerted on the stents but removal is often preceded by the stents falling out spontaneously. At the time of removal it is important to explain to patients that this procedure is not usually painful and, if resistance is felt, the stents will be left a further day and the process repeated.

APPLIANCE SELECTION

In the early postoperative period the stoma and ureteric stents need to be visible and easily accessible. This allows monitoring of their condition and urinary output to take place. Two-piece equipment with a clear pouch and a 'floating flange' is useful because the pouch can be easily reattached to the flange after monitoring without pressing on the patient's abdomen.

The pouch should have an integral non-return inner section which prevents collection of urine in the upper half of the pouch. This minimises pooling of urine around the stoma and thus helps preserve

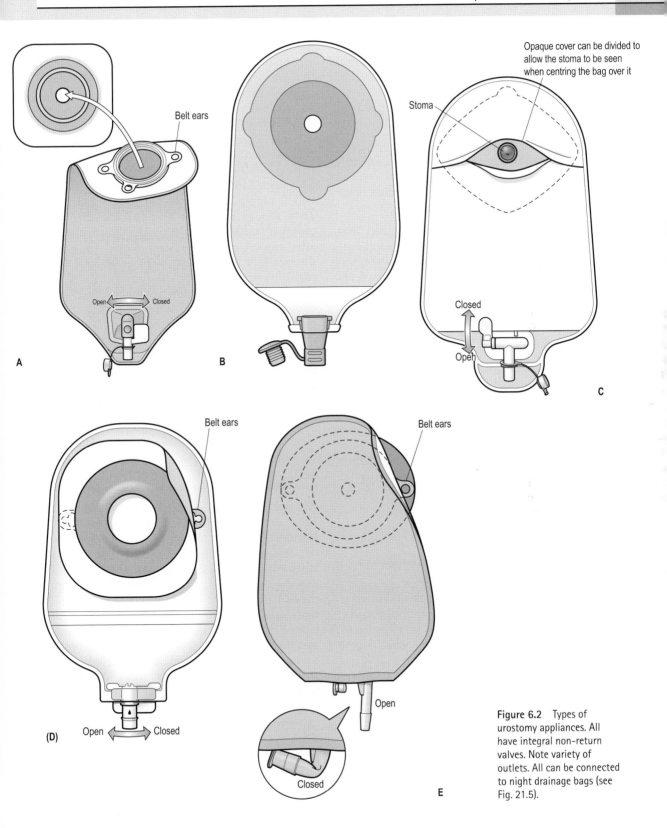

Belt ears

Open ⟷ **Closed**

A

B

Opaque cover can be divided to
allow the stoma to be seen
when centring the bag over it

Stoma

Closed

Open

C

Belt ears

Open ⟷ **Closed**

(D)

Belt ears

Open

Closed

E

Figure 6.2 Types of
urostomy appliances. All
have integral non-return
valves. Note variety of
outlets. All can be connected
to night drainage bags (see
Fig. 21.5).

the skin protective hydrocolloid and an intact bond with the skin. Urostomy pouches require an integral drainable tap which, if required, can be attached to a night drainage bag (see Figs 6.2 and 21.5).

Individual patient assessment is essential to help patients choose suitable equipment for their own use. Factors to consider include:

- manual dexterity
- vision
- mobility/mobility aids, e.g. wheelchair, body brace
- stature.

Consideration must be given to the fact that urostomies are constantly active and it is undesirable for patients to avoid drinking in an attempt to reduce urinary output. However, many patients find that if they routinely change equipment first thing in the morning before drinking any fluids, their output is likely to be lower than at other times of the day and this makes changing equipment easier.

Choosing equipment for ureterostomies can be particularly difficult because they are flush with the skin and so urine pools around the stoma instead of flowing down into the bag. Breakdown of skin protectives can be more rapid because the pooled urine is in contact with them, thus reducing wear time of equipment. A convex appliance, which moulds closely to the patient's contours, is useful when dealing with this situation (see also section on retraction in Ch. 21).

NIGHT DRAINAGE SYSTEMS

The greatest advantage of the night drainage system is that it enables patients to have an undisturbed night's sleep without the worry of emptying the appliance frequently. Most pouches can only contain up to 350 ml before emptying is essential. Night drainage systems have a capacity of up to 2000 ml. These days most manufacturers provide a specific night drainage system to accompany their range of appliances. Alternative high volume drainage systems can be interchanged with the use of an adapter if patients have specific needs. For example, if individuals require a particular style of connection or outlet because of reduced dexterity.

Patients need to acquire the ability to recognise when their stoma bag requires emptying without having to undress and look at it. As they mobilise they should disconnect their stoma bag from the night bag except when sleeping. This enables them to learn what the weight and bulk of their stoma bag feels like when it requires emptying, increasing the competence and confidence with which they will function.

Some hospitals use cheaper non-drainable night bags. These can be discarded daily, minimising any risk of infection through reconnection of stomal and night drainage equipment. However, patients will be supplied with drainable night bags at home. They should be taught how to look after these reusable systems before discharge. Each morning, after emptying it, the system should be washed through thoroughly using warm water and stored carefully, preventing the attachment tubing from trailing on the floor. Staining, mucus build-up or odour is an indication that a new appliance is required but, generally, use should be no longer than 2 weeks. Whilst in hospital use of a night drainage stand is essential (see Fig. 21.4). In the community many patients do not use a stand, preferring instead to lay the bag on a tray or in a plastic bag as they feel better drainage occurs this way. Some patients feel restricted when connected to night drainage systems and prefer not to use them.

SKIN PROTECTION

The first principle of protection is to defend the skin from attack by urine. Suitable products can be identified by patch testing. Disposable appliances are designed to be applied directly onto the skin surface by means of adhesion and, if at all possible, this should be maintained without additional products. Urine, due to its liquidity, has the ability to undermine even the strongest adhesive or hydrocolloid, particularly in the presence of skin creases and dips (which give less than flat body contours for equipment application), and retracted or flush stomas. Under these circumstances additional protection may be needed. Skin gel or films are useful in providing a barrier between the skin and the excoriating effect of urine. The creation of a watertight seal can be enhanced with the use of flexible hydrocolloid rings which can be easily moulded. Hydrocolloid or karaya pastes are extremely useful as they are easily moulded and provide additional adhesion for the primary appliance. Convex equipment and/or the use of supportive belts may become necessary for the patient to receive adequate wear time from the urostomy appliance. Ideally wear time should be at least 3 days. Some patients may require a combination of products to eliminate problems. Access to a knowledgeable stoma care nurse is important so patients can consider a range of products, and be shown how best to use them to manage their situation most effectively (see also Chs 4 and 21).

ODOUR AND COLOUR CHANGES

Patients need to be warned of changes that may occur with the use of certain medications and food products. Normal urine does have an aroma which is accentuated when smelt and observed in close proximity in the urostomy pouch. Whilst this smell is not usually as profound as with gastrointestinal stomas, many urostomists find their urine to be both offensive and a cause of anxiety. It is therefore important that staff are knowledgeable about these various effects of ingested products. For example, Watson (1987) reports changes from the following drugs and foods.

Drugs

Ferrous salts: turn urine black on standing
Metronidazole: initially red then turns brown
Senna: yellow brown in acid urine; yellow pink in alkaline urine
Sulphonamides: greenish blue
Antibiotics: strong offensive smell.

Foods

Oily fish: strong fishy smell often mistaken for infected urine
Beetroot: pink to dark red (depending on amount eaten)
Asparagus: cloudy urine, offensive smell
Herbs and spices: original smell passes through into urine.

URINE INFECTIONS

One of the major causes of colour or odour change is infected urine. Even before becoming symptomatic (e.g. pyrexial, loin pain, shivers/rigors, vomiting) patients may notice that their urine has become cloudy and thick with an offensive odour which is described as 'fishy' or 'ammonia-like'. Obtaining a urine sample for culture and sensitivity should be undertaken using an aseptic technique.

> **PATIENT SCENARIO 6.1**   Mrs Anne Smith is a 48-year-old woman who has had surgery for long-term incontinence. She has been complaining of feeling unwell and feverish with foul-smelling cloudy urine. Nurse Jones was asked to take a urine sample and prepared her equipment in accordance with the local policy for obtaining urine specimens from urostomies. Mrs Smith's anxiety was relieved as Nurse Jones carefully explained the procedure to her and assured her it would not be painful (her main concern).
>
> The procedure was carried out using an aseptic technique. Nurse Jones cleaned around the stomal area using normal saline. A disposable catheter (12 fg size) was inserted into the stoma to the depth of between 2.5 cm and 5 cm. Mrs Smith had been drinking plenty of fluids and therefore urine flowed readily into the sterile container. A sample volume of between 3 ml and 5 ml is required for culture. Once this amount had been obtained, Nurse Jones removed the catheter. She then applied a new urostomy appliance before disposing of the used equipment in accordance with local policy. The sample was correctly labelled and sent to the microbiology department. Mrs Smith's doctor then prescribed broad spectrum antibiotics, which would be reviewed once culture and sensitivity results had been received.

Bacterial breakdown in urine changes the pH from 6 to 7.5 (slightly acid-based), to an alkaline medium, pH 7–8, which is an ideal medium for bacterial and fungal growth. The excoriating effect of alkaline urine on the skin can be rapid. Alkaline urine can produce oxalate crystals which are often responsible for stomal bleeding and ulceration. Various treatments have proved effective in restoring the acidity to urine and to the surrounding skin area, including those described in the following paragraphs.

Acetic acid

Five per cent acetic acid (household vinegar) can be introduced into a small activity pouch or other small container and allowed to wash over the stomal area for approximately 30 minutes. This should be done at least twice a day and therefore the use of a two-piece appliance is indicated.

Gel preparations

Aci-Jel, which contains acetic acid 0.92% in a buffered base jelly (pH 4), is commonly used for gynaecological/vaginal conditions and has proved effective. It should be applied directly to the stomal mucosa at least twice daily, Patients often prefer this method, as it is less messy and time-consuming.

Ascorbic acid

Earlier studies indicated that high doses (4–12 g daily) of ascorbic acid (vitamin C) are required to produce acidification of urine (Young 1984). However, ongoing research into the effects of ascorbic acid may lead to revisions to the dosage that it is thought appropriate to prescribe. The total daily dose should be taken in smaller amounts over the 24-hour period, and is normally prescribed for no longer than 6 weeks. Advice from a pharmacist should be sought before commencing treatment as ascorbic acid may have an adverse effect on other medications (Young 1984). Patients should be monitored for any side effects, particularly gastrointestinal disturbances (Levine et al 1999).

Hippuric acid

The best-known source of hippuric acid is the cranberry. The North American wetland fruit has been intensively studied since 1933 when Fellers and others identified the bacteriostatic effect produced after metabolic breakdown on the urinary pH.

Mucus build-up in the urinary conduit provides an ideal medium for the colonisation of *Escherichia coli*. As a natural inhabitant of the gastrointestinal system and therefore of the conduit segment, *E. coli* is present in the culture of stomal urine. It is only when present in large numbers that patients become symptomatic and require treatment with antibiotics. The doses of hippuric acid required to reduce mucus production have been extensively argued (Rosenbaum et al 1989). Many patients find that 200 ml of cranberry juice twice a day, or a 100 mg capsule once daily, can be effective (Busuttil-Leaver 1996).

Recent reports advise that cranberry products should be avoided or limited when warfarin is prescribed (Committee on Safety of Medicines 2003, Suvarna et al 2003).

SEXUAL FUNCTION AFTER STOMA SURGERY

The formation of a stoma will undoubtedly have a profound effect on both the physiological and psychological wellbeing of the individual. It is important that as healthcare professionals we consider the general and specific changes undergone as a result of this surgery. Zolar (1982) suggested that nurses are ideal team members to counsel patients regarding sexual matters but it is essential that this is conducted with knowledge, expertise and a high degree of sensitivity. Knowledge of normal sexual function (reviewed by Fillingham 2004, Herbert 1996) is an essential prerequisite to understanding dysfunction and possible treatments.

UNDERLYING PATHOLOGY

Physical problems can arise both generally or locally and their nature will depend on the type and extent of the operation as a whole rather than stoma formation only (see also Chs 3, 5). Radical pelvic surgery creates difficulties in sexual function and response in men and women. This includes:

- *nerve damage* – of the superficial and deep nerves
- *vascular damage* – affecting engorgement and lubrication
- *tissue damage* – causing tenderness, reduced space and increased likelihood of prolapse.

MALES

Pelvic nerve damage to the sympathetic and parasympathetic nerves, particularly after cystourethrectomy, will undoubtedly result in erectile difficulties:

- damage to blood vessels reduces the blood supply to the corpus cavernosum and therefore tumescence cannot be maintained
- ejaculation is affected because of surgical damage to the sphincter at the base of the bladder
- sexual desire and orgasm often remain intact due to the circulating testosterone levels.

Research has shown that it is extremely important to counsel the patient and partner together regarding why their erectile dysfunction has occurred and also to explore the alternatives to penetrative sex (Lloyd et al 1988). After cystectomy men may be able to induce orgasm without erection during masturbation. Initially this may be regarded by the couple as an unnatural phenomenon and therefore unacceptable or even harmful. Gaining understanding that there is a sensoric and psychogenic component to the orgasmic process may give permission to the couple to accept and enjoy it and thus alleviate stress.

Erectile failure

Erectile dysfunction or failure is defined as the inability to sustain an erection sufficiently rigid to allow sexual intercourse to take place. The physiology of erection is a complex mechanism. Radical surgery causes damage to the parasympathetic nerve pathway and therefore vasodilation of the arterioles of the penis will not occur. The cavernous tissue will fail to engorge and the penis remains flaccid.

Treatment for erectile failure includes:

- vacuum therapy
- injection therapy
- intra-urethral vasodilating medication
- penile implants
- oral medication.

Vacuum pump

This consists of a cylinder, pump and constriction rings. The flaccid penis which has been previously lubricated with gel is placed inside the cylinder (Fig 6.3). The pump, either hand or battery operated, is activated and creates negative pressure. This action achieves vascular engorgement by 'pulling' blood into the penis. To maintain the erection the constriction ring is slipped from the cylinder onto the base of the penis and intercourse can take place. The constriction ring should be removed after 30 minutes to prevent any complications.

The benefits of the vacuum pump are that it will not interfere with other treatments, it may be used only when desired, can improve natural erections in some cases and claims over a 90% success rate. This form of treatment mostly benefits those couples in a stable relationship or individuals who could not contemplate further invasive surgery or self-injection therapy.

Injection therapy

Self-injection treatment is often favoured by single men as a satisfactory and less obtrusive method of overcoming their erectile dysfunction. A vasoactive drug (e.g. prostaglandin E1 (alprostadil), or moxisylyte hydrochloride) is injected into the

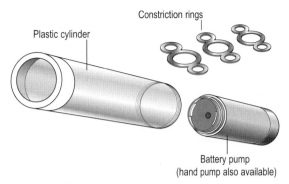

Figure 6.3 Vacuum pump.

corpus cavernosum with a fine gauge needle. Doses are titrated according to the individual's needs but ideally the erection should last about one hour. The drugs are dispensed in a single use pack. The effect of the drug is to cause relaxation of arterial and trabecular smooth muscle. The cavernous arteries dilate and the corpus cavernosum relaxes and engorgement with blood occurs. The benefits of injection therapy for many men/couples is that it is relatively less obtrusive than other methods of gaining an erection, normal body temperature is maintained and a greater degree of rigidity can be achieved.

Patients should be given written instructions which should include:

- dosage to be used per injection
- frequency with which it can be used
- method of storage
- how to recognise when medical help is required
- how and where to obtain immediate medical advice and treatment, including an emergency telephone number to contact.

It is important that men both understand and are willing to comply with these instructions as inappropriate use can have serious consequences (Gray 1992).

Priapism   A prolonged erection (i.e. over 4 hours) is a medical emergency and if this occurs men must obtain medical treatment as a matter of urgency. Prompt treatment is crucial to prevent necrosis or irreparable scarring of the cavernosal tissue. Specialised hospital treatment is likely be required, particularly if initial measures to relieve the erection are unsuccessful and a penile prosthesis may need to be considered.

Intra–urethral vasodilating medication

MUSE (medicated urethral system of erection) is a sterile single-use transurethral system for the delivery of alprostadil, contained in a tiny pellet, into the male urethra. As with injection therapy, the absorbed alprostadil causes vasodilation of blood vessels in the erectile tissues of the corpus cavernosum and an increase in cavernosal artery blood flow, resulting in the penis becoming rigid. Patients should receive written instructions similar to those given for injection therapy.

Penile implants

Stoma patients often regard implants as the last choice of treatment for their erectile difficulties. This is due to the invasive nature of the surgery and the fact that they have previously undergone extensive surgical procedures. Implant types are described as malleable or inflatable.

Malleable implants (Fig. 6.4)   These enable men to have an erection suitable for intercourse by bending their prosthesis (which has been implanted into their corpus cavernosum) so that it can be suitably positioned for sex and subsequently bent back into a comfortable position for concealment.

Preoperative treatment is concerned with reducing the possibility of postoperative infection and therefore prophylactic antibiotics are given routinely.

Inflatable implants   Cosmetically, inflatable penile implants are far easier to adjust to than malleable implants. Flaccidity is maintained when an erection is not desirable and patients often find this more acceptable than concealment. The implants, which are placed into the cavernosal tissue, are hollow. Fluid from a reservoir in the abdomen is transferred to the implant by using a pump inserted into the

scrotum. When fluid enters the implant, rigidity occurs and is sustained for intercourse to take place. To return the fluid to the reservoir the release bar on the pump is pressed and the penis returns to its flaccid state (Fillingham 2004).

There is an increased risk of infection with this surgical procedure. Additionally, individual choice may be restricted due to the high cost and the need for more extensive surgery with the inflatable prosthesis.

Oral medication

Sildenafil, vardenafil and tadalafil are oral therapies for erectile dysfunction. In order to be effective sexual stimulation is required. Whilst enhancing the smooth muscle relaxant affects of nitric oxide their main effect is to inhibit the release of phosphodiesterase type 5 (PDE5), which is the initiating chemical for causing detumescence (see also Ch. 5; Moreland et al 1998). Further research is required to identify the efficacy of these drugs with patients who have had radical pelvic surgery as this group has been minimally investigated to date (Dinsmore 2004, Kalsi & Kell 2004, Rutherford & Duffy 1999).

FEMALES

When radical cystectomy is performed the bladder, urethra, ovaries, fallopian tubes, uterus and cervix are removed. Additionally, the anterior upper third of the vagina is often removed. After such extensive surgery it may take months before the full impact of the surgery is realised. By this time medical follow-up may be relatively infrequent. It can be useful to explicitly state to patients that it is often only when people are regaining their physical health and normal lifestyle some months after surgery that other concerns become important. Patients should be encouraged to raise issues with their stoma care nurse at later stages in their rehabilitation.

The blood vessel damage resulting from radical cystectomy can cause a reduction to the lubrication of the vagina, vaginal tightness, and occasionally adhesions across the vagina. The effect of this may lead to dyspareunia (painful intercourse) or vaginismus (spasm). Dyspareunia may be helped by suggesting a change from the missionary position and the use of additional lubrication, e.g. KY jelly (see Patient scenario 5.3 in Ch. 5). Vaginismus may result from physiological or psychological trauma. It is important to diagnose and treat the underlying cause. Referral to an experienced sex therapist who

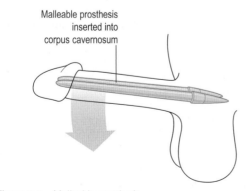

Malleable prosthesis inserted into corpus cavernosum

Figure 6.4   Malleable prosthesis.

will incorporate counselling, relaxation methods and the use of vaginal dilators in the treatment offered is valuable (Adler 1989, Biswas & Ratnam 1995).

FERTILITY AND PREGNANCY

Having a urinary stoma is not in itself a contraindication to fertility or to becoming pregnant, particularly if surgery was carried out because of congenital abnormalities or incontinence. Surgery for these conditions is usually less invasive and damaging to local nerve and blood supplies. For the male patient it may be necessary to consider sperm banking prior to surgery as, even if erectile function is regained, retrograde ejaculation may occur.

Women with urostomies have highlighted several factors regarding their pregnancies:

- Pregnancy testing – urine samples taken from the conduit have led to false negatives or false positives. This can occur if reabsorption of electrolytes and hormones has taken place, thus altering the concentration of human chorionic gonadotrophin.

- Ultrasound scan – the presence of ileal loop and ureters makes this difficult especially when attempting to assess parietal diameters.
- Urinary tract infection – pyelonephritis may induce premature labour and therefore any infections should be treated with antibiotics immediately.
- Hormone changes – as with urinary tract infection, the hormonal changes often give rise to leakage and management difficulties. Frequent changes of style of appliance and the use of subsidiary products may be necessary.

Although this chapter has specifically described care of patients who have a urinary stoma, several of the treatments related to sexual function can also be helpful for individuals who have undergone other radical pelvic surgery. Additionally, knowledgeable management entails providing a supportive environment as this is essential for both the physical and psychological wellbeing of patients (Jeffries et al 1995, Stott 2000). A wide range of supportive approaches to use with the material here when caring for people with urinary stomas are discussed in Chapters 1, 4–9, and 19–22.

References

Adler E 1989 Vaginismus – its presentation and treatment. British Journal of Sexual Medicine Nov: 420–424

Biswas A, Ratnam S S 1995 Vaginismus and outcome of treatment. Annals of the Academy of Medicine, Singapore 24(5):755–758

Blackley P 2004 Practical stoma wound and continence management, 2nd edn. Research Publications Pty, Vermont, Victoria, Australia

Bricker E M 1950 Bladder substitution after pelvic evisceration. Surgical Clinics of North America 30:1151

Brooke B N 1952 The management of an ileostomy including its complications. Lancet ii:102–104

Busuttil-Leaver R 1996 Cranberry juice. Professional Nurse 11:525–526

Committee on Safety of Medicines 2003 Possible interaction between warfarin and cranberry juice. Current Problems in Pharmacovigilance 29:8

Dinsmore W 2004 Treatment of erectile dysfunction. International Journal of STD and AIDS. 15(4):215–221

Fellers C R, Redmon B C, Parrott E M 1933 Effect of cranberries on urinary acidity and blood alkali reserve. Journal of Nutrition 6:455–463

Fillingham S, Fell S 2004 Urological stomas. In: Fillingham S, Douglas J Urological nursing, 3rd edn. Churchill Livingstone, Edinburgh, p 207–225

Fillingham S 2004 Penile disorders. In: Fillingham S, Douglas J Urological nursing, 3rd edn. Churchill Livingstone, Edinburgh, p 227–244

Gray M 1992 Genitourinary disorders. Mosby, St Louis, MO, p 258–274

Herbert R A 1996 Reproduction. In: Hinchliff S M, Montague S E, Watson R Physiology for nursing practice, 2nd edn. Baillière Tindall, London, p 679–734

Jeffries E, Butler M, Cullum R et al 1995 A service evaluation of stoma care nurses' practice. Journal of Clinical Nursing 4 (4):235–242

Kalsi J, Kell P 2004 Update on oral treatments for male erectile dysfunction. Journal of European Academy of Dermatology and Venereology 18(3):267–274

Levine M, Rumsey S C, Baruwala R et al 1999 Criteria and recommendations for vitamin C intake. Journal of the American Medical Association 281(15):1415–1423

Lloyd E E, Toth L L, Perkash I 1988 Vacuum tumescence: an option for spinal cord injured males with erectile dysfunction. Presented to the Association of Rehabilitation Nurses – Annual Conference, Las Vegas, NV, Abstract.

Moreland R B, Goldstein I, Traish A 1998 Sildenafil, a novel inhibitor of phosphodiesterase type 5 in human corpus cavernosum smooth muscle cells. Life Sciences 62:309–318

Rosenbaum T P, Shah P J R, Rose G A, Lloyd-Davis R W, 1989 Cranberry juice and the mucus production in entero-uroplasties. Neuro-Urology and Urodynamics 8(4): 55; 344–345

Rutherford D, Duffy F J 1999 Current treatment of impotence: Viagra and other options. British Journal of Nursing 8(4):235–241

Stott C A 2000 Management of patients with urinary diversions. In: World Council of Enterostomal Therapists congress proceedings. Hollister International, Libertyville, IL, p 22–26

Suvarna R, Pirmohamed M, Henderson L 2003 Possible interaction between warfarin and cranberry juice. British Medical Journal 327:1454

Wallace D M 1970 Uretero-ileostomy. British Journal of Urology 42:529–534

Watson D 1987 Drug therapy - colour changes to faeces and urine. Pharmaceutical Journal 236:68

Young C 1984 Ascorbic acid. Journal of Enterostomal Nursing 11:157–158

Zolar M K 1982 Role preparation for nurses. In: Human sexual functioning. Nursing Clinics of North America 17(3):351–363

SECTION 2

Promoting patient–centred goals

Chapter 7

Communicating effectively

Brigid Breckman

Each patient's circumstances, needs and rehabilitative goals are individual. Effective practice involves having both a commitment to tailor what we do, and how, to patients' particular needs *and* the skills to actually do so. This includes using communication skills specifically to promote patient-centred care.

In this chapter much of the focus is on:

- principles of communication that enable us to develop a patient-centred approach
- skills that help us to follow these principles in our normal practice.

There is growing evidence that the quality of communication used to deliver stoma care is a crucial factor in patients' rehabilitation (e.g. Pringle & Swan 2001, White 1999). In the following brief outline of some recent studies it is apparent that a key factor in whether patients' wellbeing and recovery was successfully promoted was the degree to which the care provided matched patients' needs.

Black (2000) reports findings from the 1997 Montreux Study in which stoma patients completed questionnaires on their quality of life, satisfaction with medical care, and self-efficacy. These study findings, involving 5289 patients from 16 European countries, included the following:

- The biggest improvement in patients' quality of life was seen between discharge from hospital and the 3-month follow-up when they completed the questionnaires again. After that time improvements, although continuing, were not so marked.
- Patients who regarded the stoma care nurse as having a genuine interest in them had a significantly higher quality of life index (QLI) score

than those who had a poor relationship with the stoma care nurse.

- Between discharge and 3-month follow-up, if the patient's relationship with the stoma care nurse worsened, their overall QLI score increased only slightly. Where the relationship improved, there was a marked increase in their QLI score.
- Most patients had moderate levels of confidence in changing their appliance at discharge. Those who had higher levels of confidence in appliance management had higher QLI scores. At 3 months patients' QLI scores decreased if their confidence decreased and increased if their confidence in managing their appliance increased.

Pringle & Swan (2001) reported the results of a multicentre study. Patients who had undergone surgery for colorectal cancer were interviewed four times in the first year after stoma surgery. Their findings included the following:

- Patients who were dissatisfied with the level of information they were given were more likely to be depressed. This occurred whether they received more or less information than they wanted.
- More than half the patients who had little understanding of what they were told were depressed, whereas less than a quarter of the patients who said they did understand what was said were depressed.

Thompson (1998) researched patients' participation in decisions about long-term colostomy management. The aim was to determine whether the level or style of collaboration in decision-making used with these new patients would affect goal achievement and patient satisfaction. Three decision-making systems were used, one with each patient.

Patients using *the instrument system* used a formal research-based decision analysis method. Structured patient participation was high but the system did not include discussion.

Patients using *the advisory system* were given advice by an expert stoma care nurse. They were informed of stoma management options but the nurse set the goals with minimal active patient collaboration.

Patients using *the discussion system* used discussion and collaborative decision-making to set their stoma management goals.

At 18 weeks patients in the discussion and advisory groups had attained their goals to a greater extent than those in the instrument group. The

processes involved in decision-making were found to be important. The discussion group (high collaboration) expressed satisfaction because they were able to explore the nature of their stoma management decisions and express feelings. The advised group (low collaboration) were not as satisfied with the method of making decisions. However, they did achieve their stoma management goals if they had confidence in the expertise of the adviser, a satisfactory relationship with that nurse, and were given reasons for the advice.

All these studies highlight the importance of developing collaborative relationships as well as individual communication skills. We can combine these skills to engage in processes that support and promote a patient-centred style of care.

Key communication processes include:

- building and maintaining rapport
- conveying genuine interest and respect
- acquiring empathic understanding of other people's experiences and needs
- eliciting relevant information from patients and families and using it to plan, provide and evaluate care
- tailoring information and ways of giving it to individuals' particular needs
- explicitly helping patients clarify and achieve goals
- helping patients and families to clarify and resolve or minimise their problems.

We can make our care most effective when we use these processes *strategically* as the means whereby we promote the current and long-term goals we are seeking to help patients achieve. The golden rule for achieving this kind of purposeful care is to:

- use *skills* to follow *strategies* to achieve *goals*.

For example, in response to Thompson's findings cited above we might use:

skills of listening, questioning and summarising as well as information-giving as
a strategy for helping patients become involved in making decisions about their stoma management, and
our goal would be for this approach to enable patients to achieve good stoma management, and feel satisfied by engaging in this collaborative process.

The ways in which we make sense of, and respond to, what patients tell us are influenced by our beliefs. Communication, counselling, and psychotherapy models and theories each have their own concepts of how people function. These concepts underpin further beliefs as to how people can be helped to function better, and which skills and strategies should be used to do so. In combination they give us a *conceptual framework* to guide our understanding and ways of working with patients and their families. For example, Lanceley (2000) outlines some psychological theories and how their conceptual frameworks shape the approaches that might be used with cancer patients. White (1999) has used a cognitive and behavioural framework to outline several approaches that can be used with stoma patients.

The kind of frameworks likely to be most useful as we seek to communicate effectively and promote patients' wellbeing are those that have a broad conceptual base. They need to be of practical use in the different situations in which we provide stoma care, and in the limited time we have with patients. Such frameworks must also be able to help us use the key processes listed above within our normal practice. In this book, particularly in this chapter and Chapter 22, I have primarily drawn on two conceptual frameworks.

The first is Egan's (2002) model of the helping process. Egan has been developing his model since the 1970s, drawing on a range of psychological theories and research findings. His model gives us a structure we can use to work collaboratively with patients and their families to identify goals, address problems and create opportunities. He shows how various skills can be used to make these processes occur. These are key components of rehabilitative stoma care.

The second approach, neurolinguistic programming (NLP), is also not a specific communication or counselling theory. NLP involves the study of how:

- people do things well
- models, or mental maps, of how people 'do' their capabilities can be created
- experts' capabilities (e.g. skills, strategies, helpful beliefs) can be most easily learned by others
- people create and solve problems.

Early work by the originators of NLP, Bandler and Grinder, had a psychotherapeutic focus (O'Connor & Seymour 1993). They enquired how expert psychotherapists could apparently be using very different theoretical approaches and yet achieve equally effective results whilst clients of colleagues using the same theoretical approaches achieved less helpful

changes. They studied Fritz Perls, the originator of gestalt therapy; Virginia Satir, a family therapist; and Milton Erickson, a hypnotherapist. Some of the approaches these three experts all used appeared to significantly aid rapport-building and communication with their clients. We can use them in stoma care (as described later in this chapter), in cancer nursing (Rushworth 1994) and when promoting health (McDermott & O'Connor 1996a).

Since those early studies NLP has been used to identify how experts in many other fields 'do' their expertise, including education, management, business, sports and writing (e.g. Van Nagel et al 1985, McDermott & O'Connor 1996b, Dilts 1998, Hickman & Jacobson 1997). This has resulted in many NLP concepts and techniques being tried out and refined in a wide variety of contexts, enabling their usefulness to be tested in practical ways.

We can use the key processes listed above to enhance stoma care. However, if you look at the list again you will see that these are processes we can use in many personal and professional situations. The NLP approaches described in this book have been developed from studying people demonstrating these capabilities in various fields, and are being used in different contexts. This means that, in my view, they have the kind of broad base and practicality we need in stoma care.

Egan's approach and NLP are different but complementary. They can be used individually or in combination to help us develop very flexible and effective patient-centred practice. Throughout the book the patient scenarios will help you gain a sense of how concepts and skills derived from Egan's work and NLP can be used to promote specific physical and psychological wellbeing and rehabilitative goals. The actual ability to use different forms of communication strategically (i.e. as a means to an end) and effectively can best be gained through experiential learning with skilled facilitation and supervision (e.g. Egan 2002, Ellis et al 2003, Morrison & Burnard 1997).

PRINCIPLES OF COMMUNICATION

When we base our practice on the following *principles* they help us plan and provide care in a patient-centred style. There are many ways in which we can use communication skills to put principles into practice. Some principles and skills included here may be ones you already use whilst others may be less familiar. The purpose of linking particular skills to specific principles here is *not* to suggest they have to be used in this way. The aim is to give you ideas as to how these principles and skills could be used effectively. As you consider each of them you can recognise what you already do and which approaches you would like to develop further. All of these approaches help patients feel valued as individuals, and supported as they seek to achieve their rehabilitative goals. However, some members of the healthcare team will have learned to use these approaches at more advanced levels than others in the team. As with all aspects of stoma care it is important to collaborate with colleagues so these principles can be used in a coherent way with each patient and their family.

  1. *Each person has their own system or neurological pattern through which they make sense of information and situations.*

Using similar patterns in our communication with them makes it easier for:

- them to understand us
- us to understand their individual experiences and needs.

NLP provides us with several useful approaches with which to recognise how people make sense of information and their world in general, and how we can use that information to enhance our communication with them.

(a) We use our neurological senses to respond to situations and store and recall them from memory. In NLP these are called *representational systems* because we use these pathways to represent experiences:
  - sight (visual; V)
  - hearing (auditory; A)
  - feelings, including tactile and body sensations, emotions, spatial awareness (kinaesthetic; K)
  - smell (olfactory; O)
  - taste (gustatory; G).
(b) Each person has their own pattern of representational system usage arising from the ways in which they use pictures, sounds or feelings as their preferred way of thinking.
(c) When we use another person's preferred representational system(s) to respond to them we increase the likelihood that they will have an experience of being understood and will understand what we say more easily. Being on the same

wavelength in this manner increases rapport and enables us to learn and teach more effectively.
(d) There are a variety of *cues* that help us recognise which representational system someone is using at any time (O'Connor & Seymour, 1993). These are known as *accessing cues*, and include their use of words and their body language/physiology.

USE OF LANGUAGE

Whenever we speak we unconsciously choose words that indicate our internal neurological processes. Someone who is visualising information is likely to use picture-related words. People who are using their auditory sense tend to use hearing or sound-related words. People who are using their kinaesthetic or feeling neurological pathway will generally use feeling type words. With practice we can learn to notice these language cues in our everyday conversation with patients, their families, and colleagues, and thus become aware of how they are thinking and how they most easily make sense of things.

Knowledge of someone's preferred representational system(s) helps us recognise what kind of words we should use to be in the same visual, auditory or kinaesthetic system as they are. This helps them understand what we are saying more easily. With practice we can build up our own explanations of the different aspects of stoma care which patients need to learn in visual, auditory and kinaesthetic language so it becomes second nature to adapt what we want to say to fit in with another person's system.

These ideas are particularly useful when someone tells us they do not understand information. We can just repeat it but, this does not always result in greater understanding. Alternatively we can use these NLP concepts while asking where they are in that overall process of understanding. We would use the same representational system as the one we thought was signalled in that person's original language. For example:

Patient 1:	I *don't see* what you mean (V)
Nurse:	Is the *whole picture hazy* or just part of it? (V)
Patient 2:	That doesn't *ring any bells* with me (A)
Nurse:	Does any of it *sound right* or is there *no rhyme* or reason to it? (A)
Patient 3:	I *can't grasp* all of this (K)
Nurse:	Tell me *which bits fit in* with what you know so we can *tie up any loose ends* (K).

The response we then get will help us know what information needs to be re-presented; whether it would be best phrased in visual, auditory or kinaesthetic language; and whether that person might learn best if they could:

- *see* the information (e.g. use a diagram; look at key words written on a board)
- *hear* the information (e.g. on audiotape; use written as well as verbal material)
- *feel* the information (e.g. handle components; try out a new skill through using it in an experiential exercise or supervised clinical practice).

PHYSIOLOGICAL CUES

As we use our neurological pathways to think or respond to situations we unconsciously indicate which ones we are using through our body language. Visual, auditory and kinaesthetic patterns are demonstrated differently physiologically, including through our:

- eye movements
- head tilt
- position of our breathing.

Eye accessing cues are the eye movements we unconsciously make when we are making visual, auditory or kinaesthetic representations. The pattern someone uses will be consistent for them. For example, any time someone wants to recall a picture of something they have seen they may either defocus and look straight ahead, or move their eyes up to their left. Cameron-Bandler (1985) and other writers suggest that most right-handed people are likely to use the pattern of eye movements shown in Figure 7.1. Notice that the *head tilt* which can indicate representational system usage is also shown.

The *position of people's breathing* also usually signals whether they are accessing pictures, sounds or feelings as they process or recall information. Generally people are likely to demonstrate these patterns:

- high chest level breathing, often shallow and more rapid: visual representation
- nipple level: auditory, including sounds and talking to themselves (internal dialogue)
- abdominal breathing, often slower and deeper: kinaesthetic representation.

These physiological cues can be readily observed as we care for patients. They help us identify how,

specifically, each person is making sense of their situation and information they are being given. It is important to remember that people's individual physiological and language cues may not follow the general patterns given above, and that people may, consciously or unconsciously, use a combination of representational systems. The essential point is that each person will have a consistent pattern so it is possible to identify which representational system is being used when that person is exhibiting a particular cue or set of cues.

Patients have to acquire substantial amounts of information in order to learn how to live with their stoma, often in very little time and when they may be experiencing discomfort and weariness. When we recognise the neurological patterns they are using, and adapt our communication to match them, we increase the ease and speed with which they can understand what we are saying. In addition, we can unobtrusively watch people's eye movements to help us recognise when someone has finished 'processing' something we have said to them (i.e. they have completed their normal pattern of eye movements) and they are now able to attend to the next piece of information. More information on accessing cues and how these can be identified and used is given in many NLP books (e.g. O'Connor & Seymour 1993, O'Connor & McDermott 1996).

Like any skill, learning to recognise and respond to people's use of different systems takes practice. It involves responding to people's processes *and* the content of what they are saying. It is often easier to increase our recognition skills first by using situations where people are talking but we are not directly taking part in the conversation. We can learn to notice cues as colleagues engage in informal chat before a meeting as well as other situations where people are conversing near us (e.g. while queuing to pay for shopping or sitting in a bus, train or restaurant).

Listening to live (unscripted) radio interviews can help us notice language cues while live television interviews give us the chance to notice eye accessing and other physiological cues as well as to practise matching (described below). Similarly it is best initially to develop our range of visual, auditory and kinaesthetic language responses in low-key conversations where the outcome is unimportant. People who are just beginning to pay attention to a speaker's language, and the representational systems it could signal, have been known to find they have not taken in the meaning (i.e. content) of large

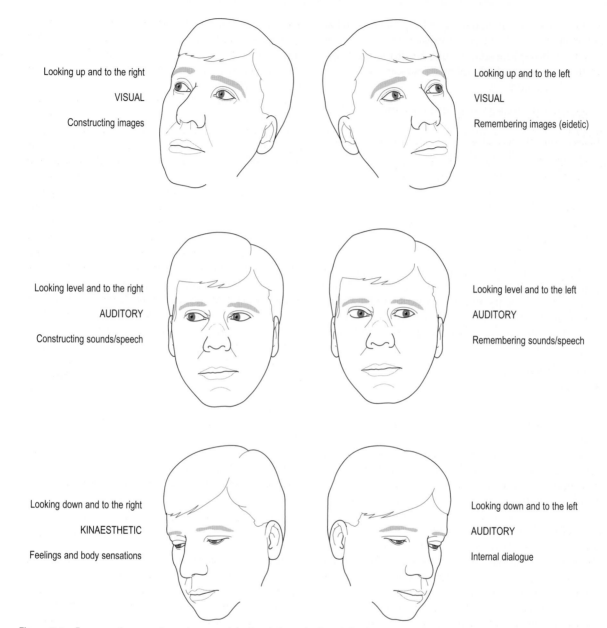

Figure 7.1   Eye accessing cues shown by many right-handed people. Eyes defocused and looking straight ahead also often indicates visualisation.

portions of what was said as they were busy trying to recognise process cues! As recognising people's use of representational systems becomes easier so our ability to pay attention to both the speaker's process and content also develops.

2. *Rapport is a relationship of trust and responsiveness to elements of someone's experience.*

This core element of effective communication can be created and maintained by recognising and acknowledging aspects of a person's experience or perception.

These aspects can be the *content* of their communication and/or the *processes* they are using.

RESPONDING TO CONTENT: BASIC AND ADVANCED LEVEL EMPATHY

Egan (2002) suggests that empathy is both a rapport-building and clarification skill which can be used at two levels to check the accuracy of our understanding of what a situation is like for the person speaking to us. The three steps are:

1. active listening in order to understand the essence of the speaker's experience
2. a tentative response in which the listener briefly conveys what they understand the core or central element of the speaker's experience to be, based on what they were told
3. observation of non-verbal and verbal cues from the speaker which indicate the degree to which they experience themselves as accurately understood.

Our willingness as listener to allow speakers to decide whether our understanding of their situation is sufficiently accurate is a powerful rapport-building process. Our intention to understand what things are like standing in the speaker's shoes is usually recognised and valued. Speakers will respond to that intention. They may confirm that we have understood accurately and go on to expand on their situation. Alternatively, they may seek to correct misunderstanding by further explanation regarding the key elements or issues in their situation. Both speaker and listener gain clarity about the situation and begin to build a shared perception of it.

With *basic level empathy* the understanding which we lay out in step 2 for the speaker to verify or correct is derived from what the speaker has actually said. It is a supremely useful skill at all stages of work with patients and families. It enables us to stay on track with them through accurate understanding and prompt them to move forward as they clarify their situation, needs and goals.

Advanced level empathy is most helpful when a trusting relationship has been established and the rapport is strong enough for the person to feel able to respond to the challenge inherent in the understanding of their situation expressed by the listener. The three steps are the same, but at this level we convey our understanding of what the speaker has only half-said or implied. (As such it is still a reflection of elements of their situation that the speaker has portrayed. We do not impose our interpretation or labelling of the situation on them.)

Empathic understanding at this advanced level needs to be expressed tentatively enough for the speaker to feel invited to verify or rectify our perception rather than dismiss or run away from it. As they consider the understanding of their situation that we have expressed, so speakers may for the first time recognise the importance and/or implications of particular elements in it. They will do this more easily if we have already demonstrated sufficient levels of respectful appropriate attention for them to accept that the purpose of this intervention is to help and support them, even though they may also feel challenged by it. Accurate advanced level empathy encourages people to further expand on their situation, thus promoting more clarification both for themselves and for their listener.

Egan (2002) suggests that generally the core elements of someone's experience for the listener to pick up will be the speaker's feelings, and the experiences and behaviours that underlie those feelings.

For example: you feel angry because they didn't take your worries seriously.

Embedded in this skill description is the idea (or model) that the components which make up people's experience of any situation are their:

- feelings
- behaviours (what they do or do not do)
- experiences (sense of what is happening to them).

Rapport is built up as the listener demonstrates understanding of what is happening in the speaker's world (the content of what they are being told verbally and non-verbally) and the meaning that the speaker derives from these three pieces which together make up the jigsaw of their experience.

RESPONDING TO PROCESS: MATCH–PACE–LEAD

When we adopt aspects of someone's behaviour this helps us step into their world and experience it more fully. In NLP this process is known as *matching*. It is a potent aid to creating rapport. The concept of rapport in NLP differs from that of Egan in that NLP suggests the experience of 'being understood' is not dependent on understanding the content of what someone is saying, but can be built up through using some of their processes to create trust and understanding. The *examples* earlier of responding to someone's language cues by using similar visual, auditory or kinaesthetic language are also examples of matching process, i.e. representational systems usage.

Ways in which we can match people include using similar:

- body posture
- breathing rate
- gestures
- rhythm and tone of voice
- language
- frequency of eye contact.

When we match one or more of someone's physiological behaviours this helps them feel attended to and acknowledged as a person. It is important to ensure that our behaviour is sufficiently similar to other people's while not mimicking them precisely (which can be experienced as disrespectful). We already do this naturally some of the time: notice people whose communication is flowing easily and you are likely to find some physiological matching is occurring too.

Our use of matching language and physiology enables us to create rapport in many different relationships and situations, even those where we do not agree with the content of what is being said. Our communication becomes more flexible and thus builds our own confidence and ability to handle a wider range of situations. As we match people we feed something of their experience through our body. It is therefore important not to match someone so closely that we take on too much of their experience, thus becoming less able to help them (e.g. by also becoming significantly depressed or angry, or hyperventilating). Instead we can use *crossover matching* where we match someone's body language with a different type of movement. *For example:* using small hand or foot movements to match the rhythm of the other person's speech. This helps us maintain rapport without landing in the hole beside them!

Both forms of matching enable us to 'walk beside' someone until they experience themselves as sufficiently understood, a prelude for becoming open to change. This is the process of *pacing* which enables us to build a bridge of trust and understanding (rapport) between another person and ourselves.

We can then *lead* them to consider different options or ideas, or alter their experience by subtly altering our verbal and non-verbal behaviours. If we have sufficiently paced them they will follow our lead and their perception/experience changes (Breckman 1992).

Match–pace–lead is a key skill for defusing tension, helping people move towards considering difficult issues or move out of being stuck in unhelpful levels of emotion, and reconsider and change unhelpful beliefs and behaviours. However, it is also a way of being with people which is beneficial to incorporate into our interactions generally because it helps us use our limited time well to develop the levels of rapport needed for concerns and problems to be expressed and dealt with as soon and as effectively as possible.

PATIENT SCENARIO 7.1   Three months after his surgery Gary Cook is talking to his stoma care nurse. He tells Mrs Reid he is pleased to be seeing her at a time when his partner, Oscar, is at work as he wants some help but does not want to upset Oscar by discussing his problems in front of him. Initially Gary had found it difficult to believe that Mrs Reid would accept Oscar and himself as partners in the same way as a heterosexual couple (Etnyre 1990). As he found she did indeed do so, his trust in her increased and he was able to be more open with her about his lifestyle and concerns. However, she notices today his body posture is tense; his eye contact is minimal, and he appears reluctant to describe his problem in any detail. He seems to be finding it difficult to ask for help so she wants to increase the levels of rapport between them, thus inviting more disclosure.

She *matches* his posture by also sitting fairly upright but with less rigidity, and keeps her eye contact intermittent. Gary's breathing is high in his chest and quite rapid and these cues of visualisation fit in with Mrs Reid's knowledge that he tends to use his visual representation system. She therefore *matches* him by using visual language (representation), telling him she understands he wants to <u>clear</u> something up and that it might help if he gave her <u>more of a picture</u> of what the problem was so that they could <u>look at it together</u>. Gary nods, and begins to talk less hesitantly. Mrs Reid has also been *cross-matching* his rapid breathing with minimal finger movements in time with his breathing, making sure her hand is within his peripheral field of vision so she can unobtrusively *pace* his breathing. As Gary continues talking she gradually slows down her finger movements, *leading* him to slow down his breathing. She also begins to relax her posture as she wants to *lead* Gary into a state of greater relaxation and rapport in order to make it easier for him to talk in detail about his problem.

Mrs Reid also draws on Egan's concept of *basic level empathy* to check with Gary intermittently that her understanding of his unfolding problem is accurate. However, while Egan (2002) suggests the core element is usually feelings much of Gary's account is in visual terms. She therefore *matches* this by also stating what she thinks are the core elements of what Gary has told her in visual language rather than kinaesthetic (feeling).

3. *Giving patient-centred information generally entails four steps.*

(a) *Eliciting relevant information from the person about themselves.* When planning their overall care this generally includes what they think about their:
   - situation
   - concerns
   - needs
   - probable tests and treatment
   - current and future lifestyles.

(b) *Using this information to consider with the patient:*
   - what information they require
   - how it can best be given
   - when to give it
   - what outcomes are expected or desired from providing this information in this manner
   - how this patient and the staff will know when these outcomes have been achieved (e.g. criteria to be met; specific patient experiences).

(c) *Providing the required information and encouraging the patient to use it.*

(d) *Evaluating with the patient whether the desired outcomes have been achieved.*

Information-giving that is shaped by this process is likely to be experienced as supportive and relevant by the patient concerned. All the skills described in this chapter can be used to gather information (see patient scenarios in Ch. 1).

4. *Information that is given to patients is most helpful to them if the content and process whereby it is given have certain qualities.*

(a) The *content* should be:
   - accurate
   - of a level and amount of detail that is in accordance with the patient's wishes
   - genuinely relevant to the patient's current and/or longer-term situation, needs and goals
   - understandable by the patient
   - specifically linked to the patient's lifestyle and goals
   - responsive to the patient's needs, concerns and questions
   - experienced as relevant and reliable by the patient.

(b) The *process* should be:
   - timely for that patient
   - conducted at a pace/speed that enables the patient to make sense of and respond to it
   - broken up into chunks of information that are of a size congruent with the patient's preferred level of detail
   - of a style that is congruent with the ways in which the patient most readily processes information
   - appropriate for the content of what is being imparted
   - congruent with the patient's personal and cultural needs for particular styles of verbal and non-verbal communication
   - flexible and responsive to the patient's needs and experiences during the information-giving process and those that might arise as a result of it.

5. *The purpose of giving information is so that the recipient can understand and utilise it in ways that are helpful to them.*

The way in which we define our purpose when giving information influences which criteria we use to decide whether we have successfully achieved it. If we only think of giving information as 'a task which we have to complete' then we are likely to focus on whether we have given someone the (right) information. We may not look for evidence as to whether the patient has understood what we said, or whether it has met their particular needs.

Assuming that giving information is 'the' way to reduce every patient's anxiety can also be unhelpful. Teasdale (1995a) reports that, for information-giving to be helpful, it must be congruent with people's normal coping styles. People with a 'monitoring' coping style need to feel in control of events.

They get this feeling from possessing information. In contrast, people with a 'blunting' coping style prefer distraction from events such as operations where they have very little control. He suggests 'blunters' can be adversely affected if overloaded with information. Helping people increase their range of coping strategies can be more helpful than automatically giving more information if patients are distressed.

One key period when we should ensure that information is appropriately provided is preoperatively. Patients often experience uncertainty and anxiety at this time. Inappropriate reassurance, or a mismatch between the level of information patients want and are given, reduces their ability to benefit from these approaches (Teasdale 1995b).

Generally patients require information that is related to:

(a) helping them deal with their situation of being in hospital and receiving medical tests and treatment, and care from nursing and other health-care staff
(b) living with a stoma.

A good starting point is to first find out how much information that patient actually wants to have. White (1999) suggests that patients can be invited to rate their levels of satisfaction with the information they have already been given, with zero equating with not at all satisfied and 100 being the most satisfied they could be. This provides a basis for discussing what additional information could be provided and how. Subsequent rating helps patients and staff monitor how well provision of information is meeting patients' needs.

Statements can be gentler forms of enquiry than direct questions. We can use them to set the scene for giving information, and signal that the purpose of giving patients such information is so that they can use it.

For example: 'Some people like a lot of information about their operation and living with a stoma and others cope best if they have less information. I would like to make sure I give you a booklet with the right level of information for you. I am wondering if one with diagrams and more detailed information would suit you best or if you would prefer one which was more general.'

Such statements invite people to collaborate in the process of getting the level of information right and, embedded in it, is the suggestion that they will then use it. Patients' verbal and non-verbal responses to

such statements can indicate whether they use monitoring or blunting coping styles as well as their informational needs. Statements can also be used as permission-givers for patients to raise issues or concerns which they may find difficult or think might be unacceptable to raise with staff (see Ch. 9), and to invite clarification from patients (Egan 2002).

Offering *constructive feedback* also entails information-giving. It is particularly useful for helping patients assess their progress in acquiring knowledge and learning to manage their own stoma care. The information or feedback is given in the form of observations about the patient's performance and/or how the nurse experiences their behaviour.

Feedback is most likely to be constructive when it meets the criteria of being:

- realistic
- specific
- descriptive rather than evaluative
- timely for the patient.

Such feedback invites people to consider the implications of what has been said and use that information to review or extend their activities.

PATIENT SCENARIO 7.2   Mrs Reid has been watching Mr Patel do his third practice change of his urostomy bag. Once he has finished and is resting comfortably she gives him information on his progress in the form of *constructive feedback*. She tells him that she noticed he generally prepared his new equipment correctly and in a more confident manner than at his last practice change. However, she also says that she noticed that he did not check that the tap of his new bag was turned off before applying it, and that she remembers he omitted this step on his previous changes as well. Mrs Reid has recognised that advising Mr Patel to check the bag tap as part of his routine equipment preparation has not led him to remember to do so now. She therefore uses feedback (rather than a reminder) this time in order to encourage him to think what the implications of his actions might be. As Mr Patel hastily checks his bag he also imagines the possible consequences of leaving the tap open, and says he now realises that routinely checking his tap is closed while preparing his bag is important.

Constructive feedback can also be a helpful way of providing information to people who do not like being given advice or who experience being given information as being told what to do. Specific descriptions of the effects of their actions on us or on a particular situation can give them sufficient 'psychological space' with which to reflect on our information rather than reject it. That in turn creates the possibility that the information can be used in a way that is more helpful for all concerned.

6. *Information gained from patients should be shared appropriately with the healthcare team. This helps staff adapt their normal practice to respond to individual patients' needs, and use complementary rather than conflicting approaches.*

Discussions between patient and nurse often start out with an implicit agreement that, as the information is to be used to deliver appropriate personal care, it will be shared with other staff involved in that patient's care. Sometimes patients then reveal information, fears and/or feelings that they felt able to tell a particular nurse but do not want other staff to know about. Patients may be comfortable with the general concept that information will be shared but feel quite different when faced with the reality of specific information being made available to all staff. Asking patients what they think about specific information being passed on, and negotiating with them how that could be documented in their records, are strategies that allow confidentiality to be maintained while relevant information is made available in a form that colleagues can use (Breckman 1986).

PATIENT SCENARIO 7.3   Mrs Boot tells Nurse Willow that she is worried about her son Terry, who has been caught shoplifting twice since she became ill. She says she feels angry and ashamed about this, and very worried about how her husband will cope with the forthcoming court proceedings and any publicity. He keeps telling her there is nothing to be concerned about and she disagrees. After discussion Nurse Willow records in Mrs Boot's care plan that she is worried about her son Terry but does not want to discuss this in detail with staff and does not want anyone questioning her husband about the problem. This alerts staff to the presence of a problem. Nurse Willow suggests that staff will want to observe for any signs that Mr or Mrs Boot want to discuss the problem and signal their willingness to listen in response to any such cues, whilst allowing Mr and

Mrs Boot to control the timing and depth of any disclosures. This information gives Mrs Boot the opportunity to consider any signals from staff as an invitation which springs from their desire to be helpful (rather than a nosy enquiry which is out of step with her expressed needs). Nurse Willow then asks Mrs Boot how she might respond to staff if she knew they were just checking she hadn't changed her mind and now wanted to talk more. This encourages Mrs Boot to use the information as she answers Nurse Willow's question, increasing the likelihood that she will also remember and use it in future interactions with staff.

7. *The purpose of teaching is to enable the recipient to gain relevant resources (e.g. knowledge, skills, understanding, awareness) with which to respond to situations and achieve their goals.*

As with principle 5 above the goal is not that knowledge has been imparted and/or skills demonstrated or described. Teaching goals are achieved when learners have gained sufficient knowledge and skills to be able to:

(a) recognise which aspects of what they have learned are relevant to use in specific situations
(b) use them when necessary and monitor the degree to which they are successful
(c) adapt their responses to deal with changing circumstances and increase the level of success with which they manage situations and problems.

8. *Teaching is most likely to promote learning if the methods used are congruent with the learner's style of learning and the material being taught is perceived by the learner as relevant to their needs.*

Most patients are still struggling with the effects of major surgery and anaesthetic when they are having to acquire substantial amounts of information and skills before discharge. They need all the help we can give them to make learning as easy as possible. When we link the elements we are teaching to specific aspects of their lifestyle and rehabilitation goals it helps them recognise they are relevant. This enhances their motivation to gain that skill or knowledge.

Asking patients how they learn best, and then using that information to adapt our teaching to their learning style, allows all concerned to use time and energy well to maximise learning. Some people use one approach for learning practical tasks and another for absorbing theoretical information, so it is wise to ask about both types of learning. As patients describe their learning experiences we are likely to gain information about their representational system usage (see principle 1 above) and the ways in which they like information presented. Some people like to learn a step at a time and build knowledge up gradually (serialist); some like to see the whole process demonstrated so they can learn it as a whole interconnected map (holist); while others may need to get an overview of the skill or material to be learned and then focus on it a little at a time (Mohanna et al 2004).

When learning does not appear to be taking place effectively we need to step back and consider the likely causes. It may be someone is in pain, or experiencing tiredness or distress and the timing of our teaching is inappropriate until these factors have been addressed. However, it may be that there is a mismatch between our style of teaching and their style of learning. Such difficulties require adoption of a more helpful teaching strategy for the particular patient either by ourselves or by a colleague.

Patients need to be able to use what they have learned flexibly. They therefore need to know:

- *why* the information or skill is relevant
- *what* they need to know and/or be able to do
- *how* to use what they are learning and, from this
- *how to use their learned resources to adapt* to changing circumstances and needs.

This style of learning requires a joint approach by patient and staff, with both being involved in the planning, achievement and evaluation of learning (e.g. Wilson & Desruisseaux 1983).

PATIENT SCENARIO 7.4 John Fletcher knows that Nurse Linden has used part of a peristomal wafer for the purpose of filling in a dip in his abdomen at one side of his stoma and thus preventing faeces from leaking along it. She has also told him that other substances such as pastes can be used to fill in dips and that, if people's abdominal shapes alter, so may any dips or creases they might have. Since he understands that the goal is to prevent leakage he can use the information he has been given to adapt his current filler strategy if necessary in the future. He feels more confident about handling changed circumstances because he has been given sufficient information to help him make decisions.

---

9. *The processes of counselling and advising are different and their use with clients is likely to result in different responses and outcomes.*

Given the implications and effects of stoma surgery it is likely that patients and their families will seek our help to resolve concerns and problems. In order to respond appropriately we need to be able to differentiate between counselling and advising, and recognise which process is more likely to help them in different situations.

Nurse (1980, p 2) cites the definition of counselling given by the Steering Committee of the Standing Committee for the Advancement of Counselling in 1969, and which is quoted below. Although more recent definitions exist, this is one that many nurses find helpful. It indicates the concept of counselling which is held whenever the term is used throughout this book:

> *Counselling is a process through which one person helps another by purposeful conversation in an understanding atmosphere. It seeks to establish a helping relationship in which the one counselled can express his thoughts and feelings in such a way as to clarify his own situation; come to terms with some new experience, see his difficulty more objectively, and so face his problem with less anxiety and tension. Its basic purpose is to assist the individual to make his own decision from among the choices available to him.*

In counselling the *client* (e.g. patient, relative) defines his concern or problem until it is sufficiently clear to him to enable him to set and achieve goals to resolve or respond to it more resourcefully. The counsellor's task is to use relevant skills and approaches for the purpose of supporting and enabling the client to make his own choices.

The underlying assumption is that *clients* have the power and responsibility to clarify and handle their situation or problem and have, or can develop, the capabilities to do this effectively. The goal is for clients to manage their situation more resourcefully.

In advice-giving it is often the *adviser* who defines the problem or concern because she selects which particular elements of a situation are relevant to ask about, pay attention to, and respond to through the advice she gives. The more energy and activities the adviser displays as she seeks to help, the more likely it is that the client will take a more passive role in defining and handling the situation.

The underlying assumption can be that, because the adviser has experience or fulfils a particular role, this means the *adviser* also has (or should have) the major responsibility and power to define and decide how best the client's situation or problem can be resolved or reduced. As this assumption is acted on so both client and adviser may experience the adviser's responsibilities and power as expanding while their sense of the client's power and responsibility becomes diminished, without any real thought or discussion as to whether this is appropriate. This can lead to the assumption by client, adviser, or both, that it is the *adviser's* responsibility to get the problem resolved and the goal then becomes that the adviser should manage the problem. This is not necessarily an appropriate or achievable outcome as it can confirm or promote the belief that the client is unable to think about and resolve problems effectively.

Neither counselling nor advising are intrinsically good or bad processes: both are generally used with the intention of helping people. The questions that are beneficial to ask before using either approach are:

- What is the goal of this interaction?
- Which process is most likely to help us achieve this goal, given the assumptions and end results that often underpin or arise from their use?
- Do I have adequate knowledge and skills to engage in this process and help the person with this issue?

The answers to these questions enable us to make choices and communicate strategically as a means of promoting desired goals. They also help us identify when we should refer patients to more informed and skilled colleagues.

10. *All the major communication processes (informing, teaching, counselling, advising) will generally need to be used at some stage to help patients in their journey through surgery to rehabilitation. The **order** in which they are used and the **combination** used can significantly affect patients' experiences and rehabilitation.*

Given that many people take about 2 years to rehabilitate it is essential that our communication should help them prepare for living with a stoma and achieving their rehabilitative goals. Almost always when we are using knowledge and skills to care for patients we also have the opportunity to inform and gently *coach* them so they develop the habit of using information to look after themselves resourcefully. We can do this effectively when we:

(a) Do not do more than 50% of the work when counselling: the more the patient does the more likely it is that the goals and strategies for achieving them will be the patient's rather than the counsellor's.

(b) Gain information from patients about their situation, concerns, needs, goals, and check the accuracy of our understanding *before* giving information or advice.

(c) Give advice sparingly. If, when asked for advice, we instead generally offer to give patients information or suggestions and tell them we would like to then discuss how this information or suggestion could be used (e.g. to act or think differently) they are more likely to expand their abilities to assess and manage both the current and future situations, and their sense of their capabilities to do so.

(d) Model explicitly for patients how we are arriving at decisions. This may be done indirectly, *for example*, as we explain to a colleague which factors we paid attention to or considered less important when assessing which type of appliance or skin care aid would be suitable in their situation while the patient can listen too.

Summarising can be a useful skill as it enables us to draw together different pieces of information, which may have been gathered separately, into a format where possible or actual connections can be considered (Egan 2002).

For example: Summarising someone's account of their situation plus summarising the relevant information which we have used to reach a position where we can give advice or suggestions can be very helpful. The explicit linkage between the information in the two summaries is a particularly useful strategy if the advice is likely to be unpalatable to the person or they generally reject advice.

When we work in these kinds of ways we help patients engage in *a four-step process:*

- *clarification and scene-setting* about what will or may happen (prompted by staff, patient, or both)
- *consideration of the input* provided by staff or through joint communication between patient and staff (e.g. explanation, demonstration, discussion)
- *early application of that input to their own situation* (e.g. new thoughts, feelings, understanding, skills)
- *consolidation and expansion* (e.g. further practice/ discussion, identification of other areas in which knowledge/skills could be used).

CONCLUSION

If the various communication skills and approaches described in this chapter and elsewhere in the book are indeed to help patients rehabilitate physically and psychologically then we must learn to use them consciously and strategically for that purpose. That means the twin goals of meeting patients' current needs *and* encouraging their long-term rehabilitation must be constantly borne in mind and promoted as an integral part of the way each member of staff works with each patient. Individually and collectively we must use skills to follow strategies to promote achievement of the small and large goals that build up over time into the kind of rehabilitation each patient desires.

References

Black P K 2000 Holistic stoma care. Baillière Tindall & RCN, Edinburgh

Breckman B 1986 Success by stages. Senior Nurse 5(3):14–16

Breckman B 1992 Using neuro-linguistic programming (NLP) to achieve individualised stoma care. World Council of Enterostomal Therapists Journal 12(4):12–18

Cameron-Bandler L 1985 Solutions. Future-Pace, San Rafael, CA

Dilts R B 1998 Modeling with NLP. Meta Publications, CA

Egan G 2002 The skilled helper, 7th edn. Brooks/Cole, Australia

Ellis R B, Gates B, Kenworthy N (eds) 2003 Interpersonal communication in nursing, 2nd edn. Churchill Livingstone, Edinburgh

Etnyre W 1990 Meeting the needs of gay and lesbian ostomates. In: World Council of Enterostomal Therapists congress proceedings. Hollister, Libertyville, IL, p 123–125

Hickman D E, Jacobson S 1997 The power process. Anglo-American Book Company, Carmarthen, Wales

Lanceley A 2000 Therapeutic strategies in cancer care. In: Corner J, Bailey C (eds) Cancer nursing: care in context . Blackwell Science, Oxford, p 120–138

McDermott I, O'Connor J 1996a NLP and health. Thorsons, London

McDermott I, O'Connor J 1996b Practical NLP for managers. Gower, Hampshire

Mohanna K, Wall D, Chambers R 2004 Teaching made easy . Radcliffe Medical Press, Abingdon

Morrison P, Burnard P 1997 Caring and communicating, 2nd edn. Macmillan Press, Basingstoke

Nurse G 1980 Counselling and the nurse, 2nd edn. HM+M Publishers, Buckinghamshire

O'Connor J, McDermott I 1996 Principles of NLP. Thorsons, London

O'Connor J, Seymour J 1993 Introducing neuro-linguistic programming, 2nd edn. Aquarian Press, London

Pringle W, Swan E 2001 Continuing care after discharge from hospital for stoma patients. British Journal of Nursing 10(19):1274–1288

Rushworth C 1994 Making a difference in cancer care. Souvenir Press, London

Teasdale K 1995a The nurse's role in anxiety management. Professional Nurse 10(8):509–512

Teasdale K 1995b Theoretical and practical considerations on the use of reassurance in the nursing management of anxious patients. Journal of Advanced Nursing 22(1):79–86

Thompson J 1998 Patient participation in decisions about longterm colostomy management. In: World Council of Enterostomal Therapists congress proceedings. Horton Print Group, Bradford, West Yorkshire, p 167–172

White C A 1999 Psychological aspects of stoma care. In: Taylor P (ed) Stoma care in the community. Nursing Times Books, London

Wilson E, Desruisseaux B 1983 Stoma care and patient teaching. In: Wilson-Barnett J (ed) Patient teaching. Churchill Livingstone, Edinburgh, p 95–118

Van Nagel C, Reese E J, Siudzinski R, Reese M 1985 Megateaching and learning-neurolinguistic programming applied to education. Southern Institute Press, Florida

Chapter 8

Towards leaving hospital

Brigid Breckman

Many patients are now discharged home between 7 and 10 days after more major operations. When such surgery includes stoma formation early discharge has substantial implications for patients and staff. Stoma patients cannot just rest at home, mobilising and resuming their normal lifestyle at a pace in keeping with bodily recovery. They are immediately faced with the challenge of managing their own stoma care. We have to prepare patients adequately to manage their stoma care in this shortened time-frame between surgery and discharge. Additionally, the methods we use must take account of the reality that patients are having to learn self-care whilst still experiencing the effects of anaesthesia, surgery, pain and analgesics. We must therefore focus our care so it actively promotes patients' acquisition of essential knowledge and skills. This includes using two approaches described in earlier chapters, and the additional approaches listed below, which are discussed in this chapter:

- helping patients relate information we give, from preoperatively onwards, to their lifestyle and needs (e.g. *patient scenarios* in Chs 1, 4, 7)
- teaching patients the principles underpinning stoma care as well as the steps (see Ch. 4)
- *enabling patients to gain capabilities* through learning:
  - what they need to know
  - what they need to be able to do
  - when and how to get physical and psychological help and support
- *helping patients to set up a system for obtaining future supplies of stomal equipment;* this includes giving them adequate amounts of stock to use in the initial period at home

• *helping patients to set up a system that will assist them to function* as easily and effectively as possible in the early weeks at home.

These preparatory activities are not separate entities but a combination which we should be helping patients and their families gain throughout the pre- and postoperative period. However, in order to evaluate patients' readiness for discharge it can be helpful to consider how well prepared they are in each separate activity as well as overall. Such detailed evaluation is useful because patients are quite often deemed medically fit for discharge from hospital before they are socially or psychologically ready to manage the practicalities of living with their stoma at home. In an environment where the pressure on beds and financial resources is intense it is important that patients and staff understand what 'adequate self-care' entails, and are committed to patients achieving it before discharge. Stating that a patient 'needs more time' before being sent home without giving reasons to justify that viewpoint is unlikely to be acceptable to administrative and medical colleagues. Patients who have difficulty recognising that they have not yet mastered the steps of an appliance change may also disregard such statements.

When specific elements of self-care (e.g. particular knowledge, skills) are identified as capabilities patients must gain before they go home these are usually recognised as relevant goals by patients, their families and staff. Time and attention can be allocated to enable patients to achieve them when all concerned accept the importance of their acquisition before discharge.

INFORMATION THAT PATIENTS NEED TO KNOW

This consists largely of information that will help patients look after their physical and psychological wellbeing adequately, and promote their rehabilitation. It therefore includes guidelines on how to recognise normal and abnormal situations and what to do if they arise. When this information is broken down into small portions for patients to acquire, it is easier for each patient and all the staff involved in their care to build up their knowledge gradually, and indicate what stage they have reached more clearly in their care plan. Learning goals should be expressed in terms of patients gaining understanding (rather

than that they were told information) as this helps us focus on whether they can recall and apply it.

> **PATIENT SCENARIO 8.1**   Mrs Jones and Nurse Ash have discussed various aspects of stoma care. Some of the goals regarding Mrs Jones' acquisition of knowledge which they have identified are that, before going home, she will *know*:
> 1. what steps are involved in changing her stomal equipment, and why each step is necessary
> 2. which order the steps need to be carried out in order to make the bag change as easy and effective as possible
> 3. how to dispose of used equipment (a) at home and (b) in a public toilet
> 4. what to do with the application for exemption from prescription charges form which she has been given
> 5. how to obtain stoma care supplies at home
> 6. when to ask for another prescription for equipment
> 7. what each item of equipment is called, and thus what to ask for when it needs replacement
> 8. what her stoma and peristomal skin look like when they are in a healthy condition
> 9. how to correctly identify situations and/or conditions when she should seek help regarding her stoma, skin condition, appliance problems/management
> 10. who to contact about the problems in point 9 and how to contact them.

It is important to identify whether patients are drivers before discharge. Insurers usually have criteria that must be met before drivers are covered following surgery. These can include the length of time that must occur following surgery or hospital discharge, or provision of evidence of fitness to resume driving such as a doctor's letter. When patients acquire this information from their insurers at an early stage it helps them plan rehabilitative activities. Usually patients can resume driving but must first recover adequately. This includes regaining sufficient ability to concentrate on and react to road conditions including emergencies. Many patients are advised not to drive before they have had their initial out patient check-up. They should specifically ask their doctor whether they can resume driving so factors such as pain and fatigue as well as their general health can be assessed in relation to driving as well as generally.

PROCESSES PATIENTS NEED TO BE ABLE TO DO

As patients develop the skills and strategies they need to carry them through the early days after they go home, so they will often also demonstrate their ability to use the knowledge they are acquiring as well as the processes. Goals related to patients' acquisition of skills are usually most helpful if they are stated as small steps, or subgoals. This helps patients and nurses check that each part of the process is being developed adeptly, and to single out problem areas at an early stage. This is particularly important because it is all too easy, meaning to be helpful, for us to step in and carry out bits of the change procedure. Ewing's (1989) research reminds us that this can result in patients not getting the practice they need to develop self-care skills before they are sent home. We must work as a team so that patients gradually increase the steps they do, while we do less and supervise more. This enables patients to gain skills without feeling overloaded by having to learn everything at once.

PATIENT SCENARIO 8.2   Mrs Boot is changing her urostomy bag with minimal help from Nurse Willow. The *goals* that Mrs Boot is working towards include the following:

Before Mrs Boot goes home she will at least twice have:

1. collected all the equipment needed to change her appliance, without reminders from anyone about any items she has forgotten
2. prepared all the equipment ready to change her appliance completely
3. removed the old stomal equipment from her body
4. cleaned around the stoma with warm water and soap, and adequately dried the skin onto which the bag will stick
5. centred her new equipment over the stoma so that it does not rub against, or lodge on the stoma itself
6. applied her new stomal appliance so it sticks firmly to her body
7. disposed of all the used equipment, including rinsing out the stoma bag
8. remembered and carried out the above steps in the correct sequence without prompting from anyone else.

Mrs Boot needs some advice as to when her appliance is well centred over her stoma, but otherwise manages all the goals well except number 7, which she has yet to learn. Nurse Willow checks whether Mrs Boot can use her knowledge of how the stoma and peristomal skin should look by asking her to say what she would observe if she was doing this bag change at home, and what condition she thinks the stoma and surrounding skin are in.

Mrs Boot and Nurse Willow are in a position to assess how well she has achieved her goals because they have been clearly stated. Nurse Willow shows Mrs Boot how to dispose of her used equipment, and suggests in the nursing care plan that Mrs Boot will require supervision for goals 5 and 7 at her next appliance change. This evaluation, coupled with all the others related to achievement of Mrs Boot's goals, aids realistic discharge planning.

Supervising patients as they learn how to dispose of stomal equipment is important. The difficulties disposal causes patients tends to be underestimated by nurses (Swan 2001). Going with patients as they practise disposing of equipment before discharge enables practical difficulties and social concerns to be addressed (Black 2000).

OBTAINING STOMAL EQUIPMENT FOR HOME USE

Many patients worry that they might have difficulties obtaining equipment at home. Helping them set up a specific supply system that is appropriate for their circumstances will increase their confidence as well as competence in this aspect of living with a stoma.

Procedures for obtaining stomal equipment vary between countries and their healthcare systems. The specific steps patients should follow will therefore depend on where they live as well as other personal circumstances. However, we can use principles which are applicable in most countries to shape how we discuss ways of obtaining equipment with patients. This will help them know what to do in their own country as well as if they need to obtain equipment elsewhere. These *principles* include the following:

1. *The amount of supplies patients are discharged with should be sufficient for the management of their stoma care between the time of discharge and the time*

when their first order of equipment can realistically be expected to be supplied.

Financial considerations as to whose budget payment of patients' initial supplies should come from can result in rules being set up regarding the specific amounts of equipment patients may be given on discharge from hospital. When these are rigidly applied it can mean patients are discharged with inadequate supplies for the time actually taken for their first equipment order to arrive. However, over-provision of supplies is also inappropriate as patients' stoma size and equipment needs may well alter during the initial weeks after discharge, necessitating a change in their equipment.

2. *The length of time taken to obtain an order for stomal equipment varies according to the supply system used. Patients' preferred supply system and its normal time-frame must therefore be identified before calculations are made as to the amount of equipment with which they should be discharged.*

3. *The system whereby patients' equipment is paid for will influence the equipment they are supplied with (i) on discharge and (ii) in subsequent orders.*

In many countries stomal equipment is paid for via an insurance system. This may limit the make, type and/or amounts of equipment that patients can receive. Availability of equipment also varies in different countries, and this should be ascertained from the manufacturer. Some patients have to purchase their own equipment. Clear information on costs must be tactfully provided to help them realistically assess what equipment they can afford to use at the time of discharge and in the future.

Patients who are UK residents and who have a *permanent* stoma do not have to pay prescription charges for stomal equipment prescribed by their NHS general practitioner. People under the age of 60 need to fill in form FP92A to apply for a Medex exemption certificate, including ticking the section stating they have 'a permanent fistula' which requires an appliance. The form must be signed by the patient. Their GP or hospital doctor must also sign it (verifying that the patient does have a stoma) before following their local procedure for sending it to the Medex Issue Office. A 5-year exemption certificate will subsequently be issued to the patient. When renewal is due the Medex Issue Office contacts patients asking them to verify they still have the condition before issuing a further exemption certificate to patients under 60. When each prescription is obtained, patients should tick the relevant box to indicate they are exempt from payment for stoma care items before passing it on to whoever is going to supply them.

Patients' levels of energy and mobility are limited following their surgery. It is therefore preferable for patients to get their FP92A form completed whilst still in hospital (where a doctor is more readily available to see they do have a stoma and sign the form) rather than putting them in a position where they may have to visit their GP for verification and completion of the form. Most stoma care nurses carry FP92A forms.

Patients do not have to wait until their exemption certificate has arrived before obtaining supplies. In the rare instances where a prescription charge is made because the certificate has not yet arrived patients should obtain a receipt so they can apply for a rebate once they have received their exemption certificate.

UK residents who have a *temporary* stoma do have to pay prescription charges for stomal equipment unless they are eligible not to, for example because they are over 60 or on benefits because of low income. Obtaining a 'season ticket' for prescriptions helps patients reduce their cost.

4. *Potential systems for obtaining equipment should be discussed with patients to enable them to identify which system could best meet their needs.*

Discussion about obtaining supplies needs to be holistic rather than narrowly task-focused as patients' individual circumstances and preferences may affect the degree to which different systems can meet their needs. In the UK patients can have their prescriptions processed by a chemist, supply company, or (in some instances) the company that makes or markets their brand of equipment. They therefore should consider where they want to get their supplies from. Discussions can include:

- the reliability of the supplier (e.g. to provide a knowledgeable service and supply all the equipment in an acceptable timeframe)
- the degree to which the system of getting equipment from the supplier to their home fits in with their lifestyle
- the degree to which different types of supply system enable the nature of the equipment to be kept private when supplies are being handed over. This helps patients retain control over who knows about their surgery and the equipment they now use.

Chemists and specialist suppliers may offer advice and home delivery, as well as similar timeframes for supplying equipment and so their systems may appear similar. However, some patients find the 'cutting service' offered by some supply companies beneficial. What is important is that patients believe the choice they make is suitable for them, and know they can set up an alternative system later on if circumstances make this advisable. It is therefore helpful to tell patients about different options and then encourage them to identify what would suit them, rather than impose a system on them.

PATIENT SCENARIO 8.3   Mrs Reid is discussing ways in which patients can obtain stomal equipment after discharge with nurses attending a short stoma care course. It becomes apparent that some of the group believe all patients should get equipment from a supply company whilst others have assumed patients will use their local chemist. She wants the nurses to consider moving from an approach where they tell patients where they should obtain supplies to one where patients are informed of different systems and encouraged to identify which one would best fit in with their circumstances and needs. She uses the comments made by patients who are currently being discharged as examples of patients' differing goals and their abilities to make appropriate choices once they have the relevant information.

(Their names are given here so you can link this example with others in the book, but Mrs Reid does not give their names or substantial personal details in order to prevent their identity being recognisable from her description.)

John Fletcher wants to use his local chemist. He thinks there could be problems if equipment is delivered to his home because there won't be anyone at home to take delivery once he is back at work and as Mary works part-time. He does not want parcels left with neighbours as he is worried that he might then have to deal with questions about this ongoing delivery of parcels. His GP already runs a service whereby repeat prescriptions can be requested, and delivered to the local chemist if the patient so wishes. John says he will use this system. Initially Mary will take a photocopy of his list of equipment to their GP for his records, and a note asking for the items needed on his first prescription. She will collect John's equipment from the chemist on her way home from work. Once

John is fit he expects to collect his own equipment as, being a self-employed decorator, he can easily fit a visit to the chemist in with his working schedule.

Mr Earl has decided to use a supply company. He and his wife are elderly. He thinks it will be better if equipment is delivered to their home so neither of them has to fetch it from the chemist. He is finding it quite difficult to cut out the opening in his appliance flange, but wants to use this particular equipment. He says using a supply company which offers a cutting service will relieve his mind, as he had been worrying about how he would manage if the arthritis in his hands got worse and he could no longer prepare his own equipment.

---

5. *Patients should be able to identify their equipment in sufficient detail to enable them to order items correctly.*

Patients sometimes need to order equipment away from home, for example if they require additional supplies on holiday or when working in different locations. Most people take for granted that they know their usual size of shoes and clothes. Patients can be encouraged to view learning the details of their equipment, or routinely carrying a list when away from home over time, as a similar way of knowing about themselves.

6. *Patients should be given written lists of the equipment they are using on discharge.*

This should include:

- the manufacturer and order number for each item
- a description of items, including size where different sizes are available (e.g. gasket, belt or bag sizes)
- number of items per box/pack
- contact details of manufacturer or supplier.

Patients can be encouraged to identify what each piece of stomal equipment is called, and which item on their list matches it, as we collect the equipment with which they will be sent home. This can then be linked to discussion as to which items should be included in their initial post-discharge order. This is not necessarily the whole list. Patients may, for example, have enough belts or bag covers and only need more bags and skin care products.

Patients should have two copies of their list. They should retain one copy and give the other to their GP or supplier for reference whenever orders are made. When equipment is changed it is important to give patients new lists and remind them to give a copy of this updated information to their GP or supplier.

Patients whose English is limited can be given a list where there is space under each item for someone to translate the information into their own language. Patients with reading difficulties can have items colour coded on both boxes and lists of equipment so they can readily identify the items they require from the total listed (B Borwell, personal communication, 1999).

7. *Patients should be given sufficient information to enable them to work out when they should request more supplies in order to maintain adequate levels of equipment.*

8. *Nurses should ensure that patients are discharged with sufficient equipment to last until their first re-stocking supplies arrive.*

The amount this should be will depend on:

- the particular supply system chosen by the patient
- the speed with which those involved in operating that system are likely to fulfil their steps in the procedure, and the degree to which their activities are compatible and enable the overall procedure to take place smoothly
- the availability of the products
- the frequency with which the patient changes the equipment
- the adeptness with which the patient can prepare and use equipment without spoilage or wastage.

These factors will also influence the timeframe that patients need to allow for equipment to arrive when they order. Patients can be *coached* as to how, specifically, to work out when to order more equipment if these factors are explicitly discussed as part of the process of deciding on the amount of equipment with which they should be sent home. Once patient and nurse have calculated how long it could take to get supplies and the frequency of equipment usage, then the amount of equipment with which the patient should be sent home can be estimated.

PATIENT SCENARIO 8.4   Mrs Reid finds that, although they intend to order equipment soon after discharge, many patients are initially too weary to do this and days can go by without a prescription being obtained. Her preparation of Mr Earl for discharge includes helping him set up an initial equipment supply of 'a box in use and a box in hand' and teaching him how to calculate when he needs to order more supplies.

Mr Earl is using a two-piece appliance so, firstly, Mrs Reid shows him the box of flanges (bases) and the box of bags he will take home with him, indicating these on his list of equipment. She suggests that one task the Earls could complete now is to ask their GP for a second set of bags and flanges, thus ensuring the ordering system is set up early enough for supplies to arrive soon after he gets home. Mrs Earl takes his GP's list in to the doctor's receptionist, who arranges for a prescription of these particular items to be sent to the supply company in the stamped addressed envelope the Earls have also provided.

Secondly, Mrs Reid explains to him that the particular supply company she suggests he uses normally processes prescriptions within 48 hours of receipt but, if he wants to use their cutting service, it might be wise to allow 3 days for the supply company's activities. Mr Earl thinks he will normally post his prescription request to his GP with an envelope addressed to the supply company so that the prescription can be posted directly to the supply company. She encourages him to allow enough time to accommodate any delays in the postal system or the promptness with which his doctor completes the prescription, adding another 4 days to the overall timeframe. Given the likelihood that none of the procedure will take place at weekends Mr Earl says he will set up a schedule that includes at least 10 days for getting his supplies.

At this early postoperative stage it is difficult to know how often Mr Earl will need to change his flanges. The frequency of his changes in hospital has been more influenced by the need to give him practice in self-care than any signals that they had come to the end of their useful life. He wants to persevere with preparing his own equipment so Mrs Reid suggests he calculates on daily bag changes, with a few spare, plus alternate day flange changes. This system of calculation should give him some spare flanges per order in case he spoils any during preparation as it is likely that he will actually only need to change his flange every third or fourth day. Mr Earl now knows how many bags and flanges there are in each box, his possible rate of using each, and the timespan he should allow for between requesting and receiving prescribed equipment. This information enables him to identify when he should order more supplies, and adapt the frequency and amount of orders in line with his actual equipment usage.

In many instances the steps described in this *scenario* could be speeded up by the use of faxes and email to convey the equipment order and, where a cutting service is used, a template of the patient's stoma size. Many suppliers deliver equipment within 24 hours if they have it in stock when the order arrives (Black 2000). Once patients have set up their preferred supply system they can get more accurate information about the timeframe they should allow when obtaining future supplies.

This type of detailed preparation has several advantages. Firstly, it builds patients' confidence in their ability to manage their supply system well. Secondly, it enables nurses to identify (and justify) the amount of equipment they should give to individual patients in order that supplies from hospital and community sources are dovetailed. Thirdly, early and appropriate requesting of supplies enables doctors, supply companies, and chemists to provide prescriptions easily and efficiently via their normal system. Anxieties over running short of equipment are avoided.

GAINING HELP AND SUPPORT: STRATEGIES PATIENTS NEED TO BE ABLE TO USE

Helping patients identify supportive strategies and people should be an integral part of preparing them for going home. Many patients experience changes in mood and emotions that they describe as worrying and difficult to handle because of their intensity and/or unpredictability, and also because they are not in tune with how they usually feel and behave. Telling patients that some of these experiences may happen to them, and inviting them to think of people who might be supportive on such occasions as well as generally, can help them consider who they might request help from if they needed it. Such thinking is easier when it is not being done in the middle of a stressful occasion. This strategy therefore helps many patients feel better prepared to cope if problems do arise later. It is also helpful for patients to know that, although such experiences are a fairly common feature of many people's early months at home, they will diminish in frequency and intensity as their rehabilitation progresses.

When the question of support is raised many patients focus on identifying the kinds of support that family, friends, and others may be willing to provide. However, the crucial issue is what does each patient *need* in the way of support to help them in their individual rehabilitation. It is therefore generally more helpful to ask patients to firstly identify what kinds of support they would like to have when they go home, and then to think of who might provide those particular supportive measures. This strategy also allows patients to interpret the term 'support' in any way they wish. For some, support may mean contact with people who allow them to discuss their illness, surgery, fears, feelings and experiences. Other patients may view supportive action as help from friends to return to normal activities such as meeting for coffee, or providing a lift to and from the pub to meet colleagues after work.

Generally, the process of getting support involves individuals in:

- identifying the types of support they want
- identifying what they want/expect the results of such support to be
- identifying the degree and frequency of each type of support that they want
- identifying people from whom they would like or not like support, and the type of support they would/would not welcome from each person
- identifying strategies for getting the desired support
- learning any new strategies necessary for (a) seeking and getting the chosen types of support and (b) declining unacceptable types of support
- obtaining the supportive measures they want
- evaluating whether these supportive measures produce the end product they want.

The focus on what the patient wants supportive measures to provide him with in the first few weeks at home (e.g. comfort, confidence to go out socially, freedom to express feelings) means that he can be helped to think of a number of strategies which could provide him with the wished-for end result. This enhances the likelihood that he will get what he wants from at least one of them. Additionally, people are often more willing to provide some help when they know they are not the only person being called upon to provide it, which can be experienced as burdensome.

Pringle & Swan (2001) found that 53% of the patients in their study were still experiencing fatigue one year after surgery for colorectal cancer. It is therefore important to encourage patients to identify ways of pacing themselves and using help from others to minimise fatigue.

PATIENT SCENARIO 8.5   Mr and Mrs Earl have been talking to Nurse Beech about how they will manage when he first goes home. They have decided that one priority will be for Mr Earl not to get overtired, and to increase his activities gradually. They think Mr Earl should spend a couple of hours resting on his bed after lunch each day, for at least his first month at home. However, Nurse Beech remembers that both Mr and Mrs Earl said they had difficulty coping with visits from their neighbours. They might need help to deal with that problem or Mr Earl's 'rest' could be spent worrying about whether his wife is having difficulties with visiting neighbours. Nurse Beech therefore starts by gently asking whether this could be a situation that might arise. The Earls agree they need to find new ways of handling their neighbours' visits if he is to achieve his goal of adequate rest.

Mrs Earl has three goals: to help her husband get sufficient rest; to stop the neighbours visiting so often; to get the neighbours to visit at convenient times without feeling she is being rude to them. She has mentioned several times how guilty she feels when a neighbour visits to offer help and her inward response is an ungrateful wish that they would visit less frequently or offer the help at different times. Nurse Beech helps Mrs Earl work out ways of telling different neighbours how much she appreciates their willingness to help, and to link this to assertively asking them not to telephone or visit between 2 and 4 p.m., identifying this as one way in which they could be really helpful. Mrs Earl tries out this strategy when a friend telephones the next day to say she will be round to see them as soon as Mr Earl gets home. She was pleased with the way the friend accepted what she said, and noticed that she felt more comfortable having asked directly for what she wanted.

Mr Earl wants to work out how he can have contact with his friends without getting exhausted. He says he often doesn't realise he is getting tired until he has overdone things. With Nurse Beech's help he works out a schedule for stopping briefly at four set times a day, noticing how he is feeling, and discussing this with his nurse. This helps him recognise early physical and psychological cues which indicate that he is beginning to feel tired, and decide what he wants to do about that. As Nurse Beech documents this goal in the nursing records other staff know to encourage him to monitor himself, rather than dismiss him as a hypochondriac. Mr Earl develops some skill in realistically pacing himself, and planning rest periods between activities, which will be useful to him when he goes home. (See sections on contracting below and 'just do's' in Ch. 9 for additional strategies.)

Mr Earl says the purpose of seeing his friends is to exchange views on common hobbies and interests, and to help him feel he is getting back into the normal world and away from his illness. Further discussion reveals that several of his friends usually stay overnight when they visit because of the distance and travelling time involved. He and Mrs Earl do likewise on return visits. He realises he will not be strong enough, or able to sit for long enough to travel himself for some time after his abdomino-perineal excision of rectum. Both Mr and Mrs Earl think it would also be too tiring to have people to stay during his initial time at home. Nurse Beech encourages Mr Earl to think of other ways in which these friends could maintain contact and provide the kind of interaction he wants. After some thought he decides to write to three friends and ask each of them if they would be willing to arrange regular telephone calls with him, alternating who makes the call, instead of visiting during his first few weeks at home. He thinks this will be acceptable to his friends because it will not cost any more than the visits would have done, and because of the concern they have expressed about him since he became ill.

Many patients say they have difficulty recognising when they 'should' ask for help or support. They usually recognise when they are concerned about a situation, whether it is how they are feeling or an aspect of managing their stoma care. However, they seem to believe it is only justifiable or acceptable to ask for help if the person they seek help from classifies their concern as a problem that warrants help. This belief can stop them from seeking help, and also leaves them in a position where they continue to worry.

Before patients go home it is important to help them clarify in their own minds:

1. under what circumstances do they think they might benefit from contacting other people to obtain help and/or support

2. who they could contact
3. how they could contact these people, and when
4. how they normally stop themselves from asking for, or getting, the kinds of help and support they want.
5. how they could stop preventing themselves from getting the kind of help and support they need.

One of the most powerful tools to encourage patients to seek help when they want it is to validate their concern as important enough to warrant help. This can be done by explaining to them that if they are worried or concerned about something then that is a good-enough reason to ask for help. The issue is not, for example, whether the peristomal skin is bad enough to warrant help, or whether their fears/feelings are severe enough to justify getting help. The issue to be dealt with is that *they experience their situation as problematic, and their need is to experience their situation as less of a problem, or not of concern*. Once this concept is understood and accepted by patients and their families it encourages them to seek help at an early stage, and thus prevent their anxiety and the situation from building up to larger proportions over time.

Although some health professionals think this process could mean they become overloaded with telephone calls and requests for visits, this rarely seems to happen. What often happens is that patients, who experience that their ability to judge when they need help is accepted, come to believe they can also use the help and information they get when they identify problems. Frequently that trust in their abilities is translated into action which resolves or reduces their problem. This success gives patients information, or feedback, on the ways they assessed and managed that problem. It often increases their willingness to try these approaches first if other problems arise later, before seeking help. In other words, they become more skilled at assessing and handling problems.

When patients do not seek help, or their concerns are met with premature reassurance that all is well without establishing what exactly is problematic for the individual, then they do not get the information or coaching they need to learn how to assess similar situations that may arise later. In other words, such responses make it hard for patients to gain relevant skills with which to assess and manage problems.

Sometimes patients who are adamant while in hospital that they will not need the services of, for example, community nurses or home care assistants, realise once they are at home that such services would be beneficial. It may make it easier for them to admit that they do want help if they have a good idea of what help can be obtained from healthcare and social service personnel, and how to request it.

Patients who do not want help from such services after they go home are unlikely to listen to information about the help that could be given if they think pressure is being put on them to accept help when they do not want it. Acknowledgement that a patient's rejection of such help has been heard and accepted by staff (however reluctantly) is an *essential* first step in any provision of information. Once patients feel their point of view is understood and accepted they are likely to be more willing to listen to a brief outline of help they could get 'if they ever needed it'. Such offering of useful information about resources can result in patients who are better prepared for discharge. Additionally, staff who would have preferred to arrange help from one or more of the services may find it easier to accept and work to support patients' decisions when they know they have the information they need if they wish to request help later.

Many people stop themselves from asking for help and support in their lives by believing, and acting on, one or both of two common myths or beliefs. People with stomas are as prone to doing this as any other human being. Recognition of the processes that result from these beliefs, and of the ways in which such beliefs may be stated, is an essential first step towards encouraging patients to develop more effective methods of seeking and accepting the help that they require. The following statements are *examples* of how such beliefs may be voiced, and many similar versions exist.

I should know when the 'right' time is to contact my friend/relative/doctor/stoma care nurse, etc. so that I do not interfere with other (more important) things that they are doing.

Since the person seeking contact or help does not have a crystal ball to look into and see what others are doing they cannot identify the perfect time at which to approach that person. The end result often is either they do not attempt to make contact at all, or they upset themselves so much worrying over whether they have got the timing right that the contact is less beneficial than it could have been.

Other people should know when I want help and support without my having to tell them what I want and/or when I want it. If I have to ask for what I want it means the help or support I get is not as valuable, because it is not freely offered. Additionally, the person who I've asked for help/support from doesn't really care about me, or genuinely want to help, or they would have done so without my having to ask for it.

The central belief here is that other people can (and should) identify when someone (e.g. partner/friend/colleague/patient) needs help and what form that help or support should take, without that person indicating they want or need it.

Checking for the presence or absence of such beliefs can be a useful part of the overall discussion with patients about how they will look after themselves and promote their social, psychological and physical wellbeing when they go home.

The question 'are there any ways you stop yourself from getting help and support from family and friends?' often exposes the presence of the first belief, or a similar version of it, in the reply that is given.

A second question 'how do you feel when you get the help/support that you have asked for?' is likely to elicit a response indicating the presence or absence of the second belief.

The use of contracts can be a helpful process to encourage patients to abandon these ways of behaving and instead ask for, and value, the appropriate help and support they need and get. Acting as though they are valuable people whose needs are important also encourages people to view themselves that way.

PATIENT SCENARIO 8.6   Mrs Jones and her stoma care nurse are discussing her discharge, planned to take place in two days. Mrs Reid has discovered that Mrs Jones thinks it will be quite hard for her to keep cheerful during the day when her husband and neighbours are at work, her children at school, and she will be on her own. Mrs Reid has also noticed that Mrs Jones is hesitant about trusting her own judgement of whether her peristomal skin is in a satisfactory condition. When Mrs Jones is reminded that she can telephone Mrs Reid if she wants help or support she says she is worried that she will phone at a time when Mrs Reid is busy. Mrs Reid picks up this cue that Mrs Jones may stop herself from telephoning by trying to work out first when would be the 'right' time to phone, and asks Mrs Jones if this might happen. When Mrs Jones agrees that this is a distinct possibility Mrs Reid

tentatively suggests that this might be what Mrs Jones does when she knows she wants to telephone someone but doesn't actually do it. As the conversation continues it becomes apparent that Mrs Jones also assumes that friends and family will know when she is feeling low, and therefore know when to contact her, even though she rarely tells them how she is feeling. Mrs Jones begins to identify more clearly the beliefs and processes she sometimes uses when she knows she wants support. This helps her understand that these are some of the reasons why she often feels unsupported, and that she can take steps to change this situation.

Mrs Reid suggests that she and Mrs Jones might make *a contract* which would help each of them know what part they would play in promoting the overall goal that Mrs Jones would get support from Mrs Reid when she needed it. The *contract* they decide upon together is:

- Mrs Jones will take responsibility for recognising when she wants to contact Mrs Reid, and will telephone and ask for what she wants (e.g. advice; a listening ear while she expresses feelings).
- If Mrs Reid is not available Mrs Jones will leave a message on the office answer phone, asking for her phone call to be returned and indicating how urgent her need is.
- Additionally, Mrs Jones will *stop* trying to take responsibility for deciding whether the timing of her phone call fits in with whatever Mrs Reid is doing at that time.
- Mrs Reid will take responsibility for assessing her own situation whenever Mrs Jones telephones. She will decide whether she is really available then to talk to Mrs Jones, or whether she could give better quality attention by arranging another time when both of them could focus on Mrs Jones' situation. If the phone call comes at a time when she is not free to give adequate time and attention Mrs Reid will tell Mrs Jones this, and negotiate an alternative time with Mrs Jones.

Now that Mrs Jones has had the experience of making a contract with Mrs Reid she is in a more informed position to consider whether making contracts with other people might also be helpful. Mrs Reid encourages her to do this by asking whether she can think of other people she doesn't telephone because she can't work out the right time to do so. Mrs Jones identifies two friends with whom she used to work. She says she never knows when to phone them as she worries in case their babies are being fed or would be sleeping, and her call would disturb them.

Mrs Reid encourages Mrs Jones to think whether anything she has learned from making their contract might help her find an acceptable way of contacting Val and Joan. Mrs Jones decides that she will tell her friends that, in order for her to feel comfortable phoning them, she needs them to tell her honestly if she phones at an inconvenient time and arrange a better time instead. Mrs Reid supports this idea. She also suggests that Mrs Jones could ask for clarification about her friends' general time boundaries for ordinary (non-emergency) phone calls, such as how early in the morning and how late at night it is acceptable to phone, and whether there are regular times when they have their meals and would prefer not to be disturbed. Mrs Jones thinks

this is a good idea, saying she will phone them both during her first week at home to set this up. Mrs Reid makes a mental note to ask Mrs Jones whether she has used this strategy and what the results were when she comes for her outpatients appointment, so she can offer congratulations or further help as appropriate.

There are a number of other situations which patients often find they have to cope with in their early days at home. These are best discussed initially with patients before they leave hospital, so they have some preparation for dealing with the situations if they arise. However, these situations, and the ways patients choose to respond to them, are likely to change as rehabilitation progresses. These issues are therefore discussed in Chapter 9 as part of the overall rehabilitative process. They include helping patients deal with enquiries about their condition and surgery, and helping patients structure their time and activities to promote rehabilitation.

References

Black P K 2000 Holistic stoma care. Baillière Tindall and RCN, Edinburgh

Ewing G 1989 The nursing preparation of stoma patients for self-care. Journal of Advanced Nursing 14:411–420

Pringle W, Swan E 2001 Continuing care after discharge from hospital for stoma patients. British Journal of Nursing 10(19):1274–1288

Swan E 2001 Waste disposal for the ostomate in the community. Nursing Standard 97(40):51–52

Chapter 9

Towards rehabilitation

Brigid Breckman

Rehabilitative stoma care involves helping patients deal with the combined effects of their total surgery; their condition and the degree to which it has been treated; and the presence and management of their stoma. The aim of this approach is that patients will achieve their rehabilitative goals and experience their lives as being of good quality. As more research studies identify the experiences of patients and their families during and after stoma surgery their findings are changing our perception of:

- the qualities and capabilities we must demonstrate in order for our care to aid patients' rehabilitation
- the information and skills that patients should normally acquire in order to promote their recovery and handle problems effectively.

MAXIMISING RECOVERY

Black (2000) reported that patients in the Montreux Study who regarded their stoma care nurse as having a genuine interest in them had a significantly higher quality of life index (QLI) score than those who had a poor relationship with the stoma care nurse. Between discharge and 3-month follow-up analysis showed that if the patient's relationship with the stoma care nurse worsened, their overall QLI score increased only slightly. Where the relationship improved there was a marked increase in their QLI score. Confidence in changing their appliance also affected patients' QLI score. At 3 months patients whose confidence in appliance management decreased also had decreased QLI scores. Patients feeling increased confidence in appliance changes also had higher QLI scores.

Patients are likely to believe we are genuinely interested in them when we enquire about their normal lifestyle and rehabilitative goals and help them gain knowledge and skills required to achieve them. Explicitly teaching patients and their families to use knowledge and skills strategically in order to achieve their chosen goals helps them develop a greater sense of control over their situation as well as more confident self-care abilities (Metcalf 1999). The following processes help us convey our willingness as well as ability to help people maximise their recovery.

Firstly, we can use the information in Chapters 19 and 20, and the approaches described in Chapter 7, to encourage each patient to tell us about the aspects of their lifestyle they want to resume or change as they rehabilitate. This process helps staff and patient *create a shared mental map* of what 'rehabilitation' could be like for that individual. We use this map to inform our care and patients' rehabilitative activities, and to monitor whether these are enabling patients to achieve their chosen goals.

Secondly, we should *link information and skills we are teaching patients to specific goals or aspects of their lives* as an integral part of our teaching, so we enable them to understand how one relates to the other (e.g. Nurse Ash's work with Mrs Jones – Patient scenario 8.1 in Ch. 8).

Thirdly, we can explicitly *demonstrate how we are using knowledge* to inform our decisions so patients get a real sense of what this capability is like in action (e.g. use of summarising, Ch. 7).

Fourthly, we can *coach patients to apply knowledge and skills* by asking them how, specifically, they might use particular information and skills to achieve a goal or manage a potential problem that they have identified (e.g. Mrs Reid's work with Mrs Jones – Patient scenario 8.6 in Ch. 8).

The first three steps of this process can be used whenever we are providing stoma care, with the fourth step being added as patients acquire sufficient knowledge to be able to apply it (e.g. Nurse Willow's work with Mrs Boot – Patient scenario 8.2 in Ch. 8).

The experience of discovering that you or your partner has an illness necessitating such major surgery can be bewildering for both. Northouse et al (1999) studied patients with colonic cancer and their spouses. How and when they responded to the cancer and its implications varied between patients and spouses, reminding us that our timing of the information and support we give must be tailored to people's individual needs. Patients wanted more preparation and better discharge teaching on colo-

stomy management. Both patients and spouses wanted more guidance on:

- the expected course of recovery
- how to manage their changing roles and responsibilities at different stages of rehabilitation
- the type of treatments that would be given
- strategies to manage complications.

We require a substantial knowledge and skill base if we are to meet the needs of patients and their families like those in Northouse et al's research. Information must be conveyed helpfully for people to be able to understand it, particularly if they may experience it as 'bad news' or a 'difficult' issue. The approaches listed above and those discussed in Chapter 7 can all be used to support and inform relatives as well as patients, as indicated in several of the *patient scenarios*.

The quality of the information we give and the ways in which we give it have substantial implications for patients' subsequent wellbeing. Pringle & Swan (2001) found that patients who were dissatisfied with the information they were given (whether this was a lot or a little) were more likely to experience depression postoperatively. More than half of the patients who had little understanding of what they were told were depressed, compared to less than a quarter of the patients who said they had understood what they were told. This means we must ensure patients find the *amount* of information they are given as well as *what* they are told is congruent with what they think they need, and easy to understand and use.

When patients and families recognise we are linking information and skills to their lifestyle and rehabilitative goals it becomes easier for them to accept their relevance. People take in information better if we provide it with the level of detail they prefer. In neurolinguistic programming (NLP) this is known as 'chunk size' (Dilts 1994, p 197). It is easier to give people the amount of information that is right for them if we identify whether they like more specific, detailed information (small chunk) or generalised, less detailed descriptions or overviews (large chunk). *For example,* we can explicitly ask patients preoperatively how much detail they would like in the information booklet they are given before surgery *and* whether their partner likes 'lots of specific detail or a more general overview without much detail'. Their response enables us to identify the best style of booklet for them and an alternative one for their partner if they prefer different chunk sized material. Subsequently we can adapt information that each individual requires so it is provided in the style best suited to their needs.

The amount of information and skills patients deem it necessary to acquire also depends on what they think rehabilitation entails. In the past it was often assumed that if physical rehabilitation occurred then psychological rehabilitation would generally happen as well. However, research indicates that many patients who are engaging in a range of family, social and work activities also say that their feelings about themselves and their stomas remain problematic to them about a year after their operation (Wade 1989, Pringle & Swan 2001). This is hardly surprising given that most people take a couple of years to come to terms with major loss, and that stoma surgery entails a number of losses (see Ch. 20). However, it sends an unmistakable message that the ways in which rehabilitation is promoted and monitored must actively support the achievement of both physical and psychological recovery.

Given the speed with which patients undergo surgery and are discharged home, and the physical and psychological demands on them during that period, the goal of helping them manage the situation they are in *and* prepare to rehabilitate themselves may seem overly ambitious. However, it is also true that stoma patients have minimal contact with the healthcare team during the 1–2 years it takes many people to rehabilitate fully. Our help and support during that period, however expert and committed, will be intermittent. The daily task of promoting and achieving rehabilitation lies in the hands of individual patients and any family and friends who support them. We have a responsibility to use the time when we are most in contact with them (in hospital and their initial weeks at home) to ensure patients get the kind of preparation they say they need. This preparation must go beyond providing information and helping patients begin to gain skills as isolated capabilities. It is essential that we help them learn *to use knowledge and skills purposefully to achieve key rehabilitative processes*. These include:

- managing their stoma care
- planning and pacing their gradually increasing activities so they promote their chosen rehabilitative goals and lifestyle
- monitoring their physical and psychological progress towards rehabilitation
- recognising problems and obtaining help to resolve or manage them effectively.

PROMOTING SELF-EFFICACY

Bekkers et al (1996) studied the role of self-efficacy in stoma patients' adaptation process. They focused on patients' expectations of their ability to perform stoma care. They found that patients who developed confidence in their ability to manage stoma care as well as competence had fewer psychosocial problems in their first year after surgery. White (1999) suggests that, in addition to helping patients acquire skills, their confidence levels should be monitored. Patients can be encouraged to keep a diary recording their levels of confidence in completing specific steps of stoma care. This helps them notice progress as well as alerting patients and healthcare staff to areas where further help is needed.

In most situations people draw on previous experiences to help them deal with current events. This helps us make sense of what is, or should be, happening and enables us to use knowledge and skills that we feel confident can help us. However, planning and pacing activities after major surgery, and working out how these will aid achievement of their longer-term goals, are new experiences for many patients. McVey et al (2001) found that patients having stoma surgery for cancer experienced lower personal control. When we help patients plan activities and thereby achieve goals that promote their recovery they generally gain more than an ability to complete particular tasks. They enhance their ability to manage their lives and any problems more resourcefully. This increases many patients' sense of personal control and confidence.

A balance is needed so we prepare patients sufficiently for difficulties they are most likely to encounter whilst avoiding making them unduly anxious. There is evidence that problems are common in the first few months after surgery and that substantial numbers of patients continue to report difficulties a year after their operation. Many of the problems which Wade found that patients were experiencing in 1989 were also being commonly experienced a decade later by the colostomists in Pringle & Swan's (2001) research. The main ones are listed in Table 9.1.

The effects of physical symptoms on the quality of patients' lives and on their ability to engage in a normal lifestyle must not be underestimated. Wade (1989) found that patients' physical state was strongly related to their subjective appraisal of the quality of their lives, the degree to which they had resumed their social activities, and their psychological adjustment one year after having stoma surgery.

Table 9.1 Percentage of patients experiencing problems 1 year after surgery

Problem	Wade (1989)	Pringle & Swan (2001)
Pain	35.8	41.4
Severe pain	10.0	8.6
Backache	35.0	30.0
Fatigue	46.7	52.9
Flatus	68.6	54.3
Bad odour	35.0	37.2
Indigestion	24.2	21.5
Constipation	25.8	7.2
Diarrhoea	25.8	12.9
Sweating	10.8	14.3
Urinary incontinence (patients with bowel stomas)	13.3	11.5

Other symptoms were also recorded.

Rehabilitative care must therefore now *routinely* include helping patients acquire the information and capabilities they need to deal with these main areas, unless there are overriding reasons why they should be excluded from a particular patient's care. Thus sections on flatus and odour are an integral part of normal stoma care in Chapters 4, 5 and 16, and information on managing constipation and diarrhoea through dietary means is provided in patient handouts in Chapter 16 (Appendix 16.1). These problems are also discussed in Chapter 21.

PACING ACTIVITIES THROUGH TIME AND ENERGY MANAGEMENT

With approximately half of all patients reporting fatigue a year after surgery (Table 9.1) it is important to help patients manage the way they use their time and energy effectively. This includes helping them plan realistic rehabilitative goals, and pace and monitor how they are achieving them. The concept of *'just do's'* can be used to help patients learn to specifically monitor their levels of activity and rest, especially in the first few weeks at home. A *'just do'* is something a person engages in before they meet their own needs (e.g. for a rest; cup of tea; contact with a friend). Examples include: 'I'll just put the washing on; clear the table; clean the bedroom; put that shelf up; trim the hedge; wash my hair … before I ….' An enquiry about an individual patient's just do's usually elicits a reluctant grin and examples of their personal preferences!

Patients who find it difficult to look after their own needs or view them as equally important as other people's needs may benefit from making a specific *contract* with a member of staff or family member. *For example*: 'I will not do more than two just do's together without then having 15 minutes looking after my own needs for (e.g.) rest/relaxation/time to think or enjoy a book or some music'. It is important for us to indicate we take a contract seriously. Firstly, we can promise to enquire how it is going when we next see patients. This encourages patients to monitor how they are keeping their contracts. Secondly, we should actually ask whether patients are curtailing their 'just do's' so any problems can be discussed. Changes to contracts can be made as patients' capabilities and energy levels change.

Information about patients' normal sleeping patterns and how they think they will spend their time in the early days at home can also be used to help patients and families plan sufficient rest and time to themselves coupled with some social and home activities. Encouraging patients to monitor their own energy levels and use that awareness to decide what they will or will not do can be coupled with some guidelines about sensible levels of activity. It is better to give advice about suitable and unsuitable activities *after* patients have identified how they think they might spend their time in the first few weeks at home so advice can be specifically related to their particular plans. *For example*: embargoes on moving or carrying anything heavy can be linked to patients' plans to do the shopping or use a washing machine or vacuum cleaner. They can then be encouraged to think of ways in which they could get help to complete such activities. This kind of specific discussion will enable patients to develop their skills in monitoring their energy levels and physical capabilities and matching these against the activities they want to follow. They can use these skills to reassess their needs and capabilities as these change, which is why this approach generally supports rehabilitation more effectively than a long list of do's and don'ts.

Many patients devise their own gradually extending plan of activities and follow them, particularly when they have family and friends to support and help them. It may be wise, however, to enquire in more detail whether patients in certain circumstances need more specific help. These include:

- people who have led a curtailed lifestyle for a considerable time before surgery
- the frail elderly who may have limitations in mobility and general physical stamina
- people living alone
- people who do not have family or friends to engage in or support their rehabilitative plans and activities.

Helping such patients identify and achieve specific, realistic goals and celebrate those achievements is an important part of rehabilitative care. These might include helping someone find and use a source of help (e.g. a lift in a neighbour's car to their local place of worship), or to enjoy rather than endure a social engagement with friends (e.g. finding a restaurant with really comfortable seats or a wide range of foods from which they can confidently choose a suitable meal). The concept of strokes and stroke balance (see Ch. 20) can be used to help patients accept the importance of paying attention to their psychological needs and social activities.

As Table 9.1. shows, a considerable number of patients experience pain and backache a year after surgery. It is important that healthcare staff are aware of patients' pain and accept their account of it as valid so that the implications of its presence can be assessed and suitable treatment offered (Middleton 2004). Bird (2003) provides a useful account of various pain assessment tools. It is important to identify which assessment methods particular patients find easiest to use as this differs between individuals. These should be used systematically so patients can report whether more than one type and/or location of pain is being experienced, and the degree to which pain-relieving measures are effective. Descriptions of pain and acceptance or rejection

of pain management strategies may be influenced by patients' cultural background (Henley & Schott 1999; see also Ch. 20).

Pain is often linked to experiences of fatigue and/or anxiety in that the presence of pain can lead to someone feeling more tired or more anxious. Alternatively, anxiety and over-tiredness themselves can increase the levels of pain that some patients experience. Enquiries as to when pain occurs may reveal it is generally during or after certain events or activities or at a particular time of day. This information can then be used when considering how to reduce or resolve the pain.

Patients may be taking medication prescribed by their doctor or obtained from other sources. They should be given information about how analgesics work and the dosage and frequency of administration that is therefore suitable, any side effects likely to arise from pain medication, and how these may be dealt with (see Ch. 17). When patients have such information they are then in a position to work out how they can get the maximum pain relief with the minimum side effects.

Patients may already have strategies which they tend to use to reduce pain or make it more bearable, such as using a heat pad to ease menstrual or joint pain. They can be encouraged to try out their usual strategies and assess their effectiveness for any pain experienced during their rehabilitation. Other non-invasive strategies such as diversion, guided imagery, and cutaneous stimulation can also be learned and used by nurses, patients, and their families (McCaffery & Pasero 1999, Rushworth 1994, Williams 1997). Audiocassettes that combine a relaxation exercise and messages to encourage pain reduction are available. Some self-help books provide transcripts for people to record their own messages to aid relaxation, pain relief and/or a sense of wellbeing (e.g. Battino 2001). These help some patients feel more relaxed and pain-free. Generally patients are likely to feel more confident about managing or resolving any pain if they have a variety of strategies with which to improve their situation.

HELPING PATIENTS MANAGE THOUGHTS AND QUESTIONS ABOUT THEIR SITUATION

The rehabilitative process is not an orderly progression from component (a) to component (b) and so on. Most patients find that thoughts, feelings and actions arising from one aspect of their rehabilitation affect how they feel, think and act in other areas (White 1999). Sometimes particular issues are brought sharply into focus when patients are faced with questions about their surgery or condition. These may come from neighbours, friends or family soon after they go home. Questions or assumptions by colleagues as to when, or if, they will return to work may also challenge them to examine more closely the implications of their surgery and the condition that made it necessary. Such situations can be quite difficult to handle, especially if patients have not realised they might arise, or considered how they might like to respond to them.

Before patients go home it is often helpful if we invite them to consider who might ask questions, and what kind of information they might (a) want to provide and (b) not want to give. This helps patients discuss how they can respond to such questions. It also invites them to ask for information about their condition, surgery or further treatment, and to discuss their thoughts and feelings if they so wish. Some patients welcome help to develop explanations about their surgery, stoma and/or condition which they could use if questions do arise. This can help them feel more confident about handling enquiries, as can help to develop ways of assertively refusing to give information or discuss their situation. Some patients gain sufficient confidence from discussion while others may benefit from also role-playing a situation that is likely to arise. In many instances this kind of pre-discharge discussion and topping-up of their information about their stoma, condition and/or surgery enables patients to take the first steps in coming to terms with their situation.

PATIENT SCENARIO 9.1 Nurse Beech asks Mr Earl whether he has thought about how he will cope with neighbours' enquiries related to his stay in hospital. Mr Earl says it is none of their business, and he does not want to discuss his situation with them. However, when Nurse Beech reminds him that he will still have to deal with the questions, he begins to talk of one neighbour who always wants to know every detail of people's illnesses and operations and then talks about them all around the neighbourhood. Mr Earl admits that telling this person he did not want to discuss his last operation had not stopped the neighbour continuing to ask lots of questions. After some discussion Mr Earl decides that what

he wants to tell his neighbour is that he is not willing to discuss his operation or the reasons why he had it, and that he wants his neighbour to stop asking questions about these things. Nurse Beech teaches him how to phrase this information assertively, and how to use a 'broken record' technique of repeating his wishes calmly and firmly whenever the neighbour persists with his questioning (Dickson 1982).

The following day Mr Earl discusses with his stoma care nurse what he might say about his situation to Alan, his nephew. He wants Alan to know why he has had an operation, and what that operation entailed. Mrs Reid suggests they cover these issues in two sessions, as he still gets easily tired and then finds it difficult to take in information. He chooses to start with what the operation entailed. She first asks Mr Earl to tell her what he thinks was done during his operation, explaining this is so they can identify any gaps in his information, or any bits which he hasn't really understood. She notices his assumption that removal of some of his bowel will mean he has to eat quite a curtailed diet. Although he has in fact already been told that he will be able to eat a full range of foods he obviously either has not understood or has not believed this. Mrs Reid gives Mr Earl an extra copy of the booklet about living with a colostomy for Alan. She uses the diagrams in the booklet to show Mr Earl that his operation (abdomino-perineal excision of rectum) still leaves him with most of his bowel, linking this with a brief outline of how digestion takes place. Since Mr Earl is keen to give Alan accurate information he is in a better frame of mind to hear and remember this information than he was when similar information was given preoperatively (when he was very anxious) and earlier postoperatively (when all he could think of was that food made him windy and uncomfortable). Mr Earl agrees to start trying a wider range of foods while he is still in hospital, so that he and the ward staff can assess their effects.

Rehabilitation is more likely to be aided if patients are allowed to discuss their situation and the meaning it has for them if and/or when they want to do so (O'Neill & Leedham 2001). Sometimes an issue is raised fairly openly by a patient, as in the *scenario* above of Mr Earl saying he wants to tell his nephew why he required his operation. At other times signals that patients want to discuss their situation may lie in the way they raise other topics; for example, saying they are wondering whether they should find out about their company's early retirement scheme, or asking whether they will be well enough next year to go abroad on holiday. It is important not to assume that such statements are definite indications that patients want to discuss the implications of their disease or prognosis, but rather that we should be aware that this could be a possibility.

Cues that nurses or other members of the health-care team are willing to discuss concerns are often most helpful if we give them as *statements of intent or information*, because these leave patients free to respond in a variety of ways. Each of us can develop our own cues of encouragement, depending on our willingness and ability to handle different topics and styles of interaction. The following statements are *examples* which you could use as a starting point for developing your own invitations to patients and their families:

- Quite often people find it helpful to talk over how they think their operation will affect their lives. Sometimes they talk to friends or family, or they may choose one of the staff looking after them.
- Asking any questions you want about your condition or operation is OK with me. If I don't know the answers I will say so, and we can discuss how to get that information.
- Talking through any concerns you have is an important part of the care you are entitled to get. It is not an optional extra for us to provide when the rest of the work is done.
- I'm here to listen if you want to talk. If there is not enough time now, then we can plan more time later.
- If you want to talk about your situation and how you are feeling then I'm willing to listen and help in any way I can. It is OK with me for you to talk when you are ready to, and not talk when you don't want to do so.

Beliefs about patients' rights to know about their situation, and the desirability or undesirability of discussing topics such as diagnosis, prognosis, side effects of treatment can be affected by the cultural and social backgrounds of patients, their families, and healthcare team members (see Ch. 19). The open invitation implicit in the above statements can lead patients to reveal or seek to hide complex concerns and needs. Our professional attitudes, roles and competence affect the degree to which we can handle their responses at the level they require. Thought must be given to processes we could use to ensure our actions are appropriate in such circumstances.

Many nurses and doctors say they find it difficult to take part in discussions with patients about their disease and prognosis, sexual concerns or impairment, or to allow patients to talk about how they see and feel about their circumstances. Lack of information, lack of adequate training in counselling and other facilitative responses, and uncertainty as to whose role it is to handle such discussions are often given as reasons for staff difficulties in responding to patients' needs to talk about these areas. Patients often pick up cues (particularly non-verbal ones) indicating a staff member's difficulty, but may assume that the cues are telling them that it is not permissible to talk about these topics. Some patients go on to assume that it is generally not all right to raise such topics with any nurse or doctor, and behave accordingly.

If patients are discouraged from expressing their fears and feelings, gaining the information they want, and/or discussing concerns and issues they end up with two problems. Firstly, they still have the topic or concern they wanted to raise initially. Secondly, they now have the added problem of deciding what that discouragement was meant to tell them. For example, did it imply they should have asked someone else and, if so, how do they learn who to ask? Alternatively, did the discouraging cues indicate that raising such topics or expressing such feelings or needs is an activity that will generally be unacceptable to other people, and therefore something they should not do? It can be quite difficult for a patient to muster the courage to approach any other members of the healthcare team.

If we do not have the knowledge, skills or psychological ability to meet the needs of a patient then it is important that we recognise and acknowledge this to be the position (White 1999). When this is done it frees us to discuss with patients who else might have the necessary knowledge and capabilities to help them get their needs met, and how this person or service and the patient could be brought together.

One very useful strategy for dealing with such circumstances is for us to *separate* the belief that patients should receive the information and psychological support they need from the belief that this means we must provide it ourselves. Learning to say to ourselves 'this patient has a right to the information/help they are needing *and* I do not have to provide all of it myself' can help us feel less overwhelmed or burdened by patients' requirements. It also serves as a reminder that we can fulfil our professional responsibilities by helping patients gain access to colleagues or services who can provide the kind of information or care that is required.

Generally it is helpful to say explicitly to patients that it was acceptable for them to ask for what they wanted, express how they felt, etc. This can be followed by a clear statement that we are not in a position to provide the *level* of information, help or support that the patient has asked for or we would like to see them receive. This can be coupled with an offer to discuss with them where they could get the help they require and how it could be obtained. Such statements acknowledge people's needs and indicate our desire to be helpful. They also give us a moment to get over our initial reaction at having this situation land on our plate, while preventing the patient from misinterpreting any signals of discomfort we have shown.

PATIENT SCENARIO 9.2   Six months after his abdomino-perineal excision of rectum John Fletcher has come to the hospital for his routine check-up in the outpatients department. He meets Staff Nurse Linden who looked after him when he had his operation (see Ch. 1). As he tells her how he is getting on he suddenly stops and blushes before blurting out that he has not been able to have sex with his wife since the operation and he is very upset about this. His eyes fill with tears as he says he feels he is only half the man he was, and no good to his wife now. He says he has heard from another patient that there is some operation men like him can have, and he would like to find out about it. Nurse Linden feels rather embarrassed as they are standing in a busy corridor where this conversation can easily be overheard. She is also quite anxious about how to cope with John's expression of feelings in so public a place. She finds a less public corner in the outpatients department and sits down to talk to him. She starts by saying she can see how upsetting this situation is for him, and that she believes it is important for him to get the information he needs and support to help him cope with how he is feeling. She tells him she does not have enough information about the penile implant operation to be much help to him and suggests he could talk to Mr Spender, the registrar,

about it and also clarify what his physical condition is as regards sexual ability. She offers to ask the nurse running his outpatients clinic to make sure John sees Mr Spender on this visit. This helps John Fletcher know she is taking his problem seriously and making sure he gets help.

Nurse Linden also knows she does not have either the time or the level of counselling skills she thinks John will need to help him handle his feelings about himself. She tells him she believes it is important that he gets the kind of informed support that will really help him and his wife in this situation, and that she thinks this may mean talking to someone trained to help in this area, perhaps on several occasions. She also tells John that it was fine with her that he told her about this problem but that she is not in a position to offer them the right sort of help. She suggests that once he has the information from Mr Spender he might like to talk to either Mrs Reid, his stoma care nurse, or his GP, and see if either of them could give him and his wife the right level of help. John says he feels better now she has listened to him and that he would prefer to talk to Mrs Reid when she returns from her holiday next week. He says he can ask Mr Spender for the information he wants now he knows he is the right person to ask, and Nurse Linden arranges this with the clinic nurse. Throughout their conversation Nurse Linden has used a gentle pace as she moved from one point to the next, allowing time for John to consider what she has said and comment or ask questions as he wishes. She also observes that his face and body posture are relaxing as they talk. She uses these non-verbal cues, as well as John's statement that he feels better, to evaluate that her conversation has given him enough initial help. However, his discussion with the doctor is yet to come and she does not know what the results of it might be. Before leaving him she mentions she will be on duty for the rest of the afternoon, in case he needs some more support later to tide him over until he can talk to Mrs Reid.

EVALUATING LONGER-TERM REHABILITATION

Achievement of longer-term rehabilitation is a key goal for patients. Identification of the degree to which rehabilitation is (a) being appropriately promoted and (b) achieved should therefore be included when evaluating patients' care and progress. This requires both the willingness and ability to focus on patients' experiences and the effects or outcomes our care is producing. These attributes are developed through experience as well as professional education.

Benner's (1984) research on skill development shows that inexperienced nurses focus on task completion (see Introduction to this book). As experience, knowledge and skills develop so nurses acquire the capacity to assess situations holistically and provide care that actively promotes the best outcomes for individual patients. Their commitment to provide this type and level of care grows because they recognise it is necessary for achievement of those goals/outcomes. Similar expertise and commitment is required to evaluate care in the light of patients' rehabilitative goals and experiences if we are to maximise patients' recovery.

When colleagues with such expertise describe how they collaborate with patients to evaluate their care and rehabilitation this helps others learn to do likewise. Such activities include:

- enquiring about the priorities patients give to learning particular aspects of stoma care (Persson & Fridstedt (2000)
- monitoring patients' experiences of competence and confidence in managing stoma care activities and living with a stoma (White 1999)
- reporting the effects of different approaches when teaching stoma care on patients' experience and learning (Thompson 1998)
- publishing care studies which report patients' experiences as well as the care processes used (Breckman 1986)

- using quality of life tools/questionnaires to monitor patients' wellbeing and the level of stoma care follow-up they require long term (Tappe & Johnson 2000).

The communication approaches in Chapter 7 and the collaborative styles of care described in the *patient scenarios* can help us monitor with patients the degree to which our care is supporting their current and long-term recovery. Individually and as a team, when planning, providing and documenting care we can consider the following questions:

- Are we enabling patients to identify the kind of rehabilitation they want?
- Have we accurately understood the key goals/outcomes this person wants to achieve?
- Have we identified how the patient, family and staff will recognise whether goals are being achieved or not?
- What strategies are we using to support patients' achievement of particular goals? Are they working effectively?
- Are patients learning to use the information and skills we are teaching them strategically, to promote their recovery, wellbeing and goals?
- Are our activities, and those of our patients, resulting in the outcomes they want?
- Is each individual achieving the best quality of life possible, given their surgery, condition, and any side effects resulting from them?

Whether patients' medical treatment is curative or palliative, and wherever we are providing care, these questions can help us respond constructively to their experiences and needs and keep our focus person-centred.

References

Battino R 2001 Coping. Crown House Publishing, Carmarthen, Wales

Bekkers M J, van Knippenberg F C, van den Borne H W et al 1996 Prospective evaluation of psychosocial adaptation to stoma surgery: the role of self-efficacy. Psychosomatic Medicine 58(2):183–191

Benner P 1984 From novice to expert. Addison-Wesley, Menlo Park, CA

Bird J 2003 Selection of pain measurement tools. Nursing Standard 18(13):33–39

Black P K 2000 Holistic stoma care. Baillière Tindall and RCN, Edinburgh

Breckman B 1986 Success by stages. Senior Nurse 5(3):14–16

Dickson A 1982 A woman in your own right. Quartet Books, London

Dilts R B 1994 Effective presentation skills. Meta Publications, CA

Henley A, Schott J 1999 Culture, religion and patient care in a multi-ethnic society. Age Concern, London

McCaffery M, Pasero C 1999 Pain: Clinical manual. Mosby, London

McVey J, Madill A, Fielding D 2001 The relevance of lowered personal control for patients who have stoma surgery to treat cancer. British Journal of Clinical Psychology 40(4):337–360

Metcalf C 1999 Stoma care: empowering patients through teaching practical skills. British Journal of Nursing 8(9):593–600

Middleton C 2004 Barriers to the provision of effective pain management. Nursing Times 100(3):42–45

Northouse L L, Schafer J A, Tipton J, Metivier L 1999 The concerns of patients and spouses after the diagnosis of colon cancer: a qualitative analysis. Journal of Wound, Ostomy, and Continence Nursing 26(1):8–17

O'Neill J, Leedham K 2001 Rehabilitation and long-term effects of treatment. In: Corner J, Bailey C (eds) Cancer nursing. Blackwell Science, Oxford, p 442–448

Persson E, Fridstedt G 2000 How to use an instrument to measure quality of care of a stoma patient. In: World Council of Enterostomal Therapists congress proceedings. Hollister, Libertyville, IL, p 160–162

Pringle W, Swan E 2001 Continuing care after discharge from hospital for stoma patients. British Journal of Nursing 10(19):1274–1288

Rushworth C 1994 Making a difference in cancer care. Souvenir Press (E & A), London

Tappe T P, Johnson V M 2000 Quality and cost-effective patient management through research and audit. In: World Council of Enterostomal Therapists congress proceedings. Hollister, Libertyville, IL, p 201–202

Thompson J 1998 Patient participation in decisions about longterm colostomy management. In: World Council of Enterostomal Therapists congress proceedings. Horton Print Group, Bradford, West Yorkshire, p 167–172

Wade B 1989 A stoma is for life. Scutari Press, London

White C A 1999 Psychological aspects of stoma care. In: Taylor P (ed) Stoma care in the community. Nursing Times Books, London, p 89–109

Williams A C de C 1997 Psychological techniques in the management of pain. In: Thomas V N (ed) Pain: its nature and management. Baillière Tindall and RCN, London, p 108–124

SECTION 3

Additional aspects of surgery and management

Chapter 10

Care of patients with internal bowel pouches

Maddie White

Patients with some bowel conditions may undergo internal pouch formation as an alternative to conventional stoma surgery. The aims of pouch surgery are to remove patients' diseased bowel and improve bowel function, thereby enhancing their quality of life.

This chapter will outline the ileo-anal pouch, the Kock pouch and the colonic pouch and aspects of these operations that patients need to consider in order to make informed choices about their surgery. Internal urinary pouches are discussed in Chapter 12.

THE ILEO-ANAL POUCH

Restorative proctocolectomy and pouch anal anastomosis (ileo-anal pouch or Parks' pouch) is now a well-established procedure and an alternative surgical option for patients faced with the daunting prospect of losing their colon and rectum. It was first performed by Sir Alan Parks in 1986. Its aim is to eradicate disease and preserve anal function (Nicholls & Williams 2002). Avoidance of a permanent ileostomy (as created in panproctocolectomy) is achieved by creating an internal reservoir from loops of small bowel which is then stapled to the anal canal. The patient stores faeces (of small bowel consistency) in the reservoir or pouch until defecation is possible, thus preserving a body image that is socially acceptable and comparable to life before their illness. This avoidance of a permanent ileostomy may make an enormous contribution to patients' psychosocial and sexual wellbeing. Keighley (1999a) suggests this procedure is now the first line choice in the treatment of ulcerative colitis. Patients' quality of life improves as their confidence increases following surgery (Fujita et al 1992). Everett (1989) and Skarsgard et al (1989) suggest that the procedure should be performed in a specialist centre by individuals who have had adequate training and experience in order to reduce morbidity and ensure a satisfactory result for the patient.

Various designs of pouch have been constructed but for several reasons the J pouch has proved the most successful (Keighley 1999a). A 30–40 cm section of distal ileum is folded into two segments, 15–20 cm each, and a side-to-side anastomosis is performed. The apex of the J pouch is then stapled to the anal sphincters to replace the rectum (Fig. 10.1). The integrity of the pouch is then tested by inserting air or saline into the pouch through the anus and observing for a leak. If there is any suspicion of a leak, or if incomplete 'doughnuts' of bowel following removal of the stapling device are found, it will be necessary to construct a loop ileostomy to protect the anastomosis.

The entire rectum is removed down to the level of the anorectal ring. Research has shown that continence and anal sensation are preserved despite this procedure, ruling out earlier theories that the presence of rectal mucosa was necessary for continence (Keighley 1999a). Rectal preservation and mucosectomy are no longer considered vital for acceptable pouch function. Rectal excision also removes the risk of malignancy in that area and reduces intraoperative morbidity (Keighley 1999a). Although stapling techniques have simplified this procedure there are cases that may require mucosectomy and difficulties can arise with the intra-anal anastomosis. Surgeons must be adequately trained to cope with these problems and those that may occur as complications of the surgery, such as complex fistulas or revision of an anastomotic stricture (Keighley 1999a).

The question of whether or not to create a loop ileostomy to protect the anastomosis has been much debated. A satisfactory anastomosis need not be covered with an ileostomy providing there are no risk factors such as steroid administration, poor haemostasis or technical factors (Grobler et al 1992). However, many surgeons routinely perform a covering ileostomy in order to reduce the possible consequences of anastomotic leakage with its risk of pelvic sepsis (Nicholls & Williams 2002). Faecal diversion also gives the anal sphincter and ileal mucosa time to recover before intestinal continuity is restored. Closure of the loop at a later date causes

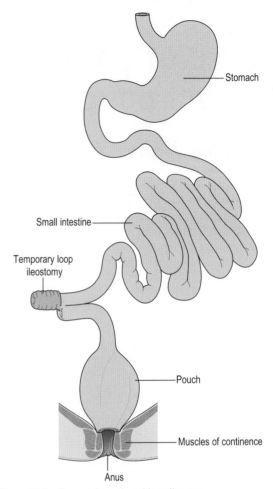

Figure 10.1   Ileo-anal pouch and loop ileostomy.

minimal morbidity (Williams et al 1989). Experiencing life with an ileostomy may be advantageous should pouch excision be necessary due to complications at a later date.

THE KOCK POUCH (CONTINENT OR RESERVOIR ILEOSTOMY)

Professor Kock in Sweden first designed this pouch in the early 1960s in order to offer patients control over incontinence of gas and faeces and in recognition of the psychological, sexual and physical dissatisfaction expressed by patients regarding their stomas (Keighley 1999b). The aim is to achieve a pouch with a capacity of between 800 and 1000 ml which is completely continent. Continence is achieved by the creation of a nipple valve, which is formed by invaginating a length of terminal ileum into the reservoir (Fig. 10.2). Intubating the pouch with a catheter three to four times a day empties the pouch, thereby reducing the necessity to wear a stomal appliance continuously. The stoma can be sited nearer the pubic area and is acceptable to many patients' perception of a normal body image, particularly as it is continent.

However, the procedure can be associated with many surgical and metabolic complications. Patients may have already had a failed ileo-anal pouch or other resections and a further 40–60 cm of ileum are then required to make the Kock pouch. Failure and removal of the pouch will therefore result in a high output stoma with potential fluid and electrolyte disturbances (Keighley 1999b). Problems experienced by patients are usually due to a leaking nipple valve, which can prolapse. Nicholls (1996) quotes a figure of 20–40% of cases in which the nipple valve fails due to desusception or dislocation. In a review of patients reported in the literature, Goldman & Rombeau (1978) found that valve dysfunction occurred in 17% of patients and was the commonest complication reported. This needs surgical correction as a local or open procedure.

COLONIC POUCH

Bowel function following rectal excision can be very poor, with patients experiencing frequency, soiling and urgency due to the lack of faecal storage capacity following removal of the rectum (Mortensen et al 1995), and a reduced resting anal pressure

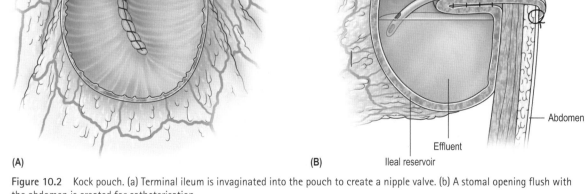

(A)   **(B)**   Ileal reservoir

Ileum
Catheter
Abdomen
Effluent

Figure 10.2   Kock pouch. (a) Terminal ileum is invaginated into the pouch to create a nipple valve. (b) A stomal opening flush with the abdomen is created for catheterisation.

(Williams 1999). Formation of a colonic pouch creates a neorectal reservoir, thereby maintaining storage capacity over both the short and long term (Mathur & Hallan 2002), at the same time preserving sphincter function. The risk of dehiscence from a colo-anal anastomosis is greater than in an ileo-anal procedure because patients are usually elderly, blood supply to the colon is less certain, and there is faecal material in the residual colon (Keighley 1996). Patients have often had radiotherapy; therefore a loop ileostomy is usually formed to protect the anastomosis (Harris et al 2002) (Fig. 10.3).

SUITABILITY FOR POUCH SURGERY

Patients must be carefully selected to undergo any type of pouch surgery as the presence of undiagnosed Crohn's disease could lead to complications such as ileal or anal disease, postoperative fistulas, sepsis, poor functional results and a high morbidity rate (Grobler et al 1993). However, the ileo-anal pouch is generally suitable for patients suffering with other conditions affecting the colon, including ulcerative colitis, familial adenomatous polyposis, megarectum, constipation and some cancers. Patients

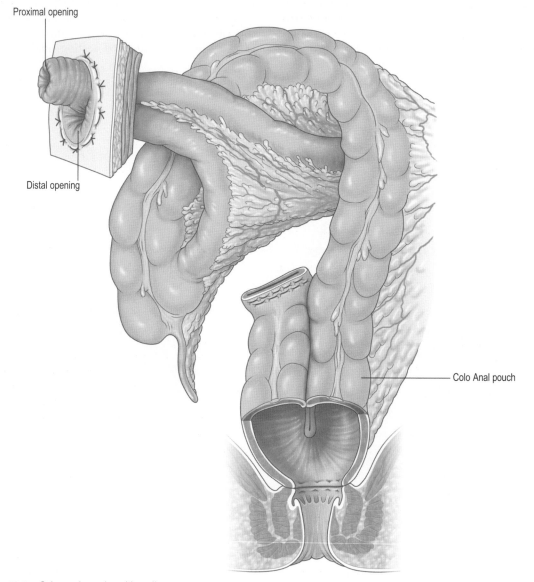

Proximal opening

Distal opening

Colo Anal pouch

Figure 10.3   Colo-anal pouch and loop ileostomy.

should have reasonable cardiopulmonary function as this is a major operative procedure. Ages of patients vary from teens to seventies and eligibility for pouch operations should be based on the suitability of their condition, level of general health, and motivation to have this type of surgery rather than a conventional stoma. Adequacy of sphincter function is also required for ileo-anal and colonic pouches (Black 2000).

A small percentage of patients, such as those undergoing emergency colectomy, can be enormously difficult to diagnose despite repeated evaluation of resected specimens (the so-called 'indeterminate colitis'). Yu et al (2000) quote a figure of 10% of cases in which the pathologist cannot definitely distinguish between ulcerative colitis and Crohn's disease as the histological features are suggestive of both conditions. However, Tjandra & Fazio (1993) quote 'It is safe to construct an ileo-anal reservoir in patients with indeterminate colitis', based on research evidence published by Hyman et al (1991). Results from the Birmingham group suggest that the outcome is not necessarily poor despite an uncertain diagnosis (Grobler et al 1993). However, it is vital that patients are made aware of possible consequences and complications as features of Crohn's disease may appear at a later date. Some patients will take their chances if only to have the pouch for a short time. The important factor is that the patient is fully informed and it may befall the clinical nurse specialist to explain and reiterate these points.

A Kock pouch may be offered to patients who have previously had a panproctocolectomy or a failed pouch, but who no longer wish to live with a permanent stoma. It is rarely offered as a first line treatment as it can be a complicated and lengthy procedure. Patients with Crohn's disease are usually not considered suitable.

Colonic pouch surgery appears not to have been universally accepted (Mathur & Hallan 2002) and only those surgeons who have experience in creating pouches are undertaking this procedure. In one institution in the USA all patients have a pouch unless there are technical difficulties (Harris et al 2002). Patients suitable are those with a resectable tumour which does not involve the anal sphincters but requires rectal excision and are usually patients in the elderly age group due to the nature of the disease. It can also be performed for solitary rectal ulcer, megarectum and other anomalies requiring rectal excision. Previous evacuation problems after surgery appear to have been resolved with the construction of a short 5 cm pouch (Fürst et al 2002).

MAKING A CHOICE

Patients with inflammatory bowel disease may present in a variety of ways. Firstly, patients may be referred to a specialist centre for a surgical opinion. Either medical therapy has not kept the disease quiescent and surgery is now the only option, or the patient has had an emergency colectomy because of an acute exacerbation of the colitis and is now in a position to contemplate further surgery. The histology of the resected specimen must be thoroughly reviewed by the specialist surgeon and histopathologist so that surgical options can be identified and discussed with individual patients.

Secondly, there are patients who have few or no symptoms but are at risk of developing serious complications. These include people with familial adenomatous polyposis (FAP) who may develop bowel cancer as a result of an inherited disease in which the colon is lined with thousands of adenomas or polyps (Neale & Phillips 2002). These patients are usually symptom free and may find it hard to adjust to the thought of major surgery and a period of rehabilitation. Genetic testing may reveal the gene responsible for the disease as early as age 11 or 12 years; therefore surgery may be offered at a time that will fit in with school life.

Thirdly, a few patients who have had surgery including anal resection and a conventional ileostomy may no longer wish to keep their stoma and may request the Kock pouch. However, this should not be undertaken lightly. Patients should explore the reasons for wanting surgery and weigh up the risks versus the quality of life being experienced with a stoma. Nowadays patients with a diagnosis of colitis should have their anal sphincters preserved at colectomy as this leaves them with the maximum treatment options subsequently.

Some patients will have been given information about pouches prior to seeing a specialist and will come armed with questions. Others may have little insight into the true realities of life with a pouch and have high expectations of returning to 'normal'. Body image associated with ileostomy function may persuade young men or women to have a pouch.

Some patients may decide upon hearing the facts that a pouch is not the operation for them and a panproctocolectomy (or proctectomy if the colon has already been removed) is a more realistic alternative. For instance, a 65-year-old man with grown-up children simply wanted one operation so that he could get on with enjoying his retirement and considered a panproctocolectomy perfectly adequate.

Before decisions regarding surgery can be made, patients need to be given information that covers the following areas:

- bowel function with a pouch and the effect on lifestyle
- potential complications and risks arising from the surgery
- stoma management
- recovery times.

It is important that patients understand the implications of deciding to undergo pouch surgery. Information should therefore be coupled with discussing the advantages and disadvantages of particular operations (Blackley 2004, Black 2000). Meeting a patient with an established pouch can also help prospective patients and their families gain a more realistic view of what undergoing assessment, surgery, and the early postoperative period entails, as well as living with a pouch generally (Hudson & Goldthorpe 1997).

BOWEL FUNCTION

Patients need to understand that their bowel function will never be 'normal', i.e. they will never pass a normal formed stool again following ileo-anal or Kock pouch formation. The output from small bowel pouches should eventually acquire thick liquid consistency. As time passes patients will be able to defer emptying and, on average, go to the toilet three or four times a day and possibly once at night although this will vary according to factors such as dietary intake, fluid balance etc. Individuals also vary as to the level of bowel function they find acceptable. Function differs in patients who have a pouch for FAP. They may empty their pouch less regularly than those who had ulcerative colitis. Colonic pouch function varies according to the capacity of the reservoir but on average should be two or three times a day (Phillips & Williams 2002).

A high output from small bowel pouches can result in frequent visits to the toilet and the patient may require medication such as loperamide or codeine to slow bowel function and thicken effluent (see Ch. 17). Perianal soreness can be troublesome

in the early stages, requiring meticulous hygiene to prevent infection. Some patients find the function unacceptable if using the toilet frequently interferes with their lifestyle or night-time sleep. Pouch excision may be the inevitable outcome for this small group, but not until all causes for frequency have been explored.

In the early days of pouch surgery pregnant women were advised to have a caesarean section to prevent obstetric trauma to the anal sphincters which, if compromised, would lead to incontinence. However, with increasing understanding of pouch surgery and how damage can affect an individual's lifestyle, selected patients may be offered a vaginal delivery. The weight of the pregnancy in the third trimester may increase frequency of defecation and some women have reported impairment of continence (Keighley 1999a).

COMPLICATIONS

Potential complications following surgery include sepsis, anastomotic leak, impaired sexual function and unacceptable pouch function.

Small bowel obstruction

Rothenberger et al (1997) quote the incidence as between 10 and 20%, resulting from adhesions, volvulus, herniation of the bowel or torsion of the ileostomy. Obstruction may also occur following ileostomy reversal due to adhesions at the site. Treatment will be dependent on the severity of the obstruction and may result in further surgery.

Anastomotic leak

Leaks can occur after pouch construction from the ileo-anal anastomosis, colo-anal anastomosis and as a complication following ileostomy reversal (Rothenberger et al 1997). Tjandra et al (1993) reported that leakage occurred more often in patients who did not have a covering ileostomy. Other risk factors include ischaemia, anastomotic tension, corticosteroids and age-related factors (Cohen et al 1992, cited in Rothenberger et al 1997).

Sepsis and fistula formation

Nicholls & Williams (2002) tell us that, on average, pelvic sepsis of clinical significance occurs in 5–10% of patients and is usually associated with a poor outcome. It is usually due to infected haematoma or anastomotic dehiscence but the argument continues as to whether hand suturing or stapling reduces the incidence. Drainage of the collection is required, usually by the insertion of a large catheter into the pouch. It is clear, however, that a standard procedure carried out by an experienced surgeon will increase patients' chances of a trouble-free postoperative recovery.

Pouch vaginal, perianal or cutaneous fistulas will only become apparent following ileostomy reversal and can occur 6-24 months postoperatively. Causes include sepsis, ischaemia, vaginal entrapment in the staple line or Crohn's disease (Keighley 1999a). Fistulas following Kock pouch formation occur in 8-10% of patients and can be through the base of the valve causing incontinence, or from the reservoir to the abdominal wall possibly due to sutures, the use of mesh or Crohn's disease (Peiser et al 1997). A diversionary loop ileostomy above the pouch may be required.

Anastomotic stricture

Stenosis at the ileo-anal anastomosis can occur as a result of fibrosis following partial dehiscence of the join or ischaemia at the margins of the pouch and anal canal. Authors quote figures of between 9 and 30% (Dozois et al 1986, Keighley et al 1993, Marcello et al 1993 cited in Rothenberger et al 1997).

Impaired sexual function

Sexual impairment can follow operations that include pouch formation (Nicholls & Williams 2002, Phillips & Williams 2002). Key factors that influence whether impairment occurs include:

- the extent of the surgery
- the line of rectal dissection followed, and degree to which this affects the presacral nerves (which can affect ejaculation) and the autonomic nerve plexus in the lower part of the pelvis on the lateral wall (which can affect erectile ability)
- the surgeon's level of expertise.

Ileo-anal pouch surgery
Most authors report the incidence of sexual dysfunction as being less than 5% in males, the main problem being retrograde ejaculation. Impotence is unlikely when experienced surgeons carry out nerve-sparing rectal dissection. This is normally possible unless patients have dysplasia. Subclinical invasion

of cancer may then have already developed so a wider dissection will be necessary (Nicholls & Williams 2002).

Painful or difficult erections may persist for a time after surgery. Women have a 25-30% incidence of dysfunction, namely dyspareunia or faecal leakage during intercourse (Keighley 1999a). As the majority of patients undergoing ileo-anal pouch surgery are in the younger age group, sexual difficulties may prove to be a real problem. However, difficulties may be encountered by patients of all ages, and help should be offered (Salter 2002).

Colo-anal pouch surgery
This operation is less extensive than abdomino-perineal excision of rectum, and the degree of sexual impairment arising from it is also thought to be less. However, it still needs to include sufficient rectal clearance to avoid local cancer recurrence. The potential for damage to the nerves involved in sexual function therefore exists. Williams (1999) states that levels of impairment which may occur are dependent on the amount of tumour and surrounding tissues that are removed and the ability of the surgeon.

Pouchitis

This is an inflammation of the ileo-anal pouch of unknown aetiology. Incidence ranges from 9% to 34% (Pemberton 1993, cited in Keighley & Williams 1999). It is usually characterised by a sudden onset of bloody diarrhoea, incontinence and fever. Extra-intestinal manifestations of colitis which may occur include arthritis, skin and eye complications. De Silva et al (1991) suggest a non-specific inflammatory reaction in the ileal mucosa which has undergone colonic metaplasia could cause pouchitis, possibly due to poor pouch emptying. It is also suggested that pouchitis may represent undiagnosed Crohn's disease. Where patients with such symptoms respond rapidly to metronidazole this is usually taken as diagnostic of pouchitis (Fleshman et al 1988, cited in Keighley & Williams 1999).

STOMA MANAGEMENT

The loop ileostomy covering an ileo-anal pouch can be difficult to manage for several reasons. The bowel is proximal to the pouch and produces a large quantity of effluent because of its high position in the gastrointestinal pathway. Oral anti-diarrhoeal drugs help to reduce the output.

Mobilising the pouch into the pelvis (not its natural position) may cause the proximal loop to become retracted. This and a high output can make stoma management very difficult for both the nurse and the patient. Convex appliances and other accessories may be necessary in order to obtain a satisfactory seal around the stoma.

A leaking valve from a Kock pouch may require similar management as the stoma here is deliberately created to be flush with the skin. Loop ileostomies above a colonic pouch are relatively straightforward in comparison and require general stoma management as described in Chapter 4.

RECOVERY TIMES

Patients undergoing pouch surgery, particularly ileo-anal pouch construction, are often of an age to have young children, work and financial commitments. All of these are likely to be affected by the amount of time the patient needs to spend undergoing their various tests, operations and recovery. Possible consequences of having to take time out from their usual activities must be carefully considered by both patient and family as they may affect whether such surgery is desirable or realistically possible. Porrett (1996) suggests that patients who are undergoing two operations for ileo-anal pouch creation may not go back to work between the stages, which may result in 5 months away from work. Alternatively, patients can delay ileostomy closure for up to a year and resume work between operations. Black (2000) suggests that the possibility of planning surgery to fit in with patients' annual leave should be discussed with surgeons.

Factors such as previous illness prior to surgery, any postoperative complications such as sepsis, prognosis if surgery has been performed for cancer, age of the patient, and nutritional status affect the time taken for recovery. On the whole patients are advised that they will be in hospital for 10–14 days for all procedures except loop ileostomy closure. Physical recovery generally takes 2–3 months, and the time needed for individuals to adjust psychologically varies. Social factors such as housing, availability of support, and number of dependants should be taken into consideration when planning discharge. Support groups may play a role in the patient's recovery as they learn to adapt from the hospital to the home situation (Hudson & Goldthorpe 1997). Ileo-anal pouch function may take many months to settle to a level acceptable to the individual patient and they should be encouraged to persevere with delaying emptying and experimenting with dietary intake until a compromise or balance is reached.

PREOPERATIVE PREPARATION

Helping patients understand the nature of their surgery and what to expect as they undergo tests and treatment is vital (Pringle & White 1997). Good communication helps patients prepare physically and emotionally for treatment, reduce anxiety (Davis & Fallowfield 1991) and actively participate in learning activities (Heron 1990). Relevant written material which is easy to read should be provided and followed up with further explanation as necessary.

Some patients will have anal sphincter measurements carried out prior to surgery. Time is allocated for a full assessment of anal sensation and function in order that appropriate surgery may be offered. For example, patients who have had a difficult vaginal delivery in the past or who have poor squeeze and resting anal sphincter pressures may be poor candidates for ileo-anal pouch surgery as they risk being incontinent of small bowel contents. This affects peoples' quality of life and independence. Elderly patients may have reduced sphincter function due to age-related factors or other disease processes. A Kock pouch or permanent stoma may be a more realistic alternative. These issues need to be addressed during patients' outpatient appointments and in follow-up discussions with the clinical nurse specialist before a final decision can be made.

If a prospective patient wants to meet someone who has already undergone the surgery it is important to match age and gender if possible so that information gleaned is more realistic and meaningful for the patient. In Birmingham we use our own database of patients and choose those who have had a successful and acceptable outcome and who are willing to share their experience with others.

During operations surgeons occasionally find it is impossible to create a pouch. This possibility, and alternative operations which could then be performed, should be discussed with patients so they are sufficiently informed to consent to the intended pouch and alternative operations (Black 2000).

Bowel preparation prior to surgery may not be necessary. If patients already have an ileostomy, restricting their oral intake to clear fluids on the day before surgery is adequate. Colonic pouch patients are treated as any other patient undergoing large bowel resection and given laxatives according to the department's protocol.

Preoperative identification of an appropriate stoma site is important for *all* patients. For example, some patients who have had an emergency colectomy may have a poorly sited stoma and a new, appropriate stoma site should be identified. Patients undergoing ileo-anal pouch surgery should be warned that, if they return from surgery with another stoma, it will not be the same one. This will be a loop ileostomy rather than an end stoma. Kock pouch patients are sited rather lower as it is not necessary to wear an appliance permanently or have a stoma with a reasonable spout. Colonic pouch patients are sited as normal (see Ch. 4).

POSTOPERATIVE NURSING CARE

General nursing care will be similar to that required by patients undergoing other major abdominal surgery, as will basic advice about resuming normal living activities (Blackley 2004, Black 2000).

ILEO-ANAL AND COLO-ANAL POUCHES

Pouch management

In most centres a rectal tube (usually a 26–30 size Foley catheter) will be inserted into the pouch during surgery with a continuous drainage appliance attached. This is to prevent distension of the pouch and to enable flushing out of clots and mucus so they do not build up and cause discomfort. Regular irrigation with 20–30 ml normal saline two or three times daily is carried out in some centres (Blackley 2004, Hudson & Goldthorpe 1997). Removal of this tube varies between 3 and 7 days.

Following removal patients should be encouraged to empty the pouch regularly. The type of effluent will depend on the amount of residual bowel after surgery and whether a diversionary stoma was created. Colo-anal pouches are normally protected by a temporary stoma. If a loop ileostomy has been formed, patients will pass mucus anally and occasionally faeces if there is any spillage into the distal loop of the stoma.

Following ileo-anal pouch formation without a covering stoma patients will pass faeces from the pouch which to begin with will be watery and may be difficult to control. This is normal and patients must be warned to expect urgency and possibly some incontinence. However, once diet is reintroduced the output gradually thickens and patients should be encouraged to defer defecation so that they can reduce the frequency of visits to the toilet and learn to 'hold on' to pouch contents. If pouch function does not settle before discharge from hospital medication to reduce or thicken faecal output may be prescribed (e.g. codeine or loperamide). Some patients have good function immediately and are very pleased with their surgery. Other patients may not settle quite so quickly and need much reassurance and encouragement to persevere as it could take up to a year before their function is satisfactory. The ability to distinguish between the presence of gas and faeces, and which is being passed, may also be acquired sooner by some patients than others.

Patients who have been advised to use pelvic floor (Kegal) and anal sphincter exercises to strengthen their muscles should be encouraged to do so once they have sufficiently recuperated (Blackley 2004, Black 2000).

Skin care

Perianal skin care is essential. The area must be gently cleaned and protected with a barrier cream or petroleum jelly after each visit to the toilet to prevent skin excoriation and breakdown.

Diet

Patients should be advised to gradually resume a normal diet following both one- and two-stage ileo-anal pouch surgery. Dietary intake can affect output and patients may need help to adapt their meals in response to troublesome symptoms. They should be advised that omitting meals will not reduce symptoms, and given similar information on foods to that given when patients acquire a conventional ileostomy (see Ch. 16). Blackley (2004) suggests patients should be advised to eat regular meals and have 3 litres of fluid intake daily. Black (2000) reports that gelatinous sweets such as marshmallows and jelly babies are very effective in producing thicker and more manageable effluent.

Patients undergoing colo-anal pouch formation will need advice as above while they have an ileostomy. Once the stoma has been closed and food intake and bowel function resumes, dietary advice similar to that given to patients with a sigmoid colostomy will usually be helpful (see Ch. 16).

Stoma care

If a diversionary loop ileostomy has been created, patients should receive normal stoma care (see Ch. 4). A loop stoma above an ileo-anal pouch will produce large volumes of watery effluent . This can cause management problems and the patient may need to take oral 'stoppers' such as codeine phosphate on a regular basis. A temporary supportive rod may be in situ which will generally be removed 4–7 days postoperatively. Patients must gain the usual information and skills so they can manage their stoma care competently and confidently in the months between their initial operation and stoma closure.

KOCK POUCH

A Medina catheter is inserted into the pouch in theatre and stitched to the peristomal skin. This catheter is more rigid than a Foley catheter with larger holes at one end to enable drainage of small bowel contents. On average this catheter is left in for 2–3 weeks to prevent pouch distension and allow flushing. A marker placed on the catheter close to the stoma to indicate the correct position will aid subsequent monitoring of whether slippage has occurred.

Blackley (2004) suggests that 30 ml of normal saline should be irrigated via a syringe and the catheter into the pouch every 2 hours for the first 24 hours postoperatively in order to gently wash out any accumulating mucus. The period may subsequently be extended to 4-hourly. A high volume of fluid effluent is normally passed when bowel function initially resumes, and this should reduce as the absorptive capacity of the pouch improves and oral diet intake resumes.

Patients return to the ward to have the Medina catheter removed and to be taught pouch management by the clinical nurse specialist. The patient is shown the correct angle to insert the catheter through the nipple valve. Patients need to learn to recognise the feeling of pushing this tube through the valve into the pouch itself. When the pouch has been drained it is flushed out with about 30 ml of tap water (via a syringe connected to the Medina catheter). This reduces the viscosity of pouch contents and helps to ensure there is no residue left in the pouch. It can take 5-10 minutes to drain the pouch: thicker effluent takes longer to drain.

On removal of the tube a stoma cap can be worn until the next time the pouch is emptied. There is a choice between a one-piece appliance or a two-piece, which may be preferable as the pouch needs to be emptied 3–4-hourly. The Medina catheter can be washed in warm soapy water, dried, and used for many months. The principles for obtaining more equipment are the same as those described in Chapter 8.

Blackley (2004, p 247) offers several management tips:

- Difficulty with pouch intubation may be eased by:
  - relaxing tense abdominal muscles
  - lying on a bed to intubate
  - lubricating the length of the tube (water-soluble lubricants only should be used; residues from petroleum jelly based compounds may irritate pouch tissues)
  - instilling a small amount of water or air through the tube.
- Draining thick pouch contents may be helped by:
  - diluting pouch contents with tap water
  - drinking two glasses of water, prune, or grape juice and waiting a while
  - using a syringe to suck contents from the pouch.
- Diet:
  - highly fibrous foods should be avoided initially and taken sparingly
  - a balanced diet including three litres of fluids should be taken daily.

Patients should be given a detailed written instruction sheet on discharge in addition to supplies of equipment and a list of these requirements. They should also be advised to seek medical help promptly if at any time their pouch feels full and they are unable to empty it.

CONCLUSION

As surgical expertise increases and patients' expectations rise, development of high quality nursing care is essential. The effects of frequent, unpredictable bowel actions on patients' lives in the early months should not be underestimated. Such experiences may appear similar to those which patients (particularly those with ulcerative colitis) had preoperatively. They may need considerable reassurance that their new bowel system will ultimately settle into acceptable and manageable levels of activity (Black 2000, Porrett 1996).

Although pouch surgery provides less obvious alterations in body image than conventional stoma surgery, patients do still have to come to terms with having major surgery, living with altered bowel function, and the physical and psychological effects of their pre- and postoperative experiences (Salter 2002). Many of the strategies whose use with stoma patients is described in other chapters can also be used to support patients with pouches as they undergo assessment, surgery and rehabilitation.

References

Black P K 2000 Holistic stoma care. Baillière Tindall and RCN, Edinburgh

Blackley P 2004 Practical stoma wound and continence management, 2nd edn. Research Publications Pty, Vermont, Victoria, Australia

Cohen Z, McLeod R S, Stephen W et al 1992 Continuing evolution of the pelvic pouch procedure. Annals of surgery 216(4):506–512

Davis H, Fallowfield L 1991 Evaluating the effects of counselling and communication. In: Davis H, Fallowfield L (eds) Counselling and communication in health care. John Wiley, Chichester, p 287–318

De Silva H J, Millard P R, Kettlewell M et al 1991 Mucosal characteristics of pelvic ileal pouches. Gut 32(1):61–65

Dozois R R, Goldberg S M, Rothenberger D A et al 1986 Symposium: Restorative proctocolectomy with ileal reservoir. International Journal of Colorectal Disease 1:2–19

Everett W G 1989 Experience of restorative proctocolectomy with ileal reservoir. British Journal of Surgery 76(1):77–81

Fleshman J W, Cohen Z, McLeod R S et al 1988 The ileal reservoir and ileoanal anastomosis procedure: factors affecting technical and functional outcomes. Diseases of the Colon and Rectum 31(1):10–16

Fujita S, Kusunoki M, Shoji Y et al 1992 Quality of life after total proctocolectomy and ileal J pouch anal anastomosis. Diseases of the Colon and Rectum 35(11):1030–1039

Fürst A, Burghofer K, Hutzel L, Jauch K W 2002 Neorectal reservoir is not the functional principle of the colonic J-pouch. Diseases of the Colon and Rectum 45(5):660–667

Goldman S L, Rombeau J L 1978 The continent ileostomy: a collective review. Diseases of the Colon and Rectum 21:594–599

Grobler S P, Hosie K B, Keighley M R B 1992 Randomised trial of loop ileostomy in restorative proctocolectomy. British Journal of Surgery 79(9):903–906

Grobler S P, Hosie K B, Affie E et al 1993 Outcome of restorative proctocolectomy when the diagnosis is suggestive of Crohn's disease. Gut 34(10):1384–1388

Harris G J C, Lavery I J, Fazio V W 2002 Reasons for failure to construct the colonic J-pouch. What can be done to improve the size of the neorectal reservoir should it occur? Diseases of the Colon and Rectum 45(10):1304–1308

Heron J 1990 Helping the client: a creative practical guide. Sage Publications, London

Hudson J, Goldthorpe S 1997 Inflammatory bowel disease. In: Bruce L, Finlay T M (eds) Nursing in gastroenterology. Churchill Livingstone, New York, p 55–84

Hyman N H, Fazio V W, Tuckson W B, Lavery I C, 1991 Consequences of ileal pouch anal anastomosis for Crohn's colitis. Diseases of the Colon and Rectum 34(8):653–657

Keighley M R B 1996 Colorectal cancer. In: Keighley M R B, Pemberton J H, Fazio V, Parc R Atlas of colorectal surgery. Churchill Livingstone, New York

Keighley M R B 1999a Restorative proctocolectomy and ileal pouch anal anastomosis. In: Keighley M R B, Williams N S Surgery of the anus, rectum and colon, 2nd edn. W B Saunders, London

Keighley M R B 1999b Reservoir ileostomy in ulcerative colitis. In: Keighley M R B, Williams N S Surgery of the anus, rectum and colon, 2nd edn. W B Saunders, London

Keighley M R B, Grobler S, Bain I 1993 An audit of restorative proctocolectomy. Gut 34(5):680–684

Marcello P W, Roberts P L, Schoetz D S et al 1993 Longterm results of the ileoanal pouch. Archives of Surgery 128:500–503

Mathur P, Hallan R I 2002 The colonic J-pouch in colo-anal anastomosis. Colorectal Disease 4:304–312

Mortensen N J M, Ramirez J M, Takeuchi N, Smiglin Humphreys M M 1995 Colonic J pouch anal anastomosis after rectal excision for carcinoma: functional outcome. British Journal of Surgery 82:611–613

Neale K, Phillips R 2002 Familial adenomatous polyposis. In: Williams J (ed) The essentials of pouch care nursing. Whurr Publishers, London, p 27–42

Nicholls R J 1996 Surgical procedures. In: Myers C (ed) Stoma care nursing. Arnold, London, p 90–122

Nicholls R J, Williams J 2002 The ileo-anal pouch. In: Williams J (ed) The essentials of pouch care nursing. Whurr Publishers, London, p 68–98

Peiser J G, Cohen Z, McLeod R S 1997 Surgical treatment of ulcerative colitis - continent ileostomy. In: Allan R N, Rhodes J M, Hanauer S B et al (eds) Inflammatory bowel diseases, 3rd edn. Churchill Livingstone, New York

Pemberton J H 1993 The problems with pouchitis. Gastroenterology 104:1209–1211

Phillips R, Williams J 2002 The colo-anal pouch and nursing care. In: Williams J (ed) The essentials of pouch care nursing. Whurr Publishers, London, p 117–127

Porrett T 1996 Restorative proctocolectomy: the nursing implications. In: Myers C (ed) Stoma care nursing. Arnold, London, p 157–165

Pringle W K, White M C 1997 Patient Information. In: Allan R N, Rhodes J M, Hanauer S B et al (eds) Inflammatory bowel diseases, 3rd edn. Churchill Livingstone, New York

Rothenberger D A, Gemlo B T, Deen K I 1997 Complications after ileal pouch anal anastomosis. In: Allan R N, Rhodes J M, Hanauer S B et al (eds) Inflammatory bowel diseases, 3rd edn. Churchill Livingstone, New York

Salter M 2002 Sexual aspects of internal pouch surgery. In: Williams J (ed) The essentials of pouch care nursing. Whurr Publishers, London, p 180–198

Skarsgard E D, Atkinson K G, Bell G A et al 1989 Function and quality of life results after ileal pouch surgery for chronic ulcerative colitis and familial polyposis. American Journal of Surgery 157:467–471

Tjandra J J, Fazio V W 1993 Current status of ileo anal reservoirs: 1992. Journal of Enterostomal Therapy 20:56–62

Tjandra J J, Fazio V W, Milsom J W et al 1993 Omission of temporary diversion in restorative proctocolectomy – is it safe? Diseases of the Colon and Rectum 36(11):1007–1014

Williams N S 1999 Surgical treatment of rectal cancer In: Keighley M R B, Williams N S Surgery of the anus, rectum and colon, 2nd edn. W B Saunders, London

Williams N S, Marzouk D E M M, Hallan R I, Waldron D J 1989 Function after ileal pouch and stapled pouch-anal anastomosis for ulcerative colitis. British Journal of Surgery 76(11):1168–1171

Yu C S, Pemberton JH, Larson D 2000 Ileal pouch-anal anastomosis in patients with indeterminate colitis. Diseases of the Colon and Rectum 43(11):1487–1496

Chapter 11

Care of patients with an electrically stimulated gracilis neosphincter

Maddie White

Formation of a gracilis neosphincter is a relatively new operation carried out in some specialist centres. A new system of opening and closing the anal canal is created for suitable patients which they can then use to manage faecal incontinence. According to Kamm (1994) the problem of anal incontinence for gas or faeces affects up to 11% of adults and occurs frequently in 2%. Incontinence may be due to either mechanical or neurological damage. Chapman et al (2002) advocate that it is likely to be a combination of both factors. True incontinence (rather than urgency or soiling alone) may be due to obstetric injury, surgical division of sphincters, trauma and anal abuse. Other contributing factors may be rectal disease, neurological and age-related weaknesses and congenital abnormalities (Yoshioka & Keighley 1989).

The loss of anal sphincter function and subsequent faecal incontinence can have a devastating effect on the quality of people's lives. Social and sexual function may be drastically reduced due to the fear and embarrassment of having a condition that is often regarded as socially unacceptable. This can lead to social isolation. Incontinence can be managed non-surgically with medication or enemas, or biofeedback treatment, and some patients with a proven sphincter defect will benefit from a sphincter repair. However, there is a small percentage of patients who have 'end stage' faecal incontinence whose treatment until recently has usually entailed formation of a permanent stoma. Some of these patients may be eligible to have a gracilis neosphincter created. Two operations are outlined in this chapter:

- *Electrically stimulated gracilis neosphincter.* Patients use opening and closing of the neosphincter as the main process through which they eliminate faeces and maintain continence (described first).
- *Electrically stimulated gracilis neosphincter with colonic conduit.* Patients use an additional system of stimulating bowel evacuation in tandem with the neosphincter opening and closing system, known as 'the combined approach' (described later).

As the availability of these procedures becomes more widely known it is likely that patients will seek further information about them. Firstly, they may hear of them from other patients or seek information on the internet before deciding whether to ask for either operation to be considered by their doctors. Secondly, a neosphincter may have been described as an option by their medical team but the complexity of the procedure has meant they need further explanation. It is therefore important for nurses to be able to provide appropriate information about these procedures and to help patients clarify their understanding of them.

Patients who may be suitable for this kind of surgery include:

1. Incontinent patients who have a deficient anal sphincter mechanism as a result of trauma or neurogenic damage. These patients have an intact rectum and anal canal. Previous attempts at sphincter repair will have failed.
2. Some patients with anorectal agenesis where there is an absence of any functioning anal sphincter.
3. Some patients who have undergone an abdomino-perineal resection. These patients must show no evidence of recurrent disease or distant metastases if the procedure was carried out for cancer.

However, patients in groups 2 and 3 may require the combined approach (described later) rather than construction of a neosphincter on its own.

Various conditions are thought to contraindicate this operation (e.g. Keighley & Williams 1999, Wexner et al 2002). Generally, patients who are currently thought *not suitable for this operation* include those aged less than 18 or more than 80, and those who have:

- perineal or pelvic sepsis
- Crohn's disease
- unmanageable diarrhoea
- recurrent pelvic tumour or widespread malignancy
- a pacemaker in situ

- total anal agenesis
- a damaged or non-functioning gracilis leg muscle, which can include patients with neurological disease such as multiple sclerosis and spina bifida; the muscle can be tested to assess its suitability by electromyography (Keighley & Williams 1999)
- respiratory or cardiac difficulties
- severe arthritis
- previous perineal radiotherapy
- any other contraindications to chronic electrical stimulation.

As the gracilis neosphincter is a relatively new operation for faecal incontinence there are likely to be some variations in patients' preparation and treatment as improvements are sought and introduced. However, the underlying principles of treatment are likely to be similar.

ELECTRICALLY STIMULATED GRACILIS NEOSPHINCTER CREATION

A system of opening and closing the anal canal is created which will ultimately be used by the patient to control elimination. It has been described by a number of writers (e.g. Chapman et al 2002, Keighley & Williams 1999, Stuchfield & Eccersley 1999). It is important that patients understand what the lengthy overall process entails. A considerable preoperative assessment process is followed by one to three stages involving hospital admissions and outpatient visits and recuperation time. These stages can be summarised as follows.

1. First operation (Figs 11.1 and 11.2)

The gracilis leg muscle is isolated (in a manner that preserves the nerve and blood supplies of both the leg and this muscle) and is then wrapped around the anal canal with one end attached to the ischial tuberosity. The leg chosen will be the same side of the body as that where the stimulator is inserted, and these will usually be on the opposite side to the stoma (Keighley & Williams 1999, p 674).

Electrodes are placed on the main nerve to the transposed muscle and attached to a stimulator box, placed in the patient's abdomen, for subsequent use as described below. This will be postponed for 6 weeks if there are any complications (Rongen et al 2001).

If necessary, a temporary stoma is raised to divert faecal effluent from the perianal area. Stuchfield &

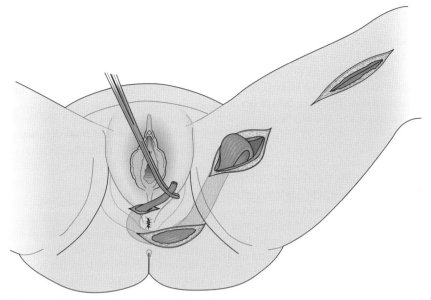

Figure 11.1   Gracilis leg muscle is wrapped around the anal canal.

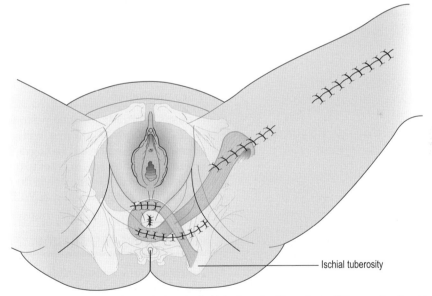

Ischial tuberosity

Figure 11.2   One end of the gracilis muscle is attached to the ischial tuberosity. The patient will have perianal and leg wounds.

Eccersley (1999) suggest a loop ileostomy is preferable if the patient does not already have a suitable stoma. Stoma management is taught prior to discharge.

2. Stimulation of the gracilis muscle to alter its action

The style of action which gracilis muscle normally has (fast twitch muscle for short bursts of action) has to be converted to the style of action which the anus normally has so that the gracilis can provide sphincter-like control (i.e. slow twitch muscle for more sustained action). Low frequency electrical stimulation of the muscle over several weeks has been found to alter the muscle physiology (Chapman et al 2002). Healing of the two perineal wounds created when positioning the gracilis around the anal canal has to take place before gracilis action conversion is started.

The conversion of the gracilis from fast twitch (fatigable) to slow twitch (fatigue resistant) muscle action is promoted by setting the electrode and stimulator system to contract the muscle for increasing lengths of time, generally over an 8-week period (Keighley & Williams 1999). It may be started before the patient is discharged and they then return on an outpatient basis for subsequent stimulation.

3. Closure of the stoma

After approximately 3 months the patient's stoma can be closed if their gracilis muscle has converted and therefore now remains contracted unless stimulated to open. Once bowel activity has resumed postoperatively they are taught to use a hand-held magnet to switch the abdominal stimulator on and off and thus enable faeces to pass out of the anal canal (Fig. 11.3).

The above summary can now be used to aid understanding of the relevance of the preoperative investigations and preparation that patients must undergo, as well as their postoperative care.

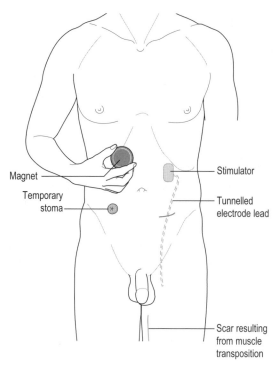

Magnet

Temporary stoma

Stimulator

Tunnelled electrode lead

Scar resulting from muscle transposition

Figure 11.3   Use of magnet to switch the abdominal stimulator on and off.

PREOPERATIVE ASSESSMENT

Assessment of patients is extremely important prior to selection for any radical procedure. All other attempts to achieve continence for these patients will have failed and their only alternative option is to have a permanent stoma. Patients will first undergo tests to establish the level of function of their anorectum and anal sphincter muscles as this information will influence decisions about their treatment options. These tests include anal manometry and video proctogram.

Anal manometry

This is the measurement of pressure within the rectum and anal canal. A probe with a balloon attached is inserted into the anal canal in order to measure the length of the canal and to record resting and squeeze pressures in the rectum. The balloon is withdrawn in stages and the pressure recorded at each stage. The patient is asked to 'squeeze' the probe and again pressure is measured in order to ascertain muscle dysfunction (Loder 1996). A tracing is recorded on graph paper and kept in the patient's notes.

Video proctogram

A quantity of radio-opaque paste which simulates faeces is inserted into the rectum. The patient attempts to defecate and radiographic screening is recorded on videotape, in order to obtain an accurate picture of function of the pelvic floor and efficiency of rectal emptying (Keighley & Williams 1999).

PREOPERATIVE PREPARATION

Patients require considerable amounts of information and careful assessment before decisions can be made as to whether this system for managing their bowels will be suitable for them. Enough time must be allowed for patients to absorb the information and have their questions answered, and for staff to check whether patients' levels of understanding are sufficient to enable them to make an informed decision about the surgery. Success cannot be guaranteed and, for some, life with a permanent stoma may be preferable. Patients should also have the opportunity to meet another person who has had this type of surgery, and to see the equipment they will need to use.

The clinical nurse specialist will also assess patients' physical and psychological ability to manage a gracilis neosphincter. Physical fitness and manual dexterity are important as the patient must be able to use the magnet, and may have to carry out colonic irrigation if the 'combined approach' is used (see later). Self-motivation is important as the procedure may be carried out in stages across several months and function may not be perfect to begin with. This has implications which patients must understand: they may be away from work or unable to fulfil their normal activities and commitments for a considerable period. During the first few months after the three stages have been completed they must learn how to use their neosphincter system effectively. They may need to experiment with diet and medication to alter faecal consistency, and may still experience some leakage of faeces and flatus. It is important for patients and their families to recognise that much support may be needed.

Patients will also need information about living with a stoma as they may have a defunctioning one for several months, as indicated earlier. Preparation and care will be similar to that outlined in earlier chapters. Generally it is more helpful to ensure patients have acquired adequate levels of information about both the neosphincter and the stoma, and then use a counselling approach to help them clarify and express concerns and make appropriate decisions (see Ch. 7).

Once admitted to hospital for their first stage operation patients require the normal preparation for major surgery in accordance with local protocols. Full bowel preparation is essential unless the patient already has a stoma (Stuchfield & Eccersley 1999). This is to prevent faecal loading or other postoperative complications.

The clinical nurse specialist will also identify and mark suitable sites for a possible temporary stoma and where the stimulator is to be implanted. Generally, the stimulator is sited in the upper abdomen on the opposite side of the body from the stoma. If the 'combined approach' is being used, siting of the colonic conduit will also be necessary (see later).

POSTOPERATIVE CARE

Nursing care is similar to that required by patients who have any major bowel procedure. Oral fluids may begin once the patient's bowel sounds return or he has passed flatus (either anally or via the stoma). Adequate fluid intake allows discontinuation of the intravenous fluids and the introduction of diet. An effective system for monitoring and controlling pain should be established.

It is essential that patients are maintained on strict bed rest for 3 days. This allows the new muscle to heal in its new setting on the ischial tuberosity (Keighley & Williams 1999) and prevent slipping of the electrode attached to it. After this, patients are encouraged to mobilise but warned not to abduct the thighs excessively (Stuchfield & Eccersley 1999). The urinary catheter may also be removed at this stage. Patients also need to be taught stoma management to promote independence.

The perineal wounds must be inspected regularly for signs of sepsis or necrosis. Once healed, the programme of stimulation of the gracilis muscle can start. This may begin before patients are discharged home and continue during their outpatient attendance every 2 weeks. The electrode and stimulator system is set to contract the gracilis neosphincter for increasing lengths of time over approximately 8 weeks so it converts to a more sustained style of action, as outlined earlier. Analgesic requirements should also be monitored as gracilis stimulation can cause tingling sensations in the muscle which some patients find difficult to tolerate. Other patients find the leg wound painful and may have reduced mobility for a while. Physiotherapy whilst the patient is in hospital helps to improve mobility and reduce complications. Sexual intercourse should be avoided during the first 6 weeks postoperatively to allow the new electrode system to become securely attached to the main gracilis muscle nerve (Stuchfield 1996).

DISCHARGE FROM HOSPITAL (1)

It is essential that patients have a contact number for the hospital for easy access to the clinical nurse specialist for advice and support. They will need time to adjust to life with a stoma. In addition they have the prospect of both further surgery to close their stoma and learning to manage their neosphincter yet to come.

CLOSURE OF THE TEMPORARY STOMA AND USING THE NEOSPHINCTER

Timing of stoma closure is usually dependent on successful conversion of the gracilis muscle so that it now normally remains contracted, occluding the anal canal unless stimulated to relax. This is tested using anorectal manometry and has generally occurred by 3 months after the original surgery. Patients are admitted for bowel preparation prior to stomal closure and restoration of bowel continuity.

Once bowel activity has resumed after stomal closure (about 4–5 days postoperatively) patients learn to operate their new system of opening and closing the bowel to control defecation:

- The contracted gracilis muscle is stimulated to relax (and thus allow anal opening) by placing a small hand-held magnet over the abdominal stimulator's position.
- The magnet switches the stimulator off and (as long as the magnet remains close to the stimulator) the gracilis will relax, enabling faeces to pass out of the anal canal.
- Once defecation is completed the magnet is removed, the stimulator resumes action, and the gracilis muscle contracts, thus closing the anal canal.

DISCHARGE FROM HOSPITAL (2)

Generally, patients are expected to resume a normal lifestyle but they are likely to need support and information to help them do so. They may need to learn ways of using diet and medication to help them develop a pattern and consistency of bowel action that can be successfully managed by their new evacuatory system. Care and protection of the perianal area is also likely to be needed in the early months. Patients may have developed a range of ways of managing their incontinence prior to receiving this new system. It will generally be helpful to review with them which of these measures are still likely to be useful and whether alternative approaches could now be used more beneficially. Psychological support as well as practical help should be provided (Hill 1996, Stuchfield & Eccersley 1999).

Stuchfield (1996) reports that magnets can affect computer equipment, discs and cassette tapes. Patients should be encouraged to identify where their magnet can be stored to retain easy access without equipment damage. Hill (1996) also reports that televisions and cameras can be affected, and clocks and watches can stop if the magnet is within 2 inches (5 cm) of them. Hill (1996) and Stuchfield (1996) also state that patients should be warned about

the possible effects of their stimulator. Although the stimulator itself should not be damaged the metal in it can show up on security equipment (e.g. at airports) and can trigger alarm systems (e.g. in stores and libraries). It may be helpful therefore for patients to carry a small card outlining the medical reasons why these events can occur so informed help can be obtained from staff involved in such situations.

The gracilis neosphincter and its stimulator system is considered robust enough to withstand most normal work and social activities including sports such as swimming, aerobics and cycling. Contact body sports are normally contraindicated because of the possibility that the electrode might become dislodged from the gracilis muscle (Stuchfield 1996).

Stuchfield & Eccersley (1999) report improvements in continence for 60% of patients, offering hope to many patients who experience a psychologically distressing and embarrassing condition.

COMPLICATIONS

Sepsis

Williams et al (1991) reported severe sepsis in 9 patients out of 32, attributable to muscle necrosis and sepsis in 3 out of 7 patients who did not have a stoma. Korsgen & Keighley's report of four cases (1995) claims no episodes of sepsis and attribute this to the fact that all patients had a defunctioning stoma. However, sepsis and muscle necrosis can destroy the muscle, requiring use of the muscle from the opposite leg, resulting in further scarring. Further surgery may be required including incision and drainage of sepsis, wound debridement and even repeat graciloplasty (Matzel et al 2001).

Stenosis

If the anal canal is already stenosed prior to the surgery, correction may be necessary before the gracilis procedure is commenced. Baeten et al (2000) suggest that muscle is wrapped around the anal canal with enough laxity to permit the placement of one or two fingers between the gracilis and the anal canal.

Technical problems

These may include lead dislodgement, poor lead positioning, neurostimulator migration and connection difficulties. All will require further surgery to amend the problem (Matzel et al 2001).

Impaired rectal evacuation

Symptoms of this may vary. Some patients experience difficulties if they do not assist evacuation and may use laxatives or suppositories to do so. Others report leakage of flatus and the use of pads to deal with minor faecal soiling. However, some patients have major problems in evacuation. This appears more likely to occur in patients who have reduced rectal sensation. It highlights the need for full assessment of rectal sensation and emptying to be carried out prior to surgery, to prevent disappointment and subsequent permanent stoma formation for the patient as reported in Korsgen & Keighley's study (1995).

Stuchfield (1997), a clinical nurse specialist in stoma care at the Royal London Hospitals NHS Trust, quotes a success rate of 50% from a series of 70 patients operated on since 1988. However, 9 patients had difficulty evacuating stool from the rectum, despite the new muscle being continent. Korsgen & Keighley (1995) report similar findings in an overview of their patients. This led to the development of the continent colonic conduit, to be performed in conjunction with the gracilis neosphincter, as a combined procedure in order to facilitate rectal emptying.

ELECTRICALLY STIMULATED NEOSPHINCTER WITH COLONIC CONDUIT

This system is often known as 'the combined approach'. It seeks to help patients achieve:

- *continence* through using a gracilis neosphincter as described earlier, and
- *regular elimination of faeces* by irrigation via a specially constructed colonic conduit. Faecal matter is irrigated through the remaining colon and rectum and passed into the toilet.

Stuchfield (1997) and Keighley & Williams (1999) suggest that patients who are likely to need this combined approach because of difficulties in evacuation can be identified and include those with:

- impaired anorectal sensation
- impairment or absence of a functioning anal sphincter (e.g. patients who have had pull-through operations for congenital abnormalities, see Chapter 13; patients who have had complex pelvic injuries)
- patients who have had an abdomino-perineal resection.

PREOPERATIVE ASSESSMENT AND PREPARATION

This includes similar physical and psychological assessment procedures to those described earlier for neosphincter formation. However, additional consideration must be given to the fact that these patients will have a permanent colonic conduit and need to undertake daily irrigations for life. Marking of suitable sites for the colonic conduit and stimulator (plus defunctioning stoma if likely to be created) is carried out. The patient is admitted 48 hours prior to surgery for full bowel preparation. Surgery will involve the following procedures:

(a) Construction of the gracilis neosphincter and implantation of hardware (as described earlier).
(b) Construction of a colonic conduit, using an intussuscepted segment of transverse colon to create an anti-reflux valve. The colon forming the conduit is tunnelled through the abdominal wall and sutured to the skin using a skin flap to prevent stenosis. There it provides a small opening for subsequent antegrade colonic irrigation. An anastomosis is performed between the ascending and transverse colon to restore bowel continuity (Fig. 11.4). At the time of surgery a catheter is inserted into the conduit and sutured in position to ensure patency.
(c) A loop ileostomy may be created to protect the conduit and graciloplasty.
(d) Gastrografin studies (conduitogram) are carried out to ensure there is no leakage from the colonic anastomoses before the catheter is removed and the patient is taught to irrigate the distal colon.
(e) Stimulation of the gracilis neosphincter is carried out as described earlier to convert its action from fast to slow twitch (fatigue resistant) action.
(f) If a defunctioning stoma has been created it is generally closed 2–3 months after the original surgery.

POSTOPERATIVE CARE

General postoperative care, management of the leg and perineal wounds, and the programme of converting the gracilis neosphincter muscle is similar to that described earlier for electrically stimulated gracilis neosphincter creation. In addition, patients are taught to irrigate their conduit. Initially they will use the catheter inserted during the operation.

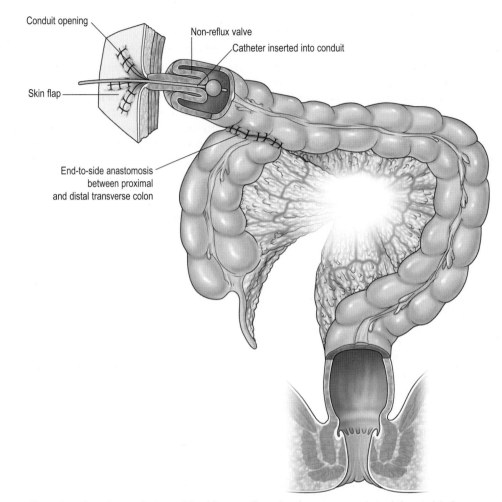

Figure 11.4 Formation of continent colonic conduit with non-reflux valve. A temporary catheter is inserted during surgery to ensure patency.

That will be removed in the outpatients department about 4 weeks after surgery and patients are then taught to intubate the conduit before their daily irrigation. Catheters are washed and reused.

Prior to irrigation the neosphincter has to be relaxed (i.e. through the stimulator being switched off) in order to allow evacuation of faeces and irrigation fluid. The magnet is held or taped over the stimulator to achieve this and, on removal, the stimulator will switch back on and the gracilis neosphincter contracts (Stuchfield 1997).

Stuchfield & Eccersley (1999) suggest:

- use of 0.5–1 litre of tepid tap water (37°C) for irrigation, using an irrigation set with a suitable size of catheter (i.e. *not* a cone), which is lubricated

- irrigation normally takes about 30 minutes, but patients with poor sphincter function may experience leakage of water per rectum for about an hour afterwards and may need to use pads
- a stoma cap or gauze dressing may be used to cover the conduit site.

It is also important that patients have easy access to help and support from staff who are familiar with this specialised type of surgery and thus can knowledgeably monitor their progress and respond to the kind of concerns and problems that patients may experience. Long-term problems include stenosis at the mucocutaneous junction, reflux of irrigation fluid into the ileum and loss of responsiveness to infused fluid (Vaizey et al 1998).

CONCLUSION

It is clear that these are relatively new procedures and that surgeons are on a learning curve. New procedural variations designed to further enhance the patient's quality of life, such as rectal augmentation in combination with the neosphincter, are being described in the literature (Williams et al 2001). As technology advances, some of the difficulties experienced should be rectified. Surgery should be carried out in a specialist centre and potential problems fully explained (Niriella & Deen 2000). However, it is evident that patient selection is of the utmost importance. Individuals must be highly motivated and prepared for the procedure to be carried out in several stages. Despite the difficulties, some patients may feel that they would rather undergo one of these procedures than have a permanent stoma, opening a further avenue of treatment designed to improve quality of life.

References

Baeten C G and the Dynamic Graciloplasty Therapy Study Group 2000 Safety and efficacy of dynamic graciloplasty for fecal incontinence: report of a prospective, multicenter trial. Diseases of the Colon and Rectum 43(6):743–751

Chapman A E, Geerdes B, Hewett P et al 2002 Systematic review of dynamic graciloplasty in the treatment of faecal incontinence. British Journal of Surgery 89(2):138–153

Hill H 1996 Dynamic anal graciloplasty. In: World Council of Enterostomal Therapists congress proceedings. Hollister, Libertyville, IL, p 22–25

Kamm M A 1994 Obstetric damage and faecal incontinence (review article). Lancet 344(8924):730–733

Keighley M R B, Williams N S 1999 Faecal incontinence In: Keighley M R B, Williams N S Surgery of the anus, rectum and colon, 2nd edn. W B Saunders, London, p 592–700

Korsgen S, Keighley M R B 1995 Stimulated gracilis neosphincter – not as good as previously thought (Report of four cases). Diseases of the Colon and Rectum 38(12):1331–1333

Loder P 1996 Physiology. In: Myers C (ed) Stoma care nursing. Edward Arnold, London, p 14–41

Matzel K E, Madoff R D, LaFontaine L J et al 2001 Complications of dynamic graciloplasty: incidence, management and impact on outcome. Diseases of Colon and Rectum 44(10):1427–1435

Niriella D A, Deen K I 2000 Neosphincters in the management of faecal incontinence. British Journal of Surgery 87(12):1617–1628

Rongen M J G M, Adang E M M, Gerritsen van der Hoop A, Baeten C G M I 2001 One step vs two step procedure in dynamic graciloplasty. Colorectal Disease 3:51–57

Stuchfield B 1996 The electrically stimulated neo-anal sphincter. In: Myers C (ed) Stoma care nursing. Arnold, London, p 146–156

Stuchfield B 1997 The electrically stimulated neoanal sphincter and colonic conduit. British Journal of Nursing 6(4):219–224

Stuchfield B, Eccersley A J P 1999 The modern management of faecal incontinence. In: Porrett T, Daniel N (eds) Essential coloproctology for nurses. Whurr Publishers, London, p 292–317

Vaizey C J, Kamm M A, Nicholls R J 1998 Recent advances in the surgical treatment of faecal incontinence. British Journal of Surgery 85(5):596–603

Wexner S D, Baeton C, Bailey R et al 2002 Long term efficacy of dynamic graciloplasty for fecal incontinence. Diseases of the Colon and Rectum 45(6):809–818

Williams N S, Patel J, George B D et al 1991 Development of an electrically stimulated neoanal sphincter. Lancet 338:1166–1169

Williams N S, Ogunbiyi O A, Scott S M et al 2001 Rectal augmentation and stimulated gracilis anal neosphincter. Diseases of the Colon and Rectum 44(2):192–198

Yoshioka K, Keighley M R B 1989. Critical assessment of the quality of continence after postanal repair for faecal incontinence. British Journal of Surgery 76:1054–1057

Chapter **12**

Care of patients with internal urinary pouches

Rachel Busuttil Leaver

The research presented by Lapides and his colleagues (1972) on intermittent, clean self-catheterisation revolutionised the way surgeons approached the diseased bladder and urinary diversions. It encouraged them to develop diversions that were more cosmetically pleasing to many patients than ileal conduits. These also reduced the risk of complications associated with conduit diversions such as renal failure, which is caused by high pressure and repeated pyelonephritis (Woodhouse 1994).

Types of internal urinary diversion include the Kock and Mainz pouches (Kock 1992, Blackley 2004), Indiana pouch (Blackley 2004) and the Mitrofanoff (Busuttil Leaver 1996a, Woodhouse 1991). The types of diversion offered by surgeons in different countries vary, as does the degree to which surgery is performed in specialist or more generalist urology departments. The Mitrofanoff tends to be the diversion of choice in the UK and is usually performed in specialist urology centres. The various operations provide patients with a system similar to that shown in Figure 12.1, comprising:

- an internal reservoir (the pouch) in which their urine collects
- a tunnel from this pouch leading to an abdominal opening (the continent stoma), which enables the pouch to be catheterised and emptied
- a non-return valve made from tissues being used to create the pouch and tunnel, which enables urine to be retained until the pouch is emptied.

A variety of tissues can be used to create the pouch, tunnel and non-return mechanism (Busuttil Leaver 1996a). The style of diversion and tissues

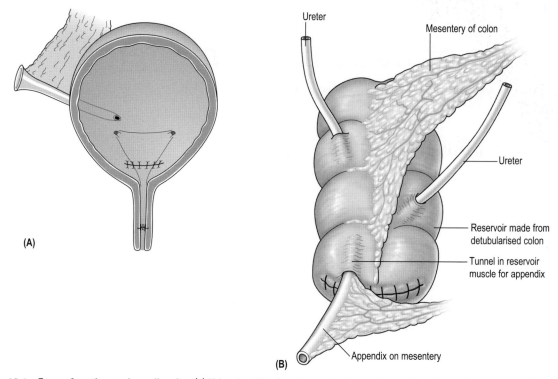

Figure 12.1   Types of continent urinary diversion. (a) Using the Mitrofanoff principle for a patient with sphincter incompetence. The appendix is used for the tunnel with the patient's native bladder as a reservoir. The bladder neck has been closed. (b) Pouch formation using colon with the appendix as tunnel. From Busuttil Leaver (2004a).

used varies in accordance with the patient's condition and the degree to which their original urinary system can be utilised in their new diversion (Woodhouse 1991). Patients do not have to wear appliances and voiding is achieved by inserting a catheter into the stoma and through the tunnel to reach the reservoir. Once the pouch is empty the catheter is removed (Fig. 12.2).

Patients may require urinary diversions for several reasons including:

- congenital problems (e.g. bladder exstrophy)
- neurological disorders affecting the bladder (e.g. myelomeningocele)
- severe incontinence
- cancer
- trauma to the bladder.

Patients may request a continent diversion because they are reluctant to consider alternatives (e.g. ileal conduit; rectal bladders). Ideally they should be given extensive information to help them decide which diversion would be the best solution for them unless there are definite medical reasons why one

type of diversion rather than another may be deemed more suitable.

Patients are *not* usually offered a Mitrofanoff type operation if they have:

- medical conditions that preclude undergoing lengthy anaesthetic (surgery may take 5 or more hours)
- impaired dexterity
- lack of understanding of, and commitment to taking care of the diversion postoperatively.

Preoperative assessment of patients' suitability to have a continent pouch is vital because inappropriate management can lead to serious or fatal consequences such as pouch rupture. Patients should be assessed for their:

- mental and physical state
- levels of motivation and commitment towards care of their pouch for life
- likely ability to cope with the very real possibility of complications, including more treatment and surgery

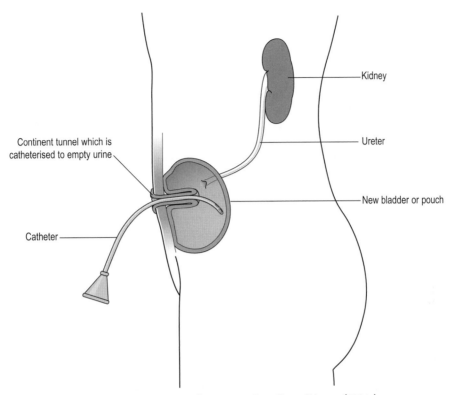

Figure 12.2   Self-catheterisation of pouch via continent urinary stoma. From Busuttil Leaver (2004a).

- ability to understand and use the substantial amount of information they will need to acquire
- likely levels of support (e.g. from family, friends)
- realistic ability to have other lifestyle commitments interrupted (e.g. work; schooling), or carried out by others (e.g. child care) for at least 3 months, as this is the minimum period they will need for surgery and recovery.

Assessment also includes providing patients, and usually their partner or carer, with sufficient information about living with an internal pouch for them to make an informed decision as to whether it is a suitable option for them. Since these operations are rarely performed as emergencies they should be scheduled to give time for such assessment to take place, and for the patient and family to reorganise their other commitments.

Before admission patients undergo many investigations such as kidney function, bladder pressure and blood tests. The results of these enable surgeons to determine what type of reconstruction the patient needs, and form a baseline set of readings against which to subsequently compare postoperative and follow-up test results (Blackley 2004, Busuttil Leaver 2004a). Patients are usually in hospital for 2 to 3 weeks for their pouch creation, followed by about 4 weeks at home. They are then readmitted to have their catheters removed and learn to catheterise their pouch.

FIRST HOSPITAL ADMISSION

PREOPERATIVE CARE

Patients require the usual preparation for surgery, including clearance of their bowel.

Siting the stoma

Even though patients do not wear an appliance over their continent stoma it is still important to site it. *The opening for an internal urinary pouch must be:*

- discreetly positioned, such as in the right iliac fossa or belly button
- in a location which is free of folds and creases in the skin

- compatible with the patient's choice of clothes and lifestyle activities
- where the patient can see and reach it for catheterisation
- able to be used easily in the position the patient adopts when catheterising the pouch, such as standing; sitting in a wheelchair (Fillingham 2004).

Siting can therefore best be achieved when patients are in their usual clothes and when they adopt probable positions in which they will catheterise their pouch as well as positions they use when engaging in normal lifestyle activities to enable potential sites to be assessed. The main difference from siting for a conventional stoma is that for an internal pouch the location is much more discreet.

POSTOPERATIVE CARE

Patients will require the normal monitoring and care given after major surgery, which may include a short stay in intensive care.

The key goals of pouch care at this stage are to ensure:

- the pouch does not stretch before it has healed properly
- urine does not leak into the peritoneum
- the tunnel leading from the abdomen to the pouch heals in a manner which ensures it will not close over once the 'stoma catheter' is removed. Tunnel healing can take 6 weeks.

In order to achieve these goals patients have two catheters draining the pouch, as well as a variety of other tubes (Fig. 12.3). It is vital that:

- The Mitrofanoff (stoma) catheter is safely anchored in place so that urine does not collect in the pouch (which could stretch it too early).
- The pouch (suprapubic) and stoma catheters are kept sufficiently clear of mucus and debris to enable drainage to occur.
- To achieve this these catheters must initially be flushed out with sterile saline twice daily to aid pouch drainage (20 ml at first, usually increasing to 100 ml after 4 days when the pouch has sufficiently healed). Proper washouts can then be commenced.
- Urinary output is monitored and recorded.
- Infection and mucus production are minimised through oral intake of cranberry juice 200 ml twice

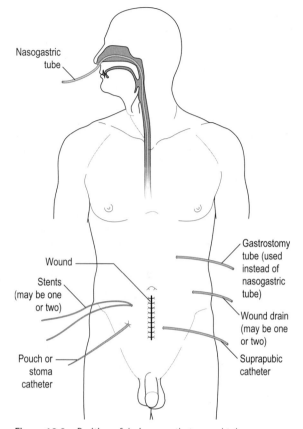

Figure 12.3 Position of drainage catheters and tubes postoperatively. From Busuttil Leaver (2004a).

daily (or equivalent capsule dosage) (Avorn et al 1994, Busuttil Leaver 1996b, Rosenbaum et al 1989). However, cranberry should be recommended with caution if patients are taking warfarin as there is some evidence of interaction between the two (Suvarna et al 2003).

Patients are normally involved in their care at an early stage so they have time to learn to manage their stomal and suprapubic catheter care confidently.

DISCHARGE

The urethral catheter is usually removed 3 to 7 days after surgery, and the ureteric stents 7 to 10 days postoperatively. Patients are discharged home with both the Mitrofanoff catheter and the suprapubic catheter in situ. Before discharge they must be taught how to look after their pouch and catheters and how to deal with more common problems such as catheter blockage; the stoma catheter falling out;

and/or catheter sites becoming infected. During this first period at home patients gain confidence in managing their catheters and urinary drainage bags and become more accustomed to the workings of their new pouch. This is good preparation for when the tubes are removed and catheterisation is started.

If the Mitrofanoff catheter inadvertently falls out it must be replaced as soon as possible to prevent the stoma from closing permanently. It can be helpful to discuss with the patient who might do this (e.g. their GP, local community or hospital staff) or whether they or a carer would have the confidence and ability to replace it. Such discussion helps patients act promptly in these circumstances and thus minimise the time occurring before catheter replacement. The alternative is to return to their specialist hospital for catheter reinsertion.

It is important that patients have a local network of support during this period at home. Community nurses can monitor how patients are coping while helping with dressings, and ensure catheters are well secured and draining adequately. Referral to the local stoma care or continence nurse specialist is often beneficial. All concerned should be aware that infection of the catheter sites and/or urine is highly likely and may require treatment by the GP. It is also essential that patients and carers understand they are welcome to contact their specialist nurse/hospital if they have any concerns.

SECOND HOSPITAL ADMISSION

Patients are readmitted 6 weeks after their original pouch surgery in order to learn how to catheterise their pouch. Discharge home should only occur once patients have both the ability and confidence to self-catheterise, and most patients gain these during a 2–3 night stay.

> **PATIENT SCENARIO 12.1**   John is a 29-year-old man with spina bifida. He is confined to a wheelchair but has some independence through driving a specially adapted car. Prior to surgery he had been incontinent of urine as well as faeces. At present he lives with his parents and does volunteer work with children. His dream is to achieve continence and become independent enough to have a flat of his own. As he has a poor short-term memory Nurse Kelly has been working closely with John and his mother to ensure he

could retain sufficient information to manage his catheters during his time at home following his initial operation. His mother had also acquired the necessary information and skills so she could support John as he completed his self-care activities.

On his second admission John and his mother told Nurse Kelly that he had coped well at home. He was keen to start catheterising his pouch but also somewhat apprehensive as when he had tried urethral catheterisation previously it had been very uncomfortable. He asked if inserting the catheter would be painful and Nurse Kelly told him that the first few catheterisations might make him feel a little sore (rather than painful) but this would quickly subside. The care she had taken to build a rapport with John and prepare him for previous events now paid dividends as John believed her assurances and visibly relaxed. Nurse Kelly then clamped off his suprapubic catheter and removed his Mitrofanoff catheter explaining that if a catheter could not be passed into the Mitrofanoff for any reason, his pouch could still be drained via the suprapubic catheter. Using her previous knowledge of how John learned best Nurse Kelly devised a pouch emptying schedule with John and his mother. By involving them at all stages she helped them build on the confidence and skills in pouch care they had already gained.

EXPANDING THE POUCH

It is important not to allow the pouch to expand too quickly. It can be painful for patients and may damage the pouch if it becomes too full too soon. A 2- or 3-hourly catheterisation regime draining volumes of 150–250 ml urine is usually well tolerated by most patients. Initially patients should be instructed to set an alarm clock to wake them at least once at night to empty their pouch. Many patients can eventually sleep through the whole night once the pouch has expanded to hold much larger volumes of urine (400–500 ml). Patients can help keep their urine volume manageable overnight by restricting their fluid intake for a couple of hours before bedtime. Some patients have enough sensation in their pouch to wake them when it needs emptying.

> **PATIENT SCENARIO 12.2**   After a slightly nervous start John was able to catheterise his pouch quite

competently, ensuring he emptied it completely by applying pressure over the pouch with one hand while twisting and turning the catheter as he pushed it in and out of the tunnel. He understood that these actions were to free the catheter of debris or mucus which might block it, and that the hand pressure would help him drain urine from any pockets or folds in the pouch. Luckily he had enough sensation to be able to identify when his pouch needed emptying. Nurse Kelly warned John that this sensation might decrease as the pouch became larger, and stressed the importance of catheterising at least every 4–6 hours and more frequently if he increased his fluid intake (e.g. when at the pub or in hot weather). She discovered John and his mother had already invested in a wrist watch with a timer and were setting it 4-hourly so John was reminded to catheterise. This sensible solution showed Nurse Kelly that John and his mother had really understood the information they had been given before and after his operation, and were well equipped to deal with any problems they might encounter. John was discharged home after 3 days knowing Nurse Kelly would see him in 8 weeks' time in the outpatients clinic when they would assess his progress.

The catheters used are usually male length size, 12–14 Charriere (Ch) Nelaton type intermittent catheters. There is a wide variety of catheters available. Patients should be encouraged to try different types and choose one which best suits their needs. They should ensure they always have spare catheters with them.

In line with catheter manufacturers' guidelines patients in the UK are normally advised not to reuse catheters. However, in some centres reuse is advocated (e.g. Blackley 2004). If patients might reuse catheters they should be advised to rinse out used catheters in hot soapy water, dry them and store them in a clean container such as a plastic or makeup bag. Nurses should familiarise themselves with local policy regarding longer storage and frequency of replacement of used catheters so that written guidelines prepared for patients reflect current practice.

Most patients do not cover their stoma between catheterisations, especially if it occupies a belly button site. However, patients should be warned that they may experience slight stomal leakage initially while the pouch expands and their new system settles down. Some patients continue to ooze mucus from the stoma and may cover it with gauze to protect their clothing.

Patients can be discharged home when they:

- can accurately identify when they need to empty their pouch
- are able to catheterise the pouch competently, and empty it completely
- have had their suprapubic catheter removed
- have an adequate timespan between catheterisations at night to obtain sufficient sleep
- know how to cleanse and store catheters if reuse may occur
- know how to obtain new equipment
- have adequate equipment for their initial period at home until orders of further supplies arrive
- have absorbed all the information they need to cope with problems
- have been given written guidelines for reference if problems arise (see Appendix 12.1).

Generally it takes upwards of 3 weeks for patients' pouches to expand to their full size. If pouch expansion is slow it can result in patients getting insufficient sleep because catheterisation several times a night is still needed. In these circumstances some patients increase the intervals between catheterisations during the day but leave a catheter taped in situ at night, connected to a night drainage bag. This temporary measure is not ideal as catheters can slip out of the pouch.

Procedures for obtaining equipment vary in different countries. In the UK the Mitrofanoff opening is classed as a stoma and therefore prescriptions of catheters and syringes are free of charge. Patients should follow the procedure for obtaining exemption from prescription charges certificates (see Ch. 8). They should be given both their usual size of Nelaton catheters and some smaller sizes for use if their stoma begins to tighten (see Appendix 12.1).

The speed with which patients' equipment is supplied varies with different suppliers. It may take as little as 24 hours with a specific supply company or 2–3 weeks via some chemists. It is therefore advisable to discuss specifically with patients how they will obtain equipment in order to ascertain how much equipment to provide on discharge (see Ch. 8).

AFTER CARE

The aim of internal pouch formation is to give patients a system of collecting a reasonable volume of urine and draining it easily through catheterisation at acceptable intervals. The system must also function in a manner which keeps the pressure in it at a sufficiently low level to prevent or minimise damage to the upper urinary tract. Woodhouse & Gordon (1994) report up to 20% of patients may have problems following pouch surgery. Woodhouse (1994) reports that common problems include:

- incontinence
- stenosis of the stoma
- urinary infections
- metabolic acidosis
- stone formation
- renal damage.

Patients are currently followed up for life with a range of tests at their clinic visits to monitor whether such complications are occurring. Most patients are happy to comply with such aftercare, feeling it is a small price to pay for having an internal system which does not require an appliance and is under their control. They should also be advised to wear a medical bracelet/pendant (e.g. Medic Alert or SOS) to indicate their condition in case of emergencies.

CONTINENT DIVERSIONS IN CHILDREN

It is rare nowadays for children to be given urostomies if they require permanent bladder reconstruction (Keeble & Lungley 1997). Urostomies are usually only performed as a temporary measure or if patients' underlying medical condition makes reconstruction impossible or unsafe. Children may have urological tests to determine what is causing their problem but treatment (unless urgent) is normally withheld until they are about 3 or 4 years old and have had the chance to gain any benefits possible from usual toilet training procedures. Reassessment at that stage establishes what treatment is needed. Conventional treatments such as intermittent self-catheterisation or use of anti-cholinergic drugs are usually tried before surgical intervention, with the aim of achieving a safe, acceptable result for the child. However, ultimately surgery may be the only option.

Like adults, children will also undergo invasive procedures such as bladder pressure and kidney function tests. It is important that staff performing such tests realise children can experience them as very traumatic, and try to help children and parents minimise difficulties. Preoperative assessment is vital with children but is also more difficult, particularly in very young children where their motivation and capability of compliance cannot be determined. Essentially it is parents' capabilities and motivation that are assessed when it is they who will be catheterising their youngster and coping with any problems. Severely disabled children may never become fully independent of parents or carers but this should not exclude them from having pouch surgery. Many parents find it more acceptable to catheterise a stoma than a urethra, particularly as their child grows older as it does not involve genital catheterisation, which might cause long-term psychological problems for the child (Kurtz et al 1996). Pouch catheterisation is also more acceptable to children's carers at school or rehabilitation centres. It allows those who can catheterise themselves independence, and more dignity for those who cannot.

The implications for children with urinary problems and/or those undergoing treatment are substantial, as are their effects on children and parents. It is essential that the style of care given by all members of the healthcare team is sensitive to the changing psychological and physical needs of children and parents, and enables them to feel well supported. Pouch surgery is time-consuming and children may undergo more than one procedure or need additional treatment. Many children lag behind their peers because of interrupted schooling. Some are bullied because they wear pads or are treated differently (e.g. having help from carers or parents in school; using teachers' toilets).

When children are too young or unable to catheterise themselves then one parent is likely to have to give up work or work part-time so they can be available to catheterise their child every 3–4 hours. The financial implications of this must be discussed and the involvement of a social worker may be beneficial. Many parents in these situations are eligible for special carers' allowances and mobility allowances for their children.

Most children take over their pouch care quite happily as they grow older, though compliance may diminish in adolescence. Some teenagers may feel that their urinary management system was foisted on them by their parents and that they had no choice of treatment.

Having a continent pouch can add to the quality of life for children born with congenital abnormalities. However, it does not take away the reality that they have problems which may affect them for the rest of their lives and they may therefore need more specialised counselling or psychosexual therapy in addition to the support given by their healthcare team. Ensuring that children have access to a counsellor or child psychologist from the very beginning is important as this gives them opportunities to talk about any problems and gain help to find the best solutions. It is too late to wait until they are adults: the damage will have been done (Busuttil Leaver 2004b). However, for most children, having a continent urinary diversion means leading a happy relatively normal life with fewer effects on their body image and quality of life than they could otherwise have experienced through their disabilities or other types of urinary diversion.

APPENDIX 12.1

Patients have a considerable amount of information to remember while learning to manage their continent urinary pouch. This should be discussed individually with patients so they can clarify points and relate it to their own situation. They can then use a handout such as the following example as a summary of key points.

Information and advice for patients

The following advice will help you manage any difficulties or concerns, and recognise when you should seek further help.

(I) If you cannot push the catheter into the tunnel:
1. use some lubricating jelly (e.g. KY) on the catheter
2. try pushing the catheter in a different direction
3. change your position (if you usually stand, lie down or sit) and now try inserting the catheter
4. try a smaller size catheter
5. if the stoma becomes sore ... stop for a few minutes and then try again
6. do not drink any more fluids.

If you manage to get the catheter in:
Leave it in. Attach it to a drainage bag, or spigot it off. Use tape to secure the catheter to your tummy. Telephone the hospital to let us know what the problem is.

(II) If you cannot empty the pouch:
1. try pushing the catheter further into the pouch
2. try coughing or pushing gently onto the pouch with your hand
3. wash out your pouch to dislodge any mucus which may be blocking your catheter
4. if it still will not drain, take out the catheter and try with a new one

Remember:
- you must contact your GP and/or the hospital immediately if unsuccessful in emptying the pouch
- it is especially important to do this if you suffer from any pain
- do not drink any more fluids.

(III) If your scar or stoma site become red; hot to touch, and painful:

1. show this to your GP. If you have an infection they will give you some antibiotics.

(IV) If you pass blood in your urine:

1. drink extra fluids to flush the blood out of your pouch
2. use a softer catheter if your usual one is too harsh and is scratching your stoma, causing the bleeding.

Remember:

*   if the bleeding persists or gets worse contact your GP and/or the hospital
*   if you have pain, leave the catheter in the pouch, attach it to a drainage bag and let the urine drain out.

(V) If your urine is smelly and thick:

1. take a sample of your urine to the GP for testing
2. drink plenty of fluids (at least 3 litres in 24 hours) to flush the pouch
3. drink an extra glass of cranberry juice
4. leave the catheter in on free drainage to let the urine drain out; you can do this only at night if you prefer.
5. catheterise more frequently so urine is not left in the pouch for long periods.

Remember:

*   contact your GP and/or the hospital immediately if you start to shiver and feel generally very unwell.

2 of 2

References

Avorn J, Monane M, Gurwitz J H et al 1994 Reduction of bacteruria and pyuria after ingestion of cranberry juice. Journal of the American Medical Association 10(271):751–754

Blackley P 2004 Practical stoma wound and continence management, 2nd edn. Research Publications, Vermont, Victoria, Australia

Busuttil Leaver R 1996a Continent urinary diversions. In: Myers C (ed) Stoma care nursing. Arnold, London, p 166–179

Busuttil Leaver R 1996b Cranberry juice. Professional Nurse 8, May: 525–526

Busuttil Leaver R 2004a Reconstructive surgery for the promotion of continence. In: Fillingham S, Douglas J Urological nursing, 3rd edn. Churchill Livingstone, Edinburgh, p 135–159

Busuttil Leaver R 2004b Psychological effect of urological problems - adolescents. In: Fillingham S, Douglas J Urological nursing, 3rd edn. Churchill Livingstone, Edinburgh, p 305–313

Fillingham S 2004 Urological stomas. In: Fillingham S, Douglas J Urological nursing, 3rd edn. Churchill Livingstone, Edinburgh, p 207–225

Keeble S, Lungley A 1997 Paediatric urology. In: Fillingham S, Douglas J Urological nursing 2nd edn. Baillière Tindall, London, p 378–411

Kock N G 1992 The evolution of the urinary bladder. In: Hohenfellner R, Wammeck R (eds) Société Internationale d'Urologie Reports - continent urinary diversion. Churchill Livingstone, Edinburgh, p 51–55

Kurtz M J, Van Zandt K, Sapp L R 1996 A new technique in independent intermittent catheterisation: the Mitrofanoff catheterisable channel. Rehabilitation Nursing 21(6):311–314

Lapides J, Diokno A C, Silber S J, Lowe B S 1972. Clean intermittent self-catheterisation in the treatment of urinary tract disease. Journal of Urology 107:458–461

Rosenbaum T P, Shah P J R, Rose G A, Lloyd-Davis R W 1989 Cranberry juice helps the problem of mucus production in enteroplasties. Neurology and Urodynamics 4(8):344–345

Suvarna R, Pirmohamed L, Henderson L 2003 Possible interaction between warfarin and cranberry juice. British Medical Journal 327:1454

Woodhouse C R J 1991 The Mitrofanoff principle for continent urinary diversion. World Council of Enterostomal Therapists Journal 11(1):12–15

Woodhouse C R J 1994 The infective, metabolic and histological consequences of enterocystoplasties. European Board of Urology-European Urology Update series. Union Européenne des Médecins Spécialistes (UEMS), Volume 3

Woodhouse C R J, Gordon E M 1994 The Mitrofanoff principle for urethral failure. British Journal of Urology 73:55–60

Chapter 13

Paediatric stoma care

Helen Johnson and Brigid Breckman

Advances in medicine and nursing in the past decade have led to changes in the way conditions in children are treated, and to the types of stoma created. Infants have their stomas for shorter periods of time and some children, such as those with spina bifida, now rarely require a conventional stoma. Continent diversions and alternative methods for managing incontinence continue to be developed, giving more choice in how bowel and urinary conditions can be managed. Stoma care and continence products also continue to be developed and knowledge of these and how they can best be used is essential if children and their parents are to have informed and supportive care.

Specialist stoma care for adults is now readily available in many countries, but currently there are few paediatric nurses working in the stoma care field. It is therefore necessary for staff in paediatric units and stoma care specialists who are not paediatric nurses to respect each other's expertise and develop ways of combining it so that children and their families have easy access to both knowledgeable, skilled stoma care and paediatric care in a system that is suited to their particular needs.

In this chapter the focus will be mainly on information and care that is required *because the patient is a child*. This includes a brief outline of the main paediatric conditions that necessitate temporary or permanent stoma formation. The types of stoma described in Chapters 3, 6, 10 and 12 are created for both adults and children, so those chapters should be read in conjunction with this one. Likewise many of the principles of practical stoma care in

Chapters 4–7 should also be applied when caring for children in addition to the care described here.

CONDITIONS REQUIRING STOMA SURGERY

IMPERFORATE ANUS

This is a congenital condition where there is no anal exit for faeces. Anomalies are normally classified as high or low depending on whether the defect lies above or below the puborectalis sling. With *high* anorectal anomalies the bowel may end as a blind pouch, and there may be a rectourethral fistula in boys or a rectovaginal fistula in girls through which faeces passes. Treatment of these defects includes creation of a temporary stoma. Full assessment is important. Fitzpatrick (1996) suggests almost two-thirds of these infants will have other abnormalities, with genitourinary and vertebral abnormalities being most common. Malformations of the cardiac, alimentary and central nervous systems can occur. Some reports have indicated that more than one sibling, parent or child in a family may be affected but Smith (1998) states that heredity has a minor or insignificant role in causing the condition.

Assessment will include establishing:

- the nature of the bowel pathway and presence or absence of fistulas
- the presence of any renal anomaly and/or fistula
- the nature of any spinal abnormality (a minimum of three sacral segments are required for normal continence).

Treatment of high anorectal anomalies is usually in three stages:

1. Formation of a colostomy to relieve clinical problems and enable faeces to leave the body freely. This may be a loop sigmoid colostomy or a divided sigmoid colostomy with a mucous fistula.
2. Corrective surgery to create a new bowel pathway linking pelvic colon and an artificially created anus, and closure of any fistulas. This is known as a posterior sagittal anorectoplasty or Peña procedure. Freeman & Bulut (1986) suggest there is physiological evidence that if the bowel is placed in the correct site before 3 months of age appropriate cortical connections may develop and the outcome for continence may be improved. However, timing of this surgery varies at different centres, with 3 months currently being usual at the first author's centre, whereas Fitzpatrick (1996) suggests that major corrective surgery is normally carried out 6-9 months after birth, to give the infant time to thrive and grow before complex surgery is done. Peña & O'Connor (1999) suggest this 'pull through' can be performed in babies over one month providing they are growing and developing normally. Approximately 7 days after this surgery, daily anal dilatations can be commenced in order to prepare the anus to accommodate passage of a normal amount of faeces.
3. Approximately 6 weeks after corrective surgery the bowel pathway is assessed via a distal loopogram and, if satisfactory, the colostomy will then be closed. The lack of a normal external sphincter makes achieving full continence difficult, with perhaps 50% of children achieving this and 25% achieving some control. The child and family may need considerable help to develop a routine which maximises bowel control (Martin 1992).

HIRSCHSPRUNG'S DISEASE

This congenital condition arises as a result of ganglion cells failing to migrate along the intestinal tract before birth. The aganglionic bowel fails to pass faeces through it adequately and the effects of this can vary from bouts of constipation or partial obstruction to total obstruction, depending on the length of bowel affected. The incidence is 1:5000 live births, with a 7% chance of other family members being affected. Fitzpatrick (1996) suggests that the areas of bowel affected by this disease are: sigmoid colon and rectum: 50%; rectal involvement only: 25%; whole colon: 5%; small intestine: 1–2%.

The disease is classified as long or short segment depending on the length of bowel affected. Assessment includes rectal suction biopsies and X-rays to establish the lack of ganglia and length of bowel affected.

Treatment of short segment Hirschsprung's disease may not involve stoma formation. Parents may be taught to perform rectal washouts once or twice daily until corrective surgery is performed.

Longer section impairment requires two or three stages of treatment.

In stage 1 a diversionary stoma will be created above the aganglionic bowel to relieve obstruction and enable adequate faecal elimination.

Stage 2 entails corrective surgery, often referred to as a 'pull-through operation'. The aganglionic bowel is resected, and ganglionic bowel is anastomosed to the anal ring in a manner which creates an adequate size of rectum (Duhamel's procedure).

Stage 3: the stoma is closed.

NECROTISING ENTEROCOLITIS

This condition mainly affects premature and low birthweight babies (Delanty 1997). The specific cause is not known, but it arises as a result of mesenteric vasoconstriction creating intestinal ischaemia and infective gangrene. Treatment is initially conservative: resting the bowel by using parenteral rather than oral feeding and giving intravenous antibiotics.

If the disease progresses and stricture or perforation occurs the diseased bowel may be resected, and a diversionary stoma created to rest the bowel beyond it. The terminal ileum is the area most commonly affected by gangrene and thus an ileostomy is usually required. If an ileo-anal anastomosis is performed because of substantial bowel damage, these children may have their stoma for 6–8 months. Closure of the stoma too early can result in diarrhoea (due to the shortened bowel), creating difficulties in preventing or treating skin damage. It can be preferable to wait until the child is taking a more solid diet and has a more solid faecal output before closing the stoma.

MECONIUM ILEUS

Cystic fibrosis is a genetically determined disease which affects intestinal, bronchial, salivary, and sweat glands and the pancreas. Approximately 10–20% of infants with cystic fibrosis are born with meconium ileus (Fitzpatrick 1999). This occurs because of a deficiency of pancreatic enzymes being released into the intestinal tract. The meconium becomes thick and adheres to intestinal mucosa, resulting in obstruction. At birth babies' abdomens are distended and the meconium is often palpable. Perforation and peritonitis can result if the obstruction is not relieved (Fitzpatrick 1996). Older children with cystic fibrosis can sometimes present with intestinal obstruction requiring stoma surgery.

Initially a hyperosmolar (Gastrografin) enema is generally given to draw fluid into the intestine and dissolve the meconium sufficiently to allow evacuation (Black 2000, Blackley 2004). If this treatment is unsuccessful a temporary loop ileostomy will be created to relieve the obstruction and enable washouts to be done via the stoma. The stoma is normally closed once the baby is thriving (Fitzpatrick 1996, 1999).

INFLAMMATORY BOWEL DISEASE

Ulcerative colitis and Crohn's disease are less common in children but have been reported in infants and older children. Conservative medical treatment is normally used initially. Surgery is used if symptoms cannot be adequately controlled (Fonkalsrud 1993). Opinions vary as to which operation should be used. Fitzpatrick et al (2002) suggest that options for children with ulcerative colitis include restorative proctocolectomy, colectomy and ileorectal anastomosis, or mucosal proctectomy and ileo-anal pull-through.

BLADDER EXSTROPHY

This is a rare and complex congenital condition affecting boys more than girls (ratio 5:2). It can vary in severity and arises because the anterior walls of the lower abdomen and bladder have failed to develop adequately before birth. The pubic bones can be widely separated and the posterior wall of the bladder bulges forward into the gap exposing the bladder mucosa, which is everted due to intra-abdominal pressure. Urine constantly dribbles from the ureteric orifices. Epispadias, a deformity of the urethra and penis, is also present and the testes are generally undescended. The specialised treatment required should be coordinated by paediatric urologists (Canning & Gearhart 1993).

Surgical repair of the abdominal wall is initially performed to try and minimise back pressure from the ureters up the urinary system, which can impair renal function. Other surgery may be staged as necessary to repair other defects such as epispadias and wide separation of the pubic bones (Malone 1994, Du Preez & Ferreira 1992). Urinary continence is usually sought by intermittent catheterisation. If a diversion is needed a Mitrofanoff pouch can be created (see Ch. 12) but children and their parents should be helped to understand that this will not necessarily resolve all problems arising from the original condition (Busuttil Leaver 1996). Artificial urethral sphincters can be used in teenage years (Kaefer et al 1997).

OTHER CONDITIONS

Small numbers of children require stoma surgery for other conditions (Black 2000, Blackley 2004, Fitzpatrick 1996, 1999).

SPECIFIC ASPECTS OF STOMA CARE

Most stomas are created in the neonatal period, often as part of quite substantial corrective surgery. Families are likely to be concerned about the nature and implications of their child's condition as a whole, and struggling to make sense of, and come to terms with the situation generally. This means that stoma-related information and care is being given when the physical and psychological demands on all concerned are considerable, and may affect child and family in many ways. Parents and grandparents may be grieving for the 'perfect' baby they have not received, and other children may experience confusion and loss as their parents' time and attention is primarily focused on the ill child (Lendrum & Syme 1992). It is therefore important that the healthcare team work closely together so that the purpose of investigations and treatment as a whole is well understood, and that information about stoma surgery and care is congruent with the overall medical treatment plan and explanations.

The weariness that comes from trying to maintain family and work commitments in tandem with hospital visits and adaptation to the child's appearance, situation and needs should not be underestimated. Approaches described in Chapters 7–9 and 22 can also be used to gain understanding of families' experiences and needs, and offer helpful support. Parents may need sensitive help to achieve a balance between spending sufficient time with their child to bond and develop a loving relationship, and having time for themselves and other family members and commitments. Where treatment is ongoing or carried out in stages over time, staff should encourage the family to develop a variety of sources of support so they have access to ongoing help and supporters do not feel overburdened.

Most of the principles of practical management of stomal appliances and skin care described in the bowel and urinary chapters are also applicable when caring for children. However, prolapse seems to be more common in children than adults (in the first author's experience) so advice about seeking medical help if this occurs and if the stoma becomes more dusky coloured and tense to touch can be given to parents and (older) children. Adaptation of principles of care includes considering:

- *how* information and care should be given in order to be appropriate for the cognitive development and capabilities of the child
- *what* information and care is required for the individual child and family
- *who* can give additional support (e.g. play specialists in hospital; community healthcare staff at home; a designated welfare assistant to help with special needs at school).

INFANTS

Generally, one-piece flexible paediatric or mini-stoma bags are more suitable for the size and shape of babies.

Babies' skin tends to dry easily so agents that are alcohol-based and/or dry the skin, such as adhesive removers and skin protective wipes, should not be used. The first author finds dry skin can be problematic with sick neonates and that general oiling of their skin, or adding a little baby oil to bath water, does not create difficulties with bag adherence as long as the excess is wiped off before completing normal stoma care. However, Fitzpatrick (1999, p 43) suggests that baby oil in the bath does prevent bags sticking.

Appropriate care and cuddling by parents should be encouraged to aid bonding and help them begin to come to terms with their baby's condition. Involvement of other family members to provide care and support is beneficial (Fitzpatrick 1996).

PATIENT SCENARIO 13.1   Mrs Reid, the stoma care nurse, was talking to Karen and Dave about how to recognise and respond to problems which could arise with their 2-week-old baby, Ben. He had undergone a hemicolectomy and formation of an ileostomy and mucous fistula for a bowel stricture following conservative treatment for necrotising enterocolitis. Ben's young parents had found it difficult initially to look at his ileostomy. They were now managing to empty and change his one-piece drainable bag quite easily, although Karen had needed repeated assurances that water would not enter his abdomen through the stoma when she first bathed him without his bag on.

Ben was likely to have his stoma for several months, spending much of this time recuperating at home. Mrs Reid had discussed his situation, and the kind of care his family would need support to provide, with their local stoma care nurse and health visitor. Their monitoring role was particularly important because prompt medical attention might be needed if problems such as dehydration, sodium imbalance, or inability to tolerate lactose arose as a result of Ben's shortened or diseased bowel. Ben was stabilised on milk-free feeds before discharge, but Karen would need additional dietary advice at weaning time if Ben still had his ileostomy and needed to continue avoiding milk products (Blackwell 1993).

Although medical follow-up would take place regularly, Mrs Reid wanted to inform Ben's parents of symptoms which would signal to them that they should seek medical help promptly rather than wait for Ben's next medical appointment. She knew it was important to achieve a balance between getting them to understand that these symptoms could indicate serious problems so help should be sought promptly without making them so anxious that they would be unwilling or unable to care for Ben at home. The symptoms she discussed were:

- increasing looseness, wateriness or volume of stomal output (could signal difficulties in digestion, e.g. with sugar, or loss of sodium requiring change of diet)
- reducing urinary output (possible sodium imbalance requiring oral or intravenous correction)
- sunken fontanelle, greyness under Ben's eyes (possible dehydration requiring oral or intravenous fluid replacements and electrolyte monitoring)
- any episode of vomiting which might be more quickly dehydrating (i.e. where there also was a high throughput of fluid via the ileostomy).

Having given Ben's parents this information Mrs Reid encouraged them to say what they would do if they noticed these symptoms under different circumstances (e.g. day or night time, if they were away from home), confirming suitable ideas. This approach helped Mrs Reid assess that Ben's parents could use their growing knowledge without undue anxiety, and the parents gained confidence in their ability to recognise and deal with problems well.

As children grow and stomal output increases their equipment will need regular reviewing. A larger capacity and adhesive area may be needed and, if the stoma size alters, a changed gasket size may be required.

AGE 6 MONTHS TO 2 YEARS

All-in-one jumpsuits/vests may prevent curious youngsters from exploring, and removing, stomal equipment!

Children of this age always prefer familiar faces so consistency in family and staff providing care is desirable to help them feel secure. Positive 'messages' about the stoma and equipment should be conveyed verbally and non-verbally during appliance changes. When parents provide skilled, confident stoma care their children accept it more readily. Simple explanations should be given at the time procedures take place, as young children live in the present and will not connect them with later events.

AGE 2 TO 5 YEARS

Children of this age are curious about their own and their friends' bodies, and may ask why they function differently. They will not have the ability to understand detailed explanations about internal body systems which they cannot see. Parents can be encouraged to offer simple explanations, bearing in mind that a child's attention span is about 10–15 minutes at 3 years, 20 minutes at 4 years, and 30 minutes at age 5 (Erwin-Toth 1996). They can also begin to involve their child in aspects of care that are suitable for the levels of hand and eye coordination and thinking which the child has developed. This also helps parents and child follow the pattern of beginning to promote self-care which would normally occur as children prepare for nursery and school attendance.

Time and opportunities should be given for parents to discuss concerns and gain additional information about help which can be provided so children can attend ordinary local schools. Liaison with school personnel may help ensure they offer informed help more knowledgeably and willingly, knowing they can call on the expertise of the parents and stoma care nurse if required.

AGE 6 TO 12 YEARS

Many children of this age group will have had their stoma for some time. It can be useful to assess their current situation and check whether parents and children need help to make the transition from the parents doing the stoma care to the child gaining the ability to manage their own care. Equipment may need changing to a style which the child can learn to manage and change, is sufficiently discreet yet robust to stand up to sporting and other activities, and has an adequate capacity to contain effluent during school lessons and social activities.

It is important that realistic goals of self-care are set so children are successful as they gradually take on more of their own stoma care. Children up to about the age of 9 can usually empty their appliance but will need prompting to do so. They also need some supervision when actually changing pouches. From age 9 onwards the majority of children with normal cognitive development and hand coordination will probably be able increasingly to care for themselves. Families are included in teaching sessions so they can offer support and reinforcement as the child acquires the ability to manage their own care competently and confidently (Erwin-Toth 1996).

Social roles and being similar to peers can be important and the child who gains a stoma during these years will need help to develop sufficient knowledge and skills to be able to adapt their stoma care to a range of situations. Books on stoma care for children and families can be used to build up their understanding and invite them to raise any concerns. Introducing the child to another child who has had similar surgery may be helpful for children and their families. Children who have had their stoma for some time can also benefit from more detailed information as their ability to understand it develops. Websites for children covering a range of health-related areas are now becoming available (Shuttleworth 2003).

ADOLESCENCE

A stoma and its management impinges on many of the areas that normally preoccupy adolescents: their developing sense of themselves physically, sexually and emotionally; their wish to be accepted as part of their chosen peer group, looking and behaving like their friends; and their need to increase the boundaries within which they can have choice and control. Absence from school due to surgery or illness can affect current studies and thus future work prospects and it is important to help teenagers maintain studies and friendships which can help them retain self-esteem and a sense of themselves as part of their normal world.

The focus of stoma care is primarily on helping the adolescent become informed and skilled in self-care so they can confidently adapt stoma management to fit in with school and social activities. It is not always easy for parents to stand back and yet signal they remain interested and available, thereby offering the kind of balanced support which enables their teenager to play a considerable role in decision-making about their treatment and care, but this can be one of the most helpful things they can do for their maturing son or daughter. Parents may need help to develop and maintain this ability, especially if thanks for it from the teenager is rare.

Adolescents who have had their stoma for a while may need to revise or increase the level of understanding they have about their stoma and condition. Generally it is wise to begin by identifying the teenager's current understanding of their condition, stoma and its management, and any concerns or questions they may have. This enables misconceptions and out-of-date information or care to be corrected before additional information is given. They may equate advice with being treated as children rather than adults. It may be more helpful to give them information and then discuss the implications and options arising from it so they can develop their abilities to make informed choices. Negotiation as to what happens to information given by adolescents is important as it signals that staff are respectful of their growing need for privacy, control and autonomy.

Common concerns include how to:

- tell friends and possible sexual partners about their condition and/or stoma
- fit their stoma and its management discreetly into sport, social, and sexual activities
- feel confident and acceptant of themselves.

Many of the skills and approaches for promoting rehabilitation in adults described in other chapters can also be used to help adolescents gain adequate knowledge and skills with which to care for themselves and make the transition to a personally and socially confident adult. Contact with other teenagers and young adults who have made this transition with a similar stoma or internal pouch can provide useful role models as well as sources of advice with 'street credibility'.

ALTERNATIVE BOWEL MANAGEMENT

Many children whose stomas have been closed after corrective surgery for congenital bowel abnormalities (such as those described earlier) may continue to have difficulties achieving continence and/or managing constipation, as may children with spina bifida. Management can often be improved by using either colonic irrigation or Malone's antegrade continence enema (ACE) technique to wash faeces out of the colon every 24–48 hours. These techniques are unsuitable for children with inflammatory bowel disease (Fitzpatrick 1996). Children with megacolon can use the ACE although washout results may not be as good.

Both techniques require children to sit on the toilet for about 40 minutes to enable their bowel to empty, so the levels of their motivation and parental support need careful assessment and children generally need to be at least 5 years old.

Each system has advantages and disadvantages. Since the rectum can be used for colonic irrigation without the preparatory surgery required for the ACE some children are advised to use colonic irrigation initially. This enables all concerned to experience the time, activities and results of a washout style of bowel management without surgery. However, children who are not mobile enough to get on and off the toilet easily may manage better with the ACE technique where they can instil fluid into the bowel via the more accessible abdominal stoma. This includes some children with spina bifida.

COLONIC IRRIGATION

The *aim* is to empty the transverse and descending colon. Most children can use a conventional irrigation set, preparing and using it in a similar manner to that described in Chapter 15 but gently inserting the lubricated cone into the rectum to instil the warmed (38°C) normal saline. After the cone is removed the child should remain on the toilet until the saline and faeces have been eliminated.

Some children with conditions affecting their anorectal area may find the Shandling enema continence catheter more useful as it has a balloon which can be inflated inside the rectum. Fitzpatrick (1996, p 195–196) suggests that the size of both catheter and balloon are too large for children under the age of 7 or those who have a very tight anus.

ANTEGRADE CONTINENCE ENEMA

Surgery entails using the appendix to create a channel between the abdominal wall and the caecum which can subsequently be catheterised and used for washouts (Malone 2004). As the caecal end is implanted in a non-refluxing manner this means the abdominal stoma remains continent. The two enema fluids are run into the bowel through the catheterised appendix channel and are eliminated rectally.

The *aim* of the ACE is to empty ascending, transverse, and descending colon. The first enema given therefore generally contains 50% enema with 50% normal saline to stimulate bowel evacuation. This is followed by a second enema which is usually of similar volume to the first one, but consists of normal saline. A small rectal tube, attached to an irrigation set or large syringe, is used to catheterise the stoma and enter the appendix channel for about 6 cm before the two enemas are given. After the tube is withdrawn the child should remain on the toilet until all the solution and faeces have been evacuated.

It may take up to a month after surgery to establish a satisfactory routine as the child resumes their normal diet and lifestyle, and enema contents and volume are adjusted to maximise evacuation and continence.

Many of the concerns about management of elimination, body image and social acceptability are just as likely to be held by children and families using these systems of bowel management, an ileo-anal pouch (see Ch. 10), or the Mitrofanoff urinary continent pouch (see Ch. 12), as those who have a conventional stoma. It is therefore important that knowledgeable care and ongoing support is readily available for them in hospital and at home (Fitzpatrick 1999, Fitzpatrick et al 2002).

References

Black P K 2000 Holistic stoma care. Baillière Tindall and RCN, Edinburgh, p 151–154

Blackley P 2004 Practical stoma wound and continence management, 2nd edn. Research Publications, Vermont, Victoria, Australia, p 35-38; 61–63

Blackwell T Y D 1993 Food and food additives intolerance in childhood. Blackwell Scientific Publications, Oxford, p 33–34

Busuttil Leaver R 1996 Continent urinary diversions – the Mitrofanoff principle. In: Myers C (ed) Stoma care nursing. Arnold, London, p 166–179.

Canning D A, Gearhart J P 1993 Exstrophy of the bladder. In: Ashcraft K W, Holder T M (eds) Paediatric surgery, 2nd edn. WB Saunders, Philadelphia, p 678–693

Delanty S 1997 Neonatal necrotizing enterocolitis. World Council of Enterostomal Therapists Journal 17(3):26–29

Du Preez N I, Ferreira M W A 1992 A study of bladder exstrophy from childhood to adolescence. In: World Council of Enterostomal Therapists congress proceedings. Hollister, Libertyville, IL, p 84–86

Erwin-Toth P 1996 The holes within the whole: childhood ostomy surgery – a developmental view. In: World Council of Enterostomal Therapists congress proceedings. Hollister, Libertyville, IL, p 53–55

Fitzpatrick G 1996 The child with a stoma. In: Myers C (ed) Stoma care nursing. Arnold, London, p 180–202

Fitzpatrick G 1999 The role of the paediatric stoma care nurse. In: Taylor P (ed) Stoma care in the community. Nursing Times Books, London, p 33–56

Fitzpatrick G, Coldicutt P, Williams J 2002 Children and internal pouches. In: Williams J (ed) The essentials of pouch care nursing. Whurr Publishers, London, p 199–217.

Fonkalsrud E W 1993 Inflammatory bowel disease. In: Ashcraft K W, Holder T M (eds) Paediatric surgery, 2nd edn. WB Saunders, Philadelphia, p 440–452

Freeman N V, Bulut M 1986 'High' anorectal anomalies treated by early 'neonatal' operation. Journal of Paediatric Surgery 21:218–220

Kaefer M, McLaughlin K P, Rink R C et al 1979 Upsizing of the artificial urinary sphincter cuff to facilitate spontaneous voiding. Urology 50(1):106–109

Lendrum S, Syme G 1992 Gift of tears. Routledge, London

Malone P S 1994 Bladder exstrophy and epispadias complex. In: Freeman N V, Burge D M, Griffiths D M, Malone P S (eds) Surgery of the newborn. Churchill Livingstone, Edinburgh

Malone P S J 2004 The antegrade continence enema procedure. British Journal of Urology International 93(3):248

Martin J 1992 Imperforate anus – achieving continence. In: World Council of Enterostomal Therapists congress proceedings. Hollister, Libertyville, IL, p 177–178

Peña A, O'Connor K 1999 Colorectal problems in paediatric patients. In: Porrett T, Daniel N (eds) Essential coloproctology for nurses. Whurr Publishers, London, p 332–357

Shuttleworth A 2003 A health website for children. Nursing Times 99(44):18–19

Smith D 1998 Incidence, frequency of types and etiology of anorectal malformations. In: Stephens F D, Smith E D (eds) Anorectal malformations in children. Update 1998. March of Dimes Birth Defect Foundation. Alan R Liss, New York, p 232–237

Chapter 14

Care of patients with fistulas and drain sites

Brigid Breckman

A fistula is an abnormal passage between two or more spaces. The communication can be from one hollow organ to another hollow organ or to the skin (Rolstad & Bryant 2000). The main focus in this chapter is on enterocutaneous fistulas, where communication is between intestine and skin. Blackley (2004), Keighley (1993) and Meadows (1997) suggest causes include:

- surgery in which bowel has been opened (most common)
- conditions such as Crohn's disease, diverticulitis, cancer
- bowel damage, e.g. following radiotherapy, trauma, gunshot wounds.

Care of patients with fistulas is normally complex. Reasons for this include the following:

- Fistulas affect patients physically and psychologically: there are multiple effects with which staff and patients must deal.
- Patients' situations can change frequently and/or with minimal warning, affecting their physical and psychological wellbeing. Treatment and care must therefore be flexible enough to respond to both the unpredictability and the effects of such changes.
- Staff from a range of healthcare disciplines will be involved in assessment and treatment. This requires detailed discussion so that shared goals, and strategies for achieving them, are agreed.
- Treatment is likely to take place over a substantial period of time. The effects of this on patients, their families, and staff adds to the complexity of the overall situation to be managed.

CLASSIFICATION OF FISTULAS

Forbes & Myers (1996) indicate that procedures used to assess types of fistulas are far from ideal. Different procedures provide particular elements of the information which needs to be known in order for treatment strategies to be decided. They suggest the following:

- Barium and other contrast agents will often show fistulous tracts, but obtaining sufficient information is dependent on careful screening of the contrast agent as it progresses through the intestine, and correct interpretation of the appearance of the contrast agent at different levels. A fistulogram may be obtained following injection of contrast agent via a small catheter inserted into the fistula opening.
- Abdominal ultrasound scanning is unlikely to show fistulous tracts, but may reveal areas of abnormal intestine, and abscesses.
- Contrast-enhanced computed tomography (CT scan) can demonstrate abscesses and retroperitoneal disease associated with a fistula, but frequently fails to demonstrate the fistula opening(s).
- Magnetic resonance imaging (MRI) discriminates between normal and diseased tissues and shows all fistula openings to a much greater degree than ultrasound or CT scans. It can therefore improve the level of assessment of fistulas and the surrounding area.
- Endoscopic examination rarely identifies fistula openings but can help establish whether there is underlying Crohn's disease or diverticulosis, and the sites where these are occurring.

Additional information will be obtained through monitoring the blood chemistry to establish the effects of effluent loss on the body.

This kind of detailed information is essential because the type of fistula and the presence or absence of disease or infection affects the potential of the fistula to heal through different types of management, and thus the choice of treatment that will be deemed suitable (O'Dwyer 1997).

Fistulas can be described in accordance with the type of alternative pathway for bowel contents which has been created (Blackley 2004, Cobb & Knaggs 2003).

Simple single fistula There is one connective pathway between the bowel and abdominal wall. Effluent can pass along this track as well as along the normal bowel route as long as there is no distal bowel obstruction.

Multiple fistulas These may appear as two or more unconnected openings on the abdominal wall, with effluent discharging from some or all of them. However, internally there may still be sufficient normal bowel pathway to allow effluent to also pass along that route.

Complex fistulas Here there may be single or multiple abdominal openings, but internally the normal bowel pathway has become disrupted through factors such as diseased bowel or abscess formation. Faecal effluent can leak into the abdominal cavity as well as through the fistula track to the exterior of the body.

With the first two types of fistulas, if there is no distal obstruction or major source of infection or disease, closure can more often be obtained through medical management without surgical intervention. However with complex fistulas, and in situations where there is bowel obstruction as well as a fistula, surgical intervention may be required once the patient's general condition and nutritional requirements have been stabilised.

Care also depends on the point along the patient's intestinal pathway at which the fistula occurs. Once effluent is diverted from the intestine along the fistula it will no longer go through the normal processes of digestion and fluid reabsorption. The fistula position therefore affects:

- the amount of digestion of food which can occur, and therefore the levels of nutrition patients obtain from oral intake
- the amount of fluid which can be reabsorbed back into the body from intestinal contents, and therefore the consistency and volume of fistula output
- the level of digestive enzymes which are still in the intestinal contents at the time they are diverted via the fistula, and therefore the potential corrosiveness of that effluent on the patient's body. This can include damage to internal abdominal tissues as well as skin damage as effluent passes out of the fistula onto the surrounding skin.

Generally, the earlier (higher) in the intestinal tract fistulas occur (e.g. small bowel) the more patients will require:

- substantial perifistular skin protection
- equipment which can accommodate a substantial weight and volume of effluent without leakage
- nutritional monitoring and supplementation.

The cumulative effect of all these factors on patients who are likely also to have at least some infection present, and who may have additional conditions such as Crohn's disease or cancer, should not be underestimated. Substantial physical and psychological support is normally required over what may well be an extended period of time (Cobb & Knaggs 2003, Hopkins 2001, Ross 1994).

CARE OF THE FISTULA AND SURROUNDING SKIN

Even when fistula effluent volume is low its odour and abrasiveness generally make management with appliances rather than dressings preferable (Rolstad & Bryant 2000). Key nursing objectives are therefore to:

- fit and maintain appliances so that patients are dry, comfortable, and as mobile as possible
- protect the skin around the fistula from discharge that can cause excoriation and leakage
- minimise odour
- ensure all losses are collected and their volume measured to allow deficits to be counteracted
- minimise cross-infection
- maintain the morale of the patient and family and their healthcare team.

The effects of fistula loss on patients' weight and body shape, skin condition, skin protectives and appliances can vary considerably, and the specific nature of those changing effects can be unpredictable. Treatment given to combat the nutritional effects of fistula loss, infection and any underlying disease also affects patients' bodies, healing capacity and fistula output, increasing the likelihood of unpredictability and change. Generally, if the occurrence of such changes is accepted as likely, it is easier to view them as factors to be dealt with rather than a signal that the situation is totally disastrous.

Principles of fistula care allowing free drainage into an appliance similar to those described below have been described by a number of writers (Black 2000, Blackley 2004, Meadows 1997, Rolstad & Bryant 2002).

PRINCIPLES OF FITTING EQUIPMENT

The task of fitting a leak-proof appliance which produces well-protected skin can be considered in three sections:

- preparation of the patient and equipment
- creation of a clean dry skin
- application of equipment.

Fistulas tend to leak copiously at inopportune moments as we seek to complete these tasks, interrupting our thoughts as well as our actions. The detailed descriptions here will help you and your colleagues develop a clear mental map of useful steps to take, why, and in what sequence.

Preparation of the patient and equipment

A full assessment may be required because:

- the fistula has recently occurred, creating a situation which requires management
- the patient is newly in the care of staff, and a regime for effective management has yet to be established
- the currently used fistula management is not achieving good skin protection, effluent containment and patient comfort.

Step 1   Obtain background information from the patient's records about the position of the fistula in the intestinal pathway, and the nature of effluent being passed (e.g. type, amount, consistency) to aid your assessment.

Step 2   If the patient has an appliance or dressing in place which is containing most of the fistula effluent, observe it *and leave it in place at this stage*. You will both concentrate better on exchanging information if your attention is not distracted by major leakage occurring when no system is in place to contain it.

Ask the patient about:

- the frequency, amount and consistency of fistula effluent
- measures already used to deal with leakage and their level of success.

Step 3   Prepare for a wide range of possible requirements when collecting equipment before starting the assessment. This enables the move from assessment to application of appropriate equipment to occur smoothly. Minimal delay between the two processes helps reduce patient anxiety and increases their confidence that their situation can be managed.

Equipment to have available for use following a full assessment should include:

- warm water, paper wipes for cleansing the skin, and a large rubbish container
- pen, paper/acetate for making a template, scissors for wafer/bag preparation
- a stoma measuring guide, and range of stoma and fistula appliances of different gasket sizes and styles to suit known fistula size, and likely output levels and consistency
- a range of products to create a level base for the appliance. Useful ones include hydrocolloid wafers, washers and powder, filler paste, a spatula for smoothing paste
- hypoallergenic tape for sealing, creating extra support
- a kidney dish, and protective material to prevent spillage onto the bed or patient's clothes
- suction apparatus and a hair dryer, to help produce a dry enough skin for bag adherence
- razor for hair removal
- gloves and apron to maintain normal professional policies on infection control
- an odour-containing spray.

Step 4 If there has been recent substantial and/or fluid fistula output it is advisable to co-opt a second person (e.g. colleague, the patient) to use suction apparatus to keep the perifistular area as free of effluent as possible while thorough assessment and effective application of equipment takes place. This reduces the problems that arise when one person tries to contain spillage at skin level and simultaneously prepare and apply new equipment.

Step 5 Ensure the patient is warm, comfortable, and their privacy assured for what may be quite a lengthy period.

Generally patients benefit from being told the assessment may take some time because information about their situation as a whole has to be gathered first, before decisions about bags and skin care (which are interrelated) can be made. This helps patients view the procedure as a positive, skilled measure to help them, rather than 'evidence' that the situation is unmanageable or that staff are unsure how to manage it.

Step 6 Use the following *three-stage process of assessment* to obtain the information you require in order to choose equipment that will promote good skin care and effluent containment.

First, assess the following:

- Size and number of fistulas.
- Position of the fistulas in relation to bones, body contours, wounds, scars, gullies, and the way in which these change when patients are lying down, standing and seated.
- Probable consistency, volume and corrosiveness of effluent, given the position of the fistula in the intestinal pathway and the records of effluent being passed.
- Patient's type of skin and any particular needs or problems with skin protective agents which might arise (e.g. through eczema, psoriasis, history of rapid burning in sunlight, which can indicate a sensitive skin). These should be considered in conjunction with any skin damage currently present.
- Level of expertise likely to be (a) required and (b) available in people who will be preparing and applying the skin protectives and appliances. Complex systems may be easily fitted by experienced nurses but if such expertise is rarely available when equipment needs changing then it may be wise to devise a simpler system.

Second, use the information you have gained to identify the *criteria which the equipment should fulfil*:

- the stoma or fistula bag:
  - its capacity, shape, ability to drain thinner or thicker effluent either for intermittent emptying or continuous drainage into a night drainage bag, level of odour containment
  - whether more than one bag is required (e.g. to collect drainage separately from different fistulas; to increase capacity to contain high volume output)
- the flange or gasket:
  - its size and ability to cover the fistula(s) individually or collectively
  - the size of the adhesive area required to provide sufficient adherence if the bag becomes weighted with substantial drainage
  - the depth, convexity and rigidity/flexibility of the whole flange and the gasket (ring or opening) which is required in order to fit in with the patient's contours, bones and bulges, and prevent pooling of effluent in the well of the gasket

- skin protection:
  - the level of skin protection that is required from the flange, both to prevent effluent seeping rapidly through the flange onto the skin or clothes, and to cover a substantial enough area of skin to prevent dragging or lifting of a heavy bag
  - the need for any filling and/or flattening materials to create a level surface for the skin protective wafer/flange
  - the likelihood of pain being experienced by the patient during the application or removal of equipment (e.g. because it is an alcohol-based substance going onto open skin; due to tender abdomen arising from unhealed wounds, fistulas etc.)
  - factors required for compatibility with the patient's skin type
- manageability of equipment:
  - ease of preparation, application, removal required (a) through the patient's situation; and (b) given the likely levels of expertise of staff available to provide the care
  - ease of emptying and/or connecting to a larger container required for the amount and consistency of effluent likely to be passed.

Third, assess the equipment available, so you can identify items meeting all or most of the above criteria.

Choosing which equipment to use may involve using the best immediately available equipment, and ordering of more suitable equipment for subsequent use by staff and/or patients and their families.

Step 7 Check that the equipment you gathered earlier contains all the items you now know you are likely to use. Collect additional items required.

Step 8 Check with patients whether they are familiar with the process you are about to use, or would like an explanation. Patients who are unfamiliar with the equipment or processes often benefit from an outline of the principles you will be following. Watching staff apply some filler paste here, peristomal wafer pieces there etc. in order to level abdominal contours, patients can experience this as a rather inexact or piecemeal management system (and may worry it will be an insecure system with which to contain effluent). Outlining the rationale underpinning the equipment choice and mode of application helps patients feel that control over their wayward fistula can be achieved. However,

explanations may have to be left until after equipment has been fitted if the fistula is leaking substantial amounts of effluent and/or odour, as the patient's mind will be more likely to be on these problems than on your explanation.

Step 9 Before removing a used appliance notice points where effluent seepage could occur, such as where a flange or wafer is lifting or creased and the seal with the body is lost. Remove the equipment and look at its undersurface: melted skin protectives can indicate where effluent is tracking along a crease or pooling in an abdominal dip. These areas will require filling in, so it is important to identify where exactly they are on the patient's abdomen.

Step 10 Cleanse the fistula and surrounding area gently with warm water. If the fistula is in an open wound it can be irrigated gently with syringefuls of warmed normal saline to remove effluent. Suction can be used to keep the cleansed area free from effluent. The skin should be patted gently dry using paper towels or tissues (not cotton wool, which can stick to the skin, creating subsequent difficulties in adherence of equipment).

Step 11 Select a suitable stoma or fistula bag to cover the fistula and allow easy drainage and/or connection to a larger drainage bag. Check that the hydrocolloid adhesive (now integral in most flanges/bases) is sufficient in substance and size to provide good skin protection and adherence (Fig. 14.1).

If additional skin protection and/or a product to create a flat abdominal surface is required, this should also be selected now. If possible use products which are not alcohol based to minimise patients' discomfort (Cobb & Knaggs 2003).

Step 12 Prepare a template for use as a pattern when cutting the opening in the wafer/flange to ensure it will fit snugly around the fistula or wound orifice. A clear piece of plastic or paper can be used to make the template by drawing an accurate outline of the opening to be cut on it, and then cutting it out.

Write on the template the date and which side of the opening is the patient's left and right, to help future users of it know if it is a recent pattern, and which way up it fits over the fistula (Fig. 14.2).

Use the template to cut out the wafer and/or flange. Close the bag outlet.

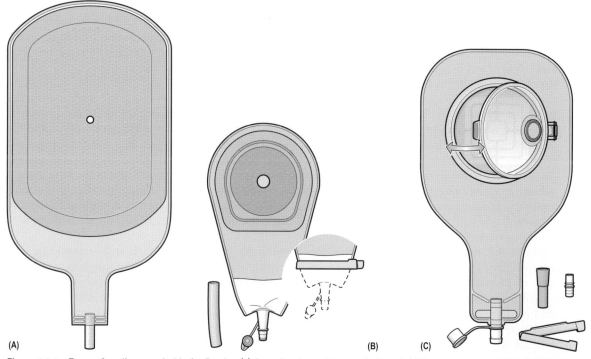

Figure 14.1 Types of appliances suitable for fistulas. (a) One-piece bag with large hydrocolloid flange area to accommodate multiple fistulas and sizeable drainage. (b) One-piece tapered bag giving choice of tube or clip outlet. (c) One-piece large drainable bag with porthole to allow access to fistula or wound area, and flatus filter. Tube or clip outlet can be used.

Step 13 Select any products you may need to use to fill in the creases and dips to create a level peri-fistular area. If using pieces of hydrocolloid wafer or rings, cut them to shape now. Use a filler paste which is fairly substantial and will harden as it dries (e.g. Stomahesive rather than Orahesive paste).

Step 14 If the fistula is very active remove the backing paper from the prepared bag, so that equipment can be speedily applied as soon as you are ready to do so.

Step 15 Decide which system of applying fillers you are going to use and prepare for it:

If the fistula is less active or you can keep the area dry using suction you can use paste and/or rings or pieces of wafer to accurately fill in and smooth out the abdominal surface first, and then apply the rest of the equipment over this base. You can get a more accurate application of skin protective fillers with this method if the area can be kept effluent-free for long enough to use it. Skin protection and prevention of leakage can be better with this method (Fig. 14.3).

If the fistula is very active it may be best to apply filler paste and/or rings to the sticky undersurface of the wafer in the appropriate positions so that when applied as an all-in-one system the paste/ring pieces squidge into the abdominal dips and creases. It is often useful to apply a thin 'worm' of paste around the hole in the wafer to help get a really snug fit around the fistula or wound opening, thus promoting maximum skin protection. It is difficult to get an entirely accurate filling in of dips with this system, but it may be the only way you can get equipment in place between fistula actions (Fig. 14.4).

With *either* of the above methods it can be helpful to line the fistula or wound orifice lightly with a pale-coloured skin protective powder (e.g. Orahesive) just before applying the other equipment. It gives added protection to the area and helps highlight the exact opening to be covered, aiding accurate equipment application.

Creation of a clean dry skin

Step 16 Complete any further skin cleansing and drying needed because of effluent leakage while

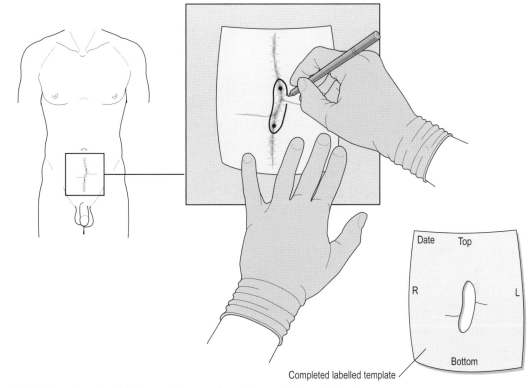

Figure 14.2   Preparing a template to use with an appliance flange or hydrocolloid wafer.

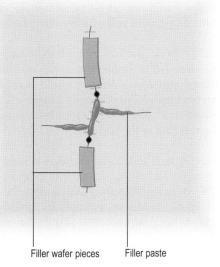

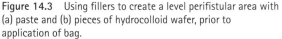
Filler wafer pieces   Filler paste

Figure 14.3   Using fillers to create a level perifistular area with (a) paste and (b) pieces of hydrocolloid wafer, prior to application of bag.

you were preparing the equipment. Use suction to contain any effluent leakage being passed. Shave area if hairs are likely to cause problems when removing or applying equipment.

Step 17   Skin that is moist, broken and/or sore can be dried using a hairdryer on a low setting. This causes less discomfort to patients and achieves a drier skin. Generally you can now apply the necessary fillers and wafers without additional skin products underneath them (see later problems section), but calamine lotion sometimes helps soothe sore skin.

Application of equipment

Step 18   Puff skin protective powder (if used) *sparingly* into the sides of the fistula or wound.

Step 19   Use a filler paste as necessary to fill in any dips and creases and create a level perifistular area.

NB: if you use a paste which contains alcohol warn patients before use that it may sting for a few seconds if being applied to broken skin. The odour

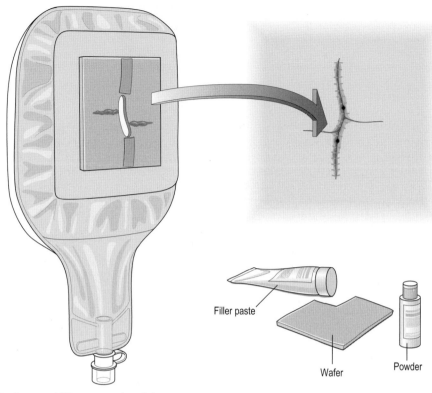

Figure 14.4 Appliance and fillers prepared as all-in-one.

(which some patients dislike) also vanishes within a few minutes of application.

Apply a small worm of paste and smooth it into place with a damp spatula or finger, adding further amounts as necessary, rather than applying too bulky a blob, some of which then has to be scraped off.

Allow the paste to dry and harden naturally, or briefly warm it with a hairdryer on a low setting to help it solidify.

Step 20 Apply any additional levelling agents, such as partial or whole washers, or pieces of wafer. If necessary add thin slivers of paste to seal any joins.

Step 21 Depending on your prepared system now apply either the all-in-one bag and flange, or the flange/base separately, ensuring the opening in it fits snugly over the fistula or wound orifice. Work from the lowest point of application towards the highest point on the abdomen, to catch any effluent spilled as you smooth it gently into place.

NB: if applying the bag separately, it may be best to just smooth the flange down lightly, and fix the bag in place so it can catch any effluent as you then press the equipment more firmly into place.

Step 22 Check carefully that all the equipment is securely bonded to the abdomen with no lifted areas or creases into which effluent could leak. Ask the patient to place a hand over the equipment to 'warm and weight it' for several minutes, encouraging good moulding to the body.

Step 23 Attach additional drainage system if used.

Step 24 Where difficulties with adherence occur it may help to encourage patients to remain in the same fairly flat position for 30–60 minutes to reduce any stress on the bonding of equipment which movement might produce. Make sure they have everything they require within reach so they can do this comfortably.

Step 25 Having cleared away the used equipment and rubbish, record the findings from your assessment and the goals of care, and describe the methods used to protect the skin and contain the effluent. Store relevant equipment and the template where it will be accessible for subsequent appliance changes.

Monitoring of equipment

It is essential to check and empty equipment regularly. Frequency of monitoring will depend on the level of fistula output and the degree to which this fills and weighs down the equipment, which puts a strain on the adhesive bonding with the patient's body. Attachment to a larger drainage bag is advisable if effluent levels are high, or occur intermittently at substantial levels. Even where such secondary drainage is used it is still important to check that drainage from the fistula bag into it is occurring freely. Discreet use of odour-containing sprays before emptying or changing equipment is desirable if the odour is unpleasant or difficult to disperse.

Accurate records of the amount and type of effluent passed should be kept so that this can be considered in conjunction with the patient's nutritional and medication needs and treatment.

PROBLEMS

Difficulties in combating infection, controlling pyrexia and maintaining a good nutritional status may arise due to the underlying cause of the fistula and/or the loss of nutriments diverted from the body before they can be absorbed. These factors can affect both the patient's situation as a whole and the local fistula area. For example, the skin condition may be altered and also the speed with which disintegration of skin protectives and filling agents takes place, requiring changes in management. A comprehensive account of fistula management strategies is provided by Rolstad & Bryant (2000). Management of common problems is outlined here.

Skin irritation (pruritus)

Patients have a distressing itch and inclination to scratch the area. This can be reduced by application of a thin layer of calamine lotion which is allowed to dry before application of their usual equipment.

Oily skin

This makes equipment lift away from the body more easily. A non-sting barrier film can be used on intact skin to create an additional 'plastic skin' before application of the usual equipment. The smooth skin must be allowed to form by waiting a few seconds before other equipment is placed over it.

Rapid disintegration of filler paste in wounds or gullies

This may mean effluent tracks along them, necessitating frequent equipment changes. Changing to a paste which hardens to a more solid consistency, or combining it with cut up strips of wafers or washers sometimes increases the time before disintegration occurs. Use of an appliance with an access porthole enables extra skin protective paste or powder to be applied between equipment changes.

Pain while equipment is being changed

Some patients have very sore skin and/or find the fistula area is highly sensitive to any form of pressure on it, such as during removal and application of equipment and skin cleansing. The thought of enduring the pain of equipment changes can lead them to refuse changes of equipment until leakage (and skin damage) is considerable, thus exacerbating the situation. In these circumstances patients require an analgesic which will act during the equipment change without subsequent longer-lasting effects. Entonox (50% nitrous oxide, 50% oxygen) can be used effectively in hospital and at home, helping patients control their pain management (Evans 2003, Lloyd Jones 2004). Once appliance changes can be pain-free, patients will usually allow them to take place as soon they are needed, reducing both physical and emotional stress.

Difficulties in collecting effluent

Collecting effluent from different openings at skin level

Fistulas can open in close proximity to each other and/or a stoma. More than one appliance can be used so effluent is contained and recorded separately. Bags with flexible faceplates are generally more suitable when they need to overlap or be sited close to each other. The principles outlined above are followed to prepare a template with openings for each orifice, and this is used to prepare a large hydrocolloid wafer or combined small wafers to create a level base. Appliances are positioned on this level base so they can be easily emptied. Base and bag can be applied separately or all-in-one.

Channelling effluent from below skin level

When fistula openings occur in a wound or gully their pooled effluent can delay wound healing and damage skin. It can be helpful to create a 'dam' so effluent is channelled to spill into an appliance rather than along the wound or gully. Strips of hydrocolloid wafer are cut and applied alternatively with small 'worms' of paste to create a dam across the wound from its base to just above skin level. Skin protectives and bags are applied in the manner described earlier, but positioned over the fistula and dam so effluent flows into the bag. Treatment of the remaining wound/gully depends on its condition (Rolstad & Bryant 2000).

Managing problems of size

One or more of the following circumstances are usually present:

- large amounts of effluent are passing from several orifices
- fistulas are lying in large wounds
- the area within which the fistulas lie is sizeable.

In these situations the management system described earlier usually requires adaptation to achieve:

- maintenance of sufficient skin protection over the extended area to prevent or minimise damage
- promotion of an environment conducive to healing
- successful management of the volume, weight and frequency of effluent being passed.

The strategies used to achieve these goals depend on:

- the particular circumstances and needs of individual patients
- the availability of equipment and expertise to use it
- the degree to which particular approaches are viewed as compatible with the ways in which the multidisciplinary team think the situation would be best managed.

Suction is often used to keep fistula and wound areas clear of effluent whilst cleansing them and preparing and applying bags. However, the issue of whether suction could be used as part of an ongoing management system should be considered separately. Input from tissue viability nurses in team discussions can be particularly helpful in reviewing options (Cardozo 2003, Weaver 2003).

Some wound management systems use intermittent or continuous suction to draw exudate from wounds and create wound environments which promote healing (Mendez-Eastman 2002, Penn & Rayment 2004). Practically speaking it would initially appear that if fistula effluent was sufficiently liquid to be suctioned away, such wound management systems could be used in fistula care. Some authorities suggest they can sometimes be used (Hess 2002, Rolstad & Bryant 2000). However, others suggest that the presence of fistulas in wounds contraindicates use of negative pressure/vacuum-assisted wound therapy systems as these can deter fistula healing and might increase fistula occurrence (Ballard & Baxter 2001, Mendez-Eastman 2002).

Rolstad & Bryant (2000) suggest that catheters inserted into fistulas act as foreign bodies and may increase output. In contrast, soft suction catheters placed in a wound bed enable effluent to be drawn away without deterring healing. This is congruent with Jeter et al's (1991) description of a system of closed suction wound drainage which was useful when fistulas were sited in areas where conventional appliance application was difficult. The *wound bed* was drained by suction and they reported rapid wound healing where the fistula output was below 800 ml in 24 hours and the patients were being fed by total parenteral nutrition. Pringle (1995) and Nishide (1997) describe adaptations of this system.

Capillary action dressings are an alternative system for drawing exudate from wounds (Russell et al 2001). Weaver (2003) reports their use as a wick to aid movement of fluid from a wound into a stoma bag. Although they may be less effective with substantial amounts of effluent than suction, their gentler action may be a useful alternative.

Blackley (2004) describes the use of parcel dressings. The perifistular skin is protected with hydrocolloid wafers. Polythene sheeting or bags are attached to the wafers with double-sided adhesives. The resultant polythene 'parcel' can be opened as required to change dressings or remove substantial drainage with suction apparatus.

The individuality of patients' circumstances has led to fistula care often being described through case studies rather than research programmes (Cleverly 1999, Gibelli et al 1999). Although some accounts may contain suggestions that conflict with others they also enable us to consider innovative thinking and practice developed in response to challenging situations.

CARE OF THE PATIENT AS A WHOLE

When fistulas initially occur the main medical focus will be on managing urgent elements (e.g. sepsis, haemorrhage), identifying the nature and extent of interrelated problems, and stabilising the patient (Rolstad & Bryant 2000). Patients with fistulas can range from being seriously to moderately ill depending on their circumstances. Thus their overall nursing care will also vary.

Patients can only benefit nutritionally from food passing through the gastrointestinal tract if it reaches the parts where it can be processed and absorbed. Diversion of gastrointestinal contents via fistulas means that material is not accessible to digestive processes which take place beyond that point. The degree to which nutritional problems could arise depends considerably on where fistulas occur and how much (if any) gastrointestinal content is not diverted but passes along the normal pathway and is processed. Where fistulas arise lower down the intestinal tract parenteral nutrition may not be necessary (O'Dwyer 1997). Where fistulas occur higher up, and result in sizeable diversion of gastrointestinal contents, parenteral feeding may be necessary. Advantages and disadvantages of enteral and parenteral nutrition, and the importance of careful assessment, are described by Burnett (2000). Management of parenteral nutrition and the move back to normal eating is discussed by Tait (2000). Wherever possible some oral feeding should occur as this helps maintain gut physiology and function (Small 2003).

Medication is usually given to enable two areas of gastrointestinal activity to function more helpfully (Small 2003). Anti-diarrhoeal drugs such as loperamide or codeine phosphate are given to reduce gut motility and thus increase the transit time for diet taken orally. These should be taken 30–60 minutes before food (Cottam 2003). Anti-secretory medication such as histamine-2 (H2)-receptor antagonists or proton pump inhibitors may be given to reduce secretion of gastric acid and thereby reduce gastrointestinal tract output (Small 2003). Somatostatin analogues (e.g. octreotide) are thought to increase the speed of small bowel fistula closure as well as inhibiting secretions from the stomach, pancreas, biliary tract and small intestine. However, octreotide appears less effective with ulcerative colitis and Crohn's disease (Rolstad & Bryant 2000).

Forbes & Myers (1996) suggest that patients with high fistulas may need a fluid intake of at least 5 litres daily but that oral fluids may have to be curtailed. This is because most ordinary drinks do not contain sodium. As they reach the intestine they stimulate the passage of sodium into the intestine, which draws large quantities of water into the bowel after it (Small 2003). Where effluent is diverted out of the body via a high fistula this prevents the reabsorption of fluid which would normally take place further along the intestine. It is important to understand the rationale for curtailment of oral fluids so that we can help patients to understand that it actively helps in their treatment, and encourage them to comply with it.

PSYCHOLOGICAL SUPPORT

Fistulas are a visible reminder that something in the patient's body has gone wrong. Their presence, unpredictable function, and the difficulties in managing and closing them successfully, creates situations that are stressful for all concerned. It is therefore essential that psychological support for patients, their families, and staff is actively built into the care process (Forbes & Myers 1996, Hopkins 2001, Keighley 1993, Ross 1994, Weaver 2003).

Nichols (2003) suggests that where psychological support is regularly being given, then supportive measures for staff should be preventative as well as responsive to stress. Reductions in professional self-esteem and morale are very real hazards for individuals and the healthcare team as fistulas can challenge nurses' and doctors' ability to fulfil their usual roles effectively over a prolonged period of time.

Patients and their families find fistulas and their situation daunting. Prolonged hospitalisation can create difficulties in fulfilling family, work and social responsibilities normally undertaken by the patient or other family members. Relatives are highly likely to need help to devise coping strategies that are suitable and effective over weeks rather than days. Time and attention to clarify and respond to relatives' needs must therefore be provided as an integral part of patients' care. As families gain confidence and the ability to cope effectively this usually enables them to respond more helpfully to the patient and the situation generally.

Patients live hour by hour with the reality of a fistula creating changes in how they look, function, feel and experience themselves as a human being. It is often difficult for them not to feel overwhelmed by their situation. Change is difficult for many people to handle, and the ever-changing dynamics of fistula care do little to help patients feel that staff are in control of the situation, and that their world will become stable and normal again (Ross 1994, Weaver 2003).

The main goals of psychological care are to prevent or minimise problems and promote the experience of being well supported in all concerned. The *principles* through which these may be achieved include:

1. Strategies for building trust, handling uncertainty and change, and resolving problems should be actively developed by the healthcare team for use between team members and with the patient and family. The style of care developed should be congruent with people's needs and coping styles (see Chs 7, 19, 20, 23).
2. Patients and their families should be helped to accept that, because the fistula and underlying condition create a changeable situation, explanations and treatment are also likely to be changeable. When patients experience situations as disastrous or unresolvable it is important to acknowledge that clearly *before* offering explanations or alternative viewpoints.
3. Patients and families should be encouraged to identify sources of support and specific kinds of help which could be beneficial, and actively helped to set these up to function over a minimum 2-month period rather than on a short-term basis (see section on stroke balance, Ch. 20). Help from a number of people may be more enthusiastically offered if each person knows they will not be asked to provide all the support, which could feel overwhelming.
4. People engaged in providing psychological support should include colleagues who are not closely affected by the demands and responsibilities engendered by direct clinical care (e.g. social workers, religious personnel, psychologists, counsellors).

Their assistance benefits patients, particularly those worrying that if they express fears and feelings to direct caregivers or question their practice, those people might become unwilling to continue providing the care on which they are so dependent. Their assistance to colleagues, both informally and through clinical and counselling supervision, can also be invaluable in providing supportive attention while clinicians consider their practice and address issues (Nichols 2003).

CARE OF MUCOUS FISTULAS AND DRAIN SITES

Where a bowel resection is protected by a temporary stoma the proximal end of the remaining rectal stump may be brought out onto the abdominal wall. This is called a *mucous fistula*. The aim is to make the end of the rectal stump readily available for subsequent surgery to restore bowel continuity (Blackley 2004). Passage of mucus from the rectal stump is fairly common. Even if mucus is minimal, dressings may be unsuitable to contain it because they still allow abdominal skin damage to occur, and do not contain odour which can be noticeably pungent. Skin protectives and small appliances or stoma caps can effectively prevent such problems, used in accordance with the principles of fistula care described earlier. Siting mucous fistulas within wound suture lines should be discouraged. There is a risk of wound contamination from the discharge. Additionally, removal of used equipment from the sensitive wound area and stitches causes patients discomfort.

Leakage from drain sites may also create skin damage, odour and discomfort for patients left with a soggy dressing. Use of skin protectives and an appliance increases patients' comfort and enables accurate monitoring of the type and amount of leakage to take place. Where drainage could be substantial (e.g. following paracentesis abdominis) a flat urostomy bag and secondary drainage may be the equipment of choice.

Patients who may have mentally prepared themselves for one stoma bag may find the presence of additional equipment distressing. Encouragement to raise any fears and feelings is important: patients may find it hard to trust staff assurances that this extra equipment should be temporary, and repeat explanations should be offered patiently and readily where needed.

References

Ballard K, Baxter H 2001 Vacuum-assisted closure. Nursing Times 97 (35) August 30: 51–52

Black P K 2000 Holistic stoma care. Baillière Tindall and RCN, Edinburgh

Blackley P 2004 Practical stoma wound and continence management, 2nd edn. Research Publications, Vermont, Victoria, Australia

Burnett C 2000 Patient assessment. In: Hamilton H (ed) Total parenteral nutrition. Churchill Livingstone, Edinburgh, p 31–53

Cardozo M 2003 A case study of holistic wound management in intensive care. British Journal of Nursing 12(11) Tissue viability supplement: S35–S42

Cleverly J 1999 Management of a fistula within a wound: a case study. World Council of Enterostomal Therapists Journal 19(3) July-September: 12–13

Cobb A, Knaggs E 2003 The nursing management of enterocutaneous fistulae: a challenge for all. British Journal of Community Nursing 8(12) Wound care supplement S32–S38

Cottam J 2003 Management of high output ileostomy following rectal excision. Gastrointestinal Nursing 1(7):19–23

Evans A 2003 Use of Entonox in the community for control of procedural pain. British Journal of Community Nursing 8(11):488–493

Forbes A, Myers C 1996 Enterocutaneous fistulae and their management. In: Myers C (ed) Stoma care nursing. Arnold, London, p 63–77

Gibelli G, Rocchi P, Guidici V 1999 Management of multiple fistulae. World Council of Enterostomal Therapists Journal 19(1):18–19

Hess C T 2002 Managing an external fistula part 2. Nursing 32(9):22–23

Hopkins S 2001 Psychological aspects of wound healing. Nursing Times 97(48):57–58

Jeter K F, Tintle T E, Chandler M 1991 A closed suction wound drainage system to enhance management of incisional and cutaneous fistulae. World Council of Enterostomal Therapists Journal 11(3):22–25

Keighley M R B 1993 Intestinal fistulas. In: Keighley M R B, Williams N S Surgery of the anus, rectum and colon, 3rd edn. WB Saunders, London

Lloyd Jones M 2004 Minimising pain at dressing changes. Nursing Standard 18(24):65–70

Meadows C 1997 Stoma and fistula care. In: Bruce L, Finlay T M D (eds) Nursing in gastroenterology. Churchill Livingstone, New York, p 85–118

Mendez-Eastman S 2002 New treatment for an old problem: negative pressure wound therapy. Nursing 32(5):58-63

Nichols K 2003 Psychological care for ill and injured people. Open University Press, Maidenhead

Nishide K 1997 Development of closed-suction pouch drainage for giant fistulae: a report on two cases. World Council of Enterostomal Therapists Journal 17(1):16–19.

O'Dwyer S T 1997 Enterocutaneous fistula: conservative and surgical management. In: Allan R N, Rhodes J M, Hanauer S B et al (eds) Inflammatory bowel diseases, 3rd edn. Churchill Livingstone, New York

Penn E, Rayment S 2004 Management of a dehisced abdominal wound with VAC therapy. British Journal of Nursing 13(4):194–201

Pringle W K 1995 The management of patients with enterocutaneous fistulas. Journal of Wound Care 4(5):211–213

Rolstad B S, Bryant R A 2002 Management of drain sites and fistulas. In: Bryant R (ed) Acute and chronic wounds, nursing management, 2nd edn. Mosby, St Louis, p 317–339

Ross J 1994 Low anterior resection vs abdomino-perineal excision: what choice? what problems? what quality? In: World Council of Enterostomal Therapists congress proceedings. Hollister, Libertyville, IL, p 124–128

Russell L, Deeth M, Jones H M, Reynold T 2001 VACUTEX capillary action dressing: a multicentre, randomised trial. British Journal of Nursing 10(11) Tissue viability supplement: 1–4

Small M 2003 Management of intestinal failure. Nursing Times 99(3) Jan 21: 52–53

Tait J 2000 Nursing management. In: Hamilton H (ed) Total parenteral nutrition. Churchill Livingstone, Edinburgh, p 137–172

Weaver B 2003 The nursing needs of a patient with a complicated abdominal wound. Professional Nurse 18(5):269–273

Chapter 15

Irrigation

Wendy Pringle

The most commonly used method of managing a colostomy in Great Britain is by spontaneous action. The improvement in odour-proof plastics, microporous adhesives and hydrocolloid skin barriers has greatly improved stoma management but, to many people, the fact that they have no control over a basic bodily function can cause anxiety and can be a barrier to a normal lifestyle. With dietary manipulation, fluid restriction and the use of drugs a colostomy may work once or twice a day but some colostomies never develop a regular evacuation pattern (Devlin et al 1971).

Irrigation was first described by Lockart-Mummery in 1927 but in earlier years factors such as inferior equipment, poor toilet facilities, lack of knowledge and expertise in the technique led to its limited popularity and many surgeons feared colonic perforation (Gabriel 1945). As knowledge and equipment improved irrigation became more widely practised in the USA (MacDonald 1991, Mullen & McGinn 1992, Williams & Johnson 1980). It appears less popular in Great Britain, with 1% of colostomists irrigating (McCahon 1999). However, it does offer patients an alternative method of managing their colostomy and one with more potential for regulating stomal action to fit in with their lives than does the conventional method of wearing a stoma pouch to contain faeces whenever they happen to be passed.

Irrigation involves instillation of water into the colon via the stoma. It is done:

- as a management procedure performed by some patients to control their faecal output

- as a method of preparing the colon for surgery or investigative procedure
- to relieve constipation.

IRRIGATION AS A MANAGEMENT PROCEDURE

The aim of colostomy irrigation is to teach the patient to effectively control their faecal output so that faeces are passed only when the colon is stimulated by the instillation of water (McPhail 2003). The purpose of irrigation is not to wash out the entire colon but to induce a reflex which brings about a peristaltic wave and evacuates faeces from the distal colon (Mullen & McGinn 1992).

SELECTION OF PATIENTS

Consideration must be given to patients' physical, psychological and social situations as irrigation will not be suitable for all patients. Writers discussing factors that make irrigation suitable for patients include Goode (1982), Laucks et al (1988), MacDonald (1991), Davis (1996), Black (2000) and McPhail (2003). Between them they suggest patients who are *suitable for irrigation* should have:

- a left-sided colostomy either in the descending or sigmoid colon, with an output of formed faeces
- no stomal stenosis, prolapse or herniation
- a good prognosis and be free from other conditions, such as diverticular disease, Crohn's disease, ulcerative colitis or irritable bowel disease
- physical ability to carry out the procedure, having good eyesight and good manual dexterity
- the ability to make an informed choice about undertaking the procedure
- good motivation towards using irrigation
- the ability to learn and carry it out independently
- private toilet facilities with running water and adequate heating.

Factors that make irrigation unsuitable have also been identified (Allen 1984, Goode 1982, Laucks et al 1988, McPhail 2003, Williams & Johnson 1980). Collectively, they suggest irrigation should *not* be considered for:

- patients with right-sided colostomies in the ascending and right transverse colon, where there is a constant liquid or semi-liquid output

- patients who are prone to diarrhoea, and/or respond as such in stressful situations
- patients with cardiac or renal disease, as potential fluid overloading may occur
- infants, where there is a greater risk of perforation (Cooney & Grosfield 1977)
- young children, who have difficulty sitting still for any length of time
- those people who would be anxious doing the procedure, or who would find it aesthetically unacceptable.

Use of irrigation in children who have undergone the ACE (antegrade continence enema) procedure is discussed in Chapter 13.

Consent to irrigate must be obtained from the patient's consultant and their general practitioner should be informed. The decision to irrigate should be made by an informed patient who has had the advantages and disadvantages of the technique clearly outlined (MacDonald 1991). Local requirements to comply with risk management procedures should be followed. These may include recording in writing that patients have been informed of potential problems and have agreed to learn irrigation, and/or patients signing a consent form before being taught irrigation (McPhail 2003). A video and a booklet (Clinimed, undated) and a factsheet produced by the British Colostomy Association (BCA 1999) are available to give additional information and act as visual aids. Introducing patients to someone who is successfully irrigating can reinforce the advantages of the technique.

A number of writers indicate the advantages of irrigation (BCA 1999, Davis 1996, Dini et al 1991, Jones 1987, Leong & Yunos 1999, MacDonald 1991, McPhail 2003, O'Bichere et al 2001, Venturini et al 1990).

Advantages:

- The patient is in control of his faecal output at a time selected by himself, and between irrigations he is continent. This in itself reduces anxiety and lessens the psychosexual stigma that comes with altered body image.
- In most cases irrigation can be done on alternate days and, if successful, it is necessary only to wear a stoma cap, instead of a conventional pouch.
- There is less bulky equipment to store, and minimal disposal problems.
- There is less potential for skin problems associated with leakage and adhesive allergies in comparison with when colostomy pouches are used.

- Irrigation equipment is available on prescription, is reusable and more economical compared to the constant use of standard colostomy pouches.
- It reduces the amount of odour and flatus.
- Fewer dietary restrictions are needed to 'control' faecal output.
- With adaptation and imagination, irrigation can be done away from home, and is suitable in hot climates, where adhesion of stoma pouches may be compromised.
- It enhances patients' confidence to pursue sport and leisure activities. Normal employment and social life can continue.
- Patients of all ages can irrigate. Venturini and others (1990) demonstrated that patients over the age of 70 (the age group to which most colostomists belong) were taught to irrigate safely and effectively.

The literature also highlights some disadvantages of irrigation (BCA 1999, Davis 1996, Jones 1987, Laucks et al 1988, McPhail 2003, Pringle 1984, Venturini 1990).

Disadvantages:

- Some people view it as an unnatural procedure which can be distasteful to perform.
- Spending up to an hour a day, at a set time, can be time-consuming and occupying a bathroom can be restrictive to other family members.
- There may be problems doing the procedure away from home.
- As mental and physical agility decline, a time may come when irrigation may no longer be possible and adaptation to natural evacuation and wearing a conventional pouch may present problems.
- There is an added risk of perforation if inappropriate equipment or techniques are used.
- Irrigation may possibly, in the long run, diminish the natural action of the bowel.

Irrigation can be taught in the early postoperative period or some months later. Some writers feel patients have enough to cope with immediately after such major surgery and irrigation should be taught after a period of recovery (Allen 1984, Davis 1996, McPhail 2003, Williams & Johnson 1980). Other writers find patients who are taught irrigation before they leave hospital benefit from daily supervised teaching and go home continent and confident (Williams & Johnson 1980, Pringle 1984). The procedure should be taught by a stoma care nurse or a designated nurse who is confident and competent in the technique (Allen 1984).

When taught in the postoperative period it is important that bowel sounds are present and that flatus has been passed. This occurs at about the seventh postoperative day. Initially 500 ml of tepid tap water (36–38°C) is used and gradually increased to 1000 ml. The quantity of water used for irrigation varies from 0.25 litre (Williams & Johnson 1981) to 1.5 litres (Goode 1982, Keighley 1999). A Danish study demonstrates that 0.5 litre gives as good a result as larger quantities and is quicker to instil (Meyhoff et al 1990). The entire irrigation procedure should take between 30 and 45 minutes. If more time is spent, careful investigation into the technique should be made.

The time of day irrigation is performed is an individual choice. It should be when the toilet is free exclusively for an hour, fitting in with patients' lifestyle (MacDonald 1991). It is important that the procedure is done at approximately the same time every day (MacDonald 1991, McPhail 2003). After meals people's gastrocolic reflex generally causes peristalsis to occur, and some patients find that irrigating after a meal takes advantage of this normal process of faecal movement along the bowel and aids elimination.

Irrigation should be performed daily for approximately 14 days (MacDonald 1991, McPhail 2003) until regulation is achieved and there are no spillages between irrigations. The procedure is then done on alternate days (McPhail 2003) and in some cases on every third day (Allen 1984). A conventional pouch is worn until the patient feels confident enough to wear a stoma cap (Black 2000). Some protective covering is essential as mucus is constantly produced by the lining of the bowel.

EQUIPMENT

There are several irrigation sets available on prescription, all having the same basic components (see list below and Fig. 15.1). The set will need replacing after about 2 years, but this will depend on how frequently irrigation is performed.

The water bag should allow clear visibility of the water level and the clamp on the tubing should be easy to regulate with one hand. The irrigation sleeve should provide a leakproof seal around the stoma and be long enough to reach into the toilet pan. Two types of irrigation sleeve are available. One has an

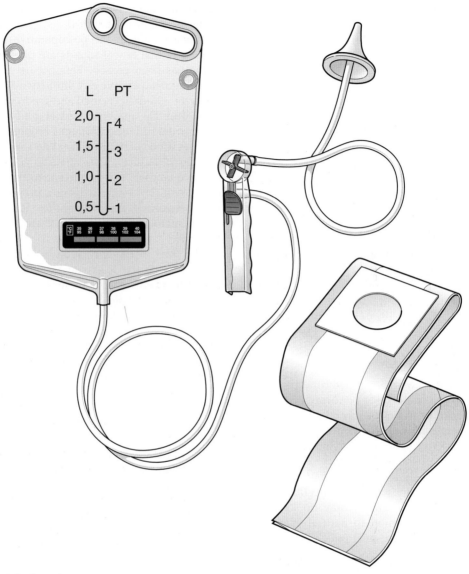

Figure 15.1   Irrigation set.

adhesive backing and is for single use. The second is attached to a plastic flange which is held in place over the stoma by an adjustable belt. This is reusable and should be replaced every 2 to 4 weeks (MacDonald 1991).

After use all the equipment should be washed in warm soapy water, rinsed, initially allowed to drip dry and then dried thoroughly. The set should be stored in a cool dry place, and replaced annually (Black 2000).

Tepid water (36–38°C) is the fluid choice: water that is too cold may overstimulate the bowel causing

cramps, and water that is too warm may cause mucosal damage (Goode 1982, Schauder 1974).

ADMINISTRATION OF A COLOSTOMY IRRIGATION

Equipment:

- Irrigation set, containing a graduated water bag, plastic tubing with regulating clamp, cone tip, irrigation sleeve (Fig. 15.1)
- Paper tissues/wipes

- Bowl of warm water
- Rubbish bag
- Stoma pouch or cap
- 1 litre of tepid tap water (36–38°C)
- Non-sterile jug
- Disposable glove
- Clothes peg.

Table 15.1 outlines the steps in the procedure and their rationale.

The criteria for discharge of patients from hospital is that they are independently able to manage the irrigation themselves. It is essential that patients' progress with learning irrigation is carefully documented so that teaching can be consistent and readiness for discharge evaluated.

> **PATIENT SCENARIO 15.1**   Mary Long is learning to irrigate following abdomino-perineal excision of rectum for cancer. She is gradually acquiring the ability to follow all the steps listed in Table 15.1. This 'standard' procedure is being adapted in response to Mary's particular circumstances. Problems and concerns are reported as separate items in her nursing care plan so they can be monitored and resolved more easily (see Appendix 15.1). Mrs Reid, her stoma care nurse, is reviewing the progress that has been made in resolving some of Mary's difficulties. She uses the care plan to make sure she checks on each concern/problem in her discussion with Mary as well as to identify any changes in her care which may be needed.

ADDITIONAL CONSIDERATIONS

The principles of giving patients sufficient equipment for discharge home, and teaching them how to obtain further supplies are similar to those described in Chapter 8.

It may be necessary to show a relative or partner the technique to give added physical and psychological support. Continued support from the stoma care nurse is essential; a home visit shortly after discharge will reinforce this and at the same time give patients the opportunity to discuss any problems. If irrigation is taught several weeks or months after surgery the same regime applies.

Irrigation can be done away from home, access to a private toilet being the basic requirement. Rubber suction hooks can be purchased to hold the water container above the toilet pan. If planning a long journey it is advisable to irrigate shortly before departure then on arrival (Aylett 1978). If travelling abroad, the irrigation set should be carried with the hand luggage, as suitcases can go astray. If the water in the country is not drinkable it should not be used for irrigation but bottled water used instead (MacDonald 1991). A supply of drainable pouches should also be available as a change in diet and temperature may cause diarrhoea, in which case irrigation should be stopped until faecal output becomes formed (Laucks et al 1988).

IRRIGATION AS A METHOD OF PREPARING THE COLON FOR SURGERY OR AN INVESTIGATIVE PROCEDURE

Prior to closure of either a loop transverse or sigmoid colostomy, or before a barium enema or colonoscopy of the distal colon, it is necessary to clear the bowel of faeces.

The *proximal* colon is prepared by giving an oral bowel cleaning solution (e.g. sodium picosulfate). This is given 24 and 16 hours before the procedure and followed by clear oral fluids. It is important that the patient has a drainable pouch over his colostomy, as liquid faeces will be passed.

The *distal* colon is prepared by irrigating water through the distal loop of the colostomy, using the technique previously described but the height of the water bag can be raised. A single use, disposable, irrigation set and cone is used for this procedure. The distal loop is usually located on the left-hand side of the stoma; a digital examination of the stoma should confirm this (McPhail 2003). The patient sits on a commode (rather than the toilet) so that the effects of the washout can be monitored. An irrigation sleeve is positioned over the colostomy so any material returned from the stoma can be observed and channelled into the commode. Sufficient tepid water is used until the fluid passed per rectum is quite clear. If there is an obstruction in the distal colon, water will not flow freely and will return via the colostomy. In this situation medical staff should be consulted as it may be necessary to give a rectal washout or disposable enema to clear the bowel distal to the obstruction, and whether the patient's overall condition allows or precludes them from undergoing such a procedure must first be ascertained.

Table 15.1   Administration of a colostomy irrigation

Action	Rationale
1 Explain the procedure to the patient	To obtain consent and cooperation
2 Prepare the bathroom/toilet	To ensure a comfortable acceptable environment
3 Ensure privacy	To avoid embarrassment to patient
4 Wash and dry hands and prepare equipment for the procedure	Although this is not a sterile procedure care should be taken to avoid unnecessary contamination
5 Fill a jug with 500 ml of tepid tap water (36–38°C)	As the bowel is not sterile there is no need to use sterile water. If the solution is too warm mucosal damage may occur. If it is too cold unnecessary cramps may occur
6 Pour the tepid water into the water container and release the regulating clamp to prime the plastic tubing	To allow the tubing to be primed and filled with water thus preventing entry of air into the colon
7 Hang the water container on a hook behind the toilet pan. The base of the bag should be at shoulder height when the patient is seated on the toilet	To allow the water to gravitate into the colostomy. If the bag is positioned any higher, abdominal cramps may occur
8 Prepare equipment for a change of stoma pouch/cap. Warm water, paper tissues/wipes, rubbish bag, stoma pouch/cap	
9 Instruct the patient to sit on the toilet pan, removing relevant clothing. Cover their legs with a blanket	To allow free access to the stoma; to ensure dignity
10 Remove the stoma pouch and wipe excess faeces from the stoma and peristomal skin	So that the stoma and skin are clean and clearly visible
11 Wash the stoma and skin with warm water and tissues and dry thoroughly	To promote cleanliness and prevent skin excoriation
12 Fit the irrigation sleeve over the stoma. The bottom end of the sleeve is placed between the patient's legs into the toilet pan	To ensure a watertight seal around the stomal area
13 At the time of the first irrigation, wearing a disposable glove, perform a gentle digital examination of the stoma (it is not necessary to do this on every occasion)	To determine the direction of the lumen of the colon and relax the stoma
14 Through the opening of the irrigation sleeve, insert the irrigation cone gently into the stoma so that a dam is made between the stoma and cone	To ensure that the water, when instilled, is retained in the colon
15 Open the regulating on/off clamp and allow the water to flow into the colon (this will take 4–5 minutes)	To allow water to run into the colon
16 When all the water has been instilled, remove the cone from the stoma, fold the top of the irrigation sleeve over and secure with a peg	To ensure there is no leakage from the top of the irrigation sleeve
17 Wait for a period of 20 minutes. Water and faeces will be evacuated from the stoma at varying intervals	To allow peristalsis to take place causing evacuation of faeces and water
18 Clean the lower end of the irrigation sleeve; fold up and clip to the top end of the sleeve	To allow the patient to leave the toilet and pursue other activities
19 After 10 minutes, when there is no further action and abdominal cramps have stopped, remove the irrigation sleeve and leave it hanging over the side of the toilet pan	
20 Clean the stoma and peristomal skin with tissues and warm water and dry	To promote cleanliness and prevent excoriation. The appliance will adhere more securely to dry skin
21 Apply a clean stoma pouch/cap	
22 Clean the irrigation sleeve (if using a reusable one) by holding it over the pan and pouring warm water from a jug into it. A shower head attachment fixed to an adjoining washbasin could also be used	To clean any faeces and mucus from the irrigation sleeve
23 Hang the sleeve, water container and tubing to initially drip dry, then dry thoroughly and store in a cool place	To prolong the life of the plastic
24 Dispose of rubbish bag	
25 Wash and dry hands thoroughly	To reduce cross-infection

IRRIGATION TO RELIEVE CONSTIPATION

Hard faeces can be initially softened by instilling warm arachis oil (130 ml) into the colostomy. It is important to check first that neither the patient nor the person who will give the oil has a nut allergy (Black 2000). The oil should remain in the bowel for sufficient time to soften and lubricate the faeces. A cone and irrigation set can be used.

An alternative system is to gently insert a 16F Foley catheter, about 8 cm into the colon via the stoma. The end of the catheter is connected to the nozzle of the plastic container containing the oil and gentle pressure applied to squeeze the oil into the colon. This should be followed 24 hours later by a routine irrigation, using 1 litre of tepid tap water. This can be repeated until the situation has been resolved. It is important to determine the cause of constipation as dietary and drug manipulation may be necessary.

CONCLUSION

Modern equipment has made irrigation a much easier procedure for patients and nurses to use. Stoma care nurses can work with hospital and community colleagues so that the levels of expertise and support which patients need while they learn to irrigate adeptly become more readily available. This will enable irrigation to become an option which more colostomists can use successfully.

APPENDIX 15.1

Table A15.1 contains excerpts from the nursing care plan for Mary Long.

References

Allen S 1984 Stoma management. Nursing 2(30):877–881

Aylett S O 1978 Colostomy care by the washout (or irrigation) technique. In: Todd I P (ed) Intestinal stomas. Heinemann, London, p 59–64

Black P K 2000 Holistic stoma care. Baillière Tindall and RCN, Edinburgh

British Colostomy Association 1999 Colostomy irrigation. BCA, Reading

Clinimed Ltd (undated) Colostomy Irrigation – A video for patients. Clinimed Ltd. High Wycombe

Clinimed Ltd (undated) Colostomy irrigation. Clinimed Ltd, High Wycombe

Cooney D E, Grosfield J L 1977 Care of the child with a colostomy. Paediatrics 59:469

Davis K 1996 Irrigation technique. In: Myers C (ed) Stoma care nursing. Arnold, London, p 136–145

Devlin H B, Plant J A, Griffen M 1971 Aftermath of surgery for anorectal cancer. British Medical Journal iii:413–418

Dini D, Venturini M, Forno G et al 1991 Irrigation for colostomized cancer patients: a rational approach. International Journal of Colorectal Disease 6(1):9–11

Gabriel W B 1945 Discussion of the management of the permanent colostomy. Proceedings of the Royal Society of Medicine 38:692–694

Goode P S 1982 Colostomy irrigation. In: Broadwell D C, Jackson B S (eds) Principles of ostomy care. C V Mosby, St Louis, p 369–380

Jones H 1987 The advantages and disadvantages of irrigation. Ostomy International June-November, 11

Keighley M 1999 Colostomy. In: Keighley M, Williams N Surgery of the anus, rectum and colon, 2nd edn. W B Saunders, London

Laucks S S 2nd, Mazier W P, Milsom J W et al 1988 An assessment of colostomy irrigation. Diseases of the Colon and Rectum 31(4):279–282

Leong A, Yunos A 1999 Stoma management in a tropical country: colostomy irrigation versus natural evacuation. Ostomy Wound Management 45(11):52–56

Lockart-Mummery P 1927 discussion on colostomy. Proceedings of Royal Society of Medicine 20:1461

McCahon S 1999 Faecal Stomas. In: Porrett T, Daniel N (eds) Essential coloproctology for nurses. Whurr, London, p 165-187

MacDonald K 1991 Colostomy Irrigation: an option worth considering. Professional Nurse 7(1):15–19

McPhail J 2003 Irrigation technique. In: Elcoat C Stoma care nursing, 2nd edn. Hollister, Reading

Meyhoff H H, Anderson B, Nielsen S 1990 Colostomy irrigation: a clinical and scintigraphic comparison between three different irrigation volumes. British Journal of Surgery 77(10):1185–1186

Mullen B D, McGinn K A 1992 The ostomy book. Bull Publishing, Palo Alto

O'Bichere A, Bossom C, Gangoli S et al 2001 Chemical colostomy irrigation with glyceryl trinitrate solution. Diseases of Colon and Rectum 44(9):1324–1327

Pringle W 1984 Colostomy irrigation. Nursing Mirror 159(8):29–31

Schauder M R 1974 Ostomy care. American Journal of Nursing 74(8):1424–1427

Venturini M, Bertelli G, Forno G et al 1990 Colostomy irrigation in the elderly: effective recovery regardless of age disease. Diseases of the Colon and Rectum 33(12):1031–1034

Williams N S, Johnson D 1980 Prospective trial comparing colostomy irrigation with 'spontaneous action' method. British Medical Journal 281:107–109

Table A15.1   Excerpts from nursing care plan of Mary Long

Date	Patient need or problem	Goal	Action	Evaluation
6 May	(1) Mary feels ignorant and anxious about the irrigation procedure and worried about doing it.	Mary feels confident and competent doing irrigation.	(a) Explain and demonstrate irrigation to Mary. (b) Gradually involve her in the procedure. (c) Supervise until Mary is confident to do own care. (d) Support and reassure Mary. (e) Give her booklet to read on irrigation.	13 May Mary feels much happier about irrigation technique and is able to undertake unaided.
6 May	(2) Mary is anxious that her perineal wound will be painful while sitting to do irrigation.	She is able to sit comfortably while doing irrigation.	(a) Sit on a cushion or pillow on a chair opposite toilet. (b) Relieve pressure by lifting buttocks from chair every 5 minutes. (c) 20 minutes after instilling water, the irrigation sleeve can be wiped, folded and clipped to the top of sleeve, allowing mobilisation.	10 May Mary is able to minimise the weight on her perineal wound and is more comfortable when irrigating.
6 May	(3) Anxious that she will have privacy in bathroom when doing irrigation.	Mary has privacy in bathroom while doing irrigation.	(a) Evaluate the best time of day the bathroom is free for one hour. As Harry leaves for work at 8.00 a.m. and Mother does not get up until 9.30 a.m. irrigation is to be done at 8.15 a.m. (b) Lock the bathroom door.	10 May That Mary will feel relaxed and secure while doing irrigation.
7 May	(4) Mary is finding it difficult to insert the cone into the stoma.	The cone is inserted into stoma without any difficulty.	(a) Ensure Mary is relaxed – deep breathing will help to relax abdominal muscles. (b) Ensure she had had full explanation of the procedure – apprehension and fear can cause tension. (c) Gently inserting a gloved finger into the stoma will relax it prior to introducing the cone (Aylett 1978, MacDonald 1991).	13 May Mary is easily able to insert cone into stoma.

(Continued)

Table A15.1 Excerpts from nursing care plan of Mary Long (Continued)

Date	Patient need or problem	Goal	Action	Evaluation
7 May	(5) Mary felt faint and light-headed during irrigation procedure.	She feels well during procedure.	(a) Ensure that there is a well-ventilated bathroom/toilet. (b) Check the water is not being instilled too quickly (Goode 1982). (c) Check the water used is not too cold (Goode 1982). (d) Advise Mary that the irrigation should not be done more than once daily, as this could result in fatigue as well as a potential fluid and electrolyte imbalance (Goode 1982).	13 May Mary is now able to undertake irrigation without feeling faint or light-headed – she felt the incident occurred because the toilet was hot and stuffy.
8 May	(6) Mary finds the water is not flowing freely into the stoma.	The water flows freely into the stoma.	(a) Check the tip of the cone is not blocked with faeces (MacDonald 1991, Davis 1996, McPhail 2003). (b) Check that the tip of the cone is not touching the lumen of the bowel – a digital examination of the stoma will indicate the direction in which to introduce the cone (Allen 1984). (c) Ensure that the patient is relaxed (Davis 1996, McPhail 2003).	12 May Mary is able to instil water into the colon over a 4–5 minute period.
8 May	(7) Mary is experiencing abdominal cramps after the water has been instilled into the stoma.	To minimise the abdominal cramps Mary may get.	(a) Ensure that the water used is not too hot or too cold (Goode 1982, Davis 1996, McPhail 2003). (b) Check that all air is expelled from the tubing (Goode 1982, MacDonald 1991). (c) Check that the water container is at shoulder height; if it is higher, the water will enter the colon at a greater pressure causing abdominal cramps (MacDonald 1991). (d) It may not be necessary to use 1 litre of water, 500 ml may be sufficient. Cramps may be a sign that the colon is ready to evacuate, the stretch reflex having been stimulated (Goode 1982).	13 May Mary is aware that she may get some abdominal cramps, as most people do prior to defecation but is aware of how to reduce them to a minimum.

(Continued)

Table A15.1 Excerpts from nursing care plan of Mary Long (Continued)

Date	Patient need or problem	Goal	Action	Evaluation
9 May	(8) Mary has leakage of water around the stoma when water is instilled.	All the water instilled via stoma into the colon with no leakage.	(a) Ensure that the tapered cone fits snugly into the stoma and is held firmly in position.	12 May Mary is aware that the cone must be held firmly into place while the water is being instilled.
11 May	(9) Mary is anxious that irrigation may not make her fully continent and that she may have spillage of faeces between irrigations.	Irrigation will ensure total continence.	(a) Check she is using 1 litre of water. (b) Check water container is at shoulder height – if higher, water is under greater pressure and will be forced along colon to the ileocaecal valve, thus water will be retained for hours and faeces passed intermittently. (c) Check Mary is aware that if she had diarrhoea, due to stomach upset, she should stop irrigating until settled. (d) Check Mary is not hurrying the procedure and not allowing adequate time for evacuation of faeces (McPhail 2003). (e) Check Mary is not on drugs that may cause diarrhoea. (f) Check that she is waiting half an hour for evacuation to take place following instillation of water.	13 May Mary is having very slight spillage of faeces between irrigations but is assured, as days progress, this will cease.
11 May	(10) Mary is aware of passing odorous flatus from stoma and feels embarrassed by this.	To help Mary learn to cope with passing flatus in public.	(a) Discuss dietary intake, encouraging sensible eating, but outlining some foods may cause more flatus and odour than others. (b) Check patient's medication as some drugs can cause excess flatus and odour. (c) Ensure Mary is using an odour-proof colostomy pouch or stoma cap, which has a flatus filter.	13 May Flatus and odour are decreased with irrigation. (William & Johnson 1980, Jones 1987). Flatulence cannot be totally eliminated but can be reduced to a minimum. Mary feels better able to cope with passing flatus, but still feels anxious that it will cause embarrassment.

(Continued)

Table A15.1 Excerpts from nursing care plan of Mary Long (Continued)

Date	Patient need or problem	Goal	Action	Evaluation
12 May	(11) Possible risk of constipation.	Mary passes a normal formed stool.	(a) Check fluid intake is at least 1½ litres daily. (b) Encourage a well-balanced high-fibre diet. (c) Encourage regular exercise. (d) Check medication. Analgesia can cause constipation and a laxative may be required.	15 May Mary is aware that the causes of constipation are the same as for those who do not have a colostomy and that the aim is to have a normal stool.
12 May	(12) No faecal return and possible retention of water following irrigations.	That water and faeces are passed following irrigation.	(a) Check the fluid intake. If the body is dehydrated water will be absorbed via the colon (Davis 1996, McPhail 2003). (b) Ensure Mary is relaxed. Nervousness can cause bowel spasm, which results in water retention. (c) A warm drink and gentle massage of the abdomen will encourage return of water and faeces (Goode 1982, McPhail 2003). (d) Suggest the wearing of a colostomy pouch following the procedure, as faeces may be returned later in the day (Goode 1982). (e) A further 150 ml of water can be instilled. Repeat the irrigation the following day.	13 May Mary understands the reasons why there is no return of faeces and can act accordingly.

Chapter 16

Dietary considerations following stoma surgery

Barbara Borwell

Eating is an experience from which most people derive gastronomic pleasure and adventure. The majority of patients are concerned that having a stoma will affect what they can eat and drink, and thus impinge not only on eating at home but also on any situations where eating and drinking occur. It is therefore important when diet is discussed with patients that both nutritional and social aspects are included in the discussion. Information and advice should be based on patients' probable physiological function (i.e. what they are likely to have retained plus what functions may be impaired/lost as a result of their particular operation). Normal physiological function and possible impairment arising from bowel surgery is described in Chapter 2.

In this chapter diet is considered in relation to:

- preoperative preparation
- the transitional postoperative period when patients resume oral intake
- general dietary considerations arising from different types of surgery and stoma
- potential nutritional problems after stoma surgery
- social considerations.

PREOPERATIVE PREPARATION

Prior to surgery it is important to assess patients' nutritional status and dietary intake to ensure their body is well prepared to aid an uncomplicated postoperative recovery. Decreased appetite can result from disease, radiotherapy and chemotherapy, surgery and taking steroids, and thus may well be experienced by some patients both before and after their operation. These can lead to weight loss, anaemia, hypoalbuminaemia and malnutrition. The usual regime of restricted food intake and bowel clearance in readiness for surgery is also likely to affect patients' nutritional status. Preoperative nutritional assessment and support will vary in accordance with the individual needs of patients and the regimes advocated by their healthcare team. Pedder (1998) describes the kind of assessments nurses should undertake with all patients while more detailed assessments for patients with gastrointestinal problems are discussed by Hamilton & Boorman (1997). Referral to a dietician may well be appropriate.

EARLY POSTOPERATIVE PERIOD

Following major abdominal surgery the gastrointestinal system requires a period of adjustment before it resumes normal peristaltic action. Patients must be monitored for evidence of returning bowel activity, such as the presence of bowel sounds and passage of flatus, to determine when oral fluids can be reintroduced. There is then a gradual transition from clear fluids towards a light, low residue diet.

Given the current encouragement to eat fibre-containing foods it is important that patients and staff understand the need to reduce these in the early period after surgery. Fibre (i.e. the indigestible portion of vegetables) affects the large intestine by increasing peristalsis, reducing gut transit time and increasing stool bulk. This is undesirable whilst the gut is healing and may also be inflamed. Patients can be encouraged to gradually introduce fibre into their diet and generally, by 2 months after surgery, to be eating a 'normal' diet which is:

(a) *High in fibre* – to increase peristalsis and faecal bulk and reduce transit time through the remaining bowel pathway.
(b) *High in fluids* – 1500–2000 ml fluid daily, depending on the fluid loss via the stoma (Iggulden 1999). Since fibre acts as a sponge, mopping up intestinal fluid, adequate fluid intake is necessary to prevent constipation, particularly in colostomists who still have much of their bowel pathway with which to reabsorb fluid.
(c) *Made up of three regular meals daily* – to help regulate stomal output.

The early postoperative period is an ideal time to review patients' eating patterns, which may have been curtailed by various factors such as their original bowel condition, dental or mouth problems, and work and social patterns of activity. Barasi (1997) suggests that patients' mental state can also affect their dietary intake.

GENERAL DIETARY CONSIDERATIONS ARISING FROM DIFFERENT TYPES OF SURGERY AND STOMA

The specific aspects of eating, drinking and digestion that individual patients and healthcare staff should consider will be largely determined by:

• the amount of bowel pathway still in place with which to digest food and absorb fluids and nutrients before elimination occurs
• any reduction in normal alimentary processes likely to occur because bowel has been excised or food no longer passes through it, as described in Chapter 2
• the effects of eliminating faeces or urine without sphincteric control which generally occur with their particular alterations in the bowel or urinary pathway, and how these can be most easily managed by dietary intake
• how problems in digestion and absorption of food and drink can be recognised and managed effectively.

Patients may have personal preferences and beliefs about foods. Dietary discussion is therefore more helpful if it includes:

• what the effects of their surgery are likely to be on digestion and stomal action, and why
• what types of foods and drinks they normally enjoy, and now think they can or cannot have (so misconceptions or previous curtailed diets can be discarded)
• any effects that their normal cultural, religious, work and lifestyle activities might have on how and when they eat, including any periods of fasting (so information can be adapted to take account of these factors)
• any conditions or medications that might require them to restrict or modify their diet
• any concerns or preferences of the individual patient.

Adequate nutrition can be maintained in almost all stoma patients since absorption from the remaining gut above their stoma can normally take place. Patients with short bowel syndrome will need specialised information and help to maximise nutritional intake and minimise the speed with which food is eliminated (Wood 1996).

CUTANEOUS URETEROSTOMY

There are no dietary restrictions but a good fluid intake is recommended to minimise urinary tract infection.

ILEAL AND COLONIC CONDUITS

Surgical techniques necessitate resection and handling of the gut (see Ch. 6). Initially flatus can be a problem and establishing a bowel action difficult. Oral fluids will be recommenced once bowel activity is sufficiently established after surgery, and a light, low fibre diet is then advisable with a gradual return to the individual's normal eating pattern.

Patients should have a fluid intake of 2.5–3 litres daily (Blackley 2004, p 181). This helps minimise urinary stasis and infection. Fluids of any type may be taken, including beer, while remembering that 'a night out' will also require more frequent emptying of their pouch! Some patients include cranberry juice as its bacteriostatic qualities are thought to reduce the risk of infection (Fillingham & Douglas 2004, Stott 2000). Diabetics should be advised to take capsules rather than juice (Stott 2000). As the effects of warfarin are being questioned, patients on warfarin should be advised to consult their doctor before taking cranberries (Suvarna et al 2003).

Ideally, patients should be encouraged to maintain an acidic urine (pH 6–7.5) as alkaline urine is associated with infections and stone formation (Fillingham & Douglas 2004). Patients should be informed that their fluid intake should be increased if their urine becomes darker and concentrated as this could indicate they are becoming dehydrated.

Patients should also be informed of foods that can affect their urine as such knowledge will prevent undue anxiety and embarrassment if changes occur. Examples include beetroot, which causes discolouration, and asparagus, which causes some odour. Further examples are given in Chapter 6.

ILEOSTOMY

People with an ileostomy can and do eat a normal diet (Bryan et al 1982). Whether there is any

impairment to normal digestion will largely depend on the amount of small bowel left to function after operation (including previous surgery), and the effects of any residual disease in the remaining bowel (e.g. Crohn's disease).

Postoperatively the nature and volume of ileostomy effluent must be monitored so that an adequate fluid balance can be maintained. Nicholls (1996, p 118) suggests that several litres of effluent containing electrolytes may be lost during the first few days of ileostomy action and replacement of sodium in particular may well be required. As patients' dietary intake increases and their remaining bowel resumes normal function so ileostomy output should decrease to a level where approximately 400–800 ml daily output can be expected, and the consistency is usually similar to toothpaste. If the bowel pathway has been shortened by more extensive resection then increased output is likely.

Water, sodium, bile salts, some fats, and vitamin B_{12} are normally absorbed in the ileum. Surgery that includes removal of some ileum as well as colon can reduce absorption of some or all of these items with subsequent nutritional implications for patients, as discussed below. The increased risk of having nutritional problems may be an ongoing one if the remaining bowel cannot take over some of these absorption functions.

Fat malabsorption

Some fat is absorbed in the terminal ileum in combination with bile salts and this may mean ileostomists cannot readily absorb a high fat intake. However, it is important that patients should incorporate moderate amounts of fat within their diet because it is a valuable source of calories and aids absorption of vitamins A, D, E and K and calcium. If there is fat malabsorption this is likely to be signalled by steatorrhoea and medical and dietary advice should be sought. If fat is reduced other sources of calories must be taken, such as sugar, jam, honey and carbohydrate foods, to ensure there is no weight loss. Calcium and vitamin supplements may be necessary (Thompson et al 1970).

Vitamin B_{12} absorption

In the stomach a substance called intrinsic factor is released which binds onto dietary vitamin B_{12}. This complex is then absorbed in the terminal ileum. Malabsorption can therefore occur if the amount of terminal ileum that has been resected leaves insufficient ileum to absorb adequate vitamin B_{12}. Wood (1996, p 85) states that vitamin B_{12} replacement therapy should be given if more than one metre of terminal ileum has been resected. This will have to be given regularly for life in order to prevent pernicious anaemia.

Fluid and electrolytes

A decrease in the levels of absorption of fluid and electrolytes may occur if patients have had some ileum as well as their colon removed. Hamilton & Boorman (1997, p 230) suggest that ileostomy patients usually require extra sodium, potassium and fluids during (at least) the first 6–8 weeks after surgery to compensate for the loss of these constituents through inadequate absorption in this early postoperative period.

Black (2000, p 178) suggests ileostomists pass 400–800 g of effluent daily, containing about 4 g of salt and 600 ml water. Additionally, quantities lost of nutrients such as potassium, magnesium, iron, zinc, fat and protein may equal those lost by the large bowel. Ileostomists should generally be advised to include enough fluids and minerals in their diet to enable sufficient to be absorbed (see Appendix 16.1, Handout A) unless they have medical conditions that contraindicate such action.

Most patients' bodies gradually adapt physiologically so that their remaining small bowel absorbs more fluid and electrolytes and their renal system works in conjunction with these changes to achieve a functional balance. This resumed function, coupled with a normal diet, will generally be sufficient for adequate levels of these constituents to be maintained under normal circumstances. However, in situations where patients may be losing extra fluids and/or electrolytes (e.g. with added sweating in hot weather; extra loss because of vomiting or diarrhoea) they should seek to replace these losses (Black 2000, Blackley 2004). There are several commercially produced electrolyte replacement solutions available and more convenient substitutes include clear fruit juices, caffeine-free carbonated drinks, weak tea with sugar, and sports drinks.

It is essential that ileostomists accept the need to take adequate amounts of fluid because they no longer have a colon reabsorbing water. Reducing fluid intake in an attempt to regulate ileostomy output should be strongly discouraged as it can lead to dehydration and can also affect electrolyte reabsorption (see Ch. 2). Ileostomists should be encouraged to check the amount and colour of urine they pass daily as a means of assessing whether their fluid levels are low. Urine should be clear, and they should pass a minimum of two full bladders of urine (a minimum total of 1000 ml) in 24 hours.

It is important to remember that conditions such as ulcerative colitis and Crohn's disease may have led this group of patients to consume a modified diet and adapt their lifestyle considerably before surgery. They may need help to identify and try out a more varied diet both at home and elsewhere. Specialist dietary advice should be sought for patients who are underweight before surgery. During the first few weeks postoperatively patients may benefit from eating a low fibre diet with extra sodium and potassium, and avoiding substantial intake of foods that are likely to increase the liquidity and/or frequency of stomal action. Meadows (1997, p 107) suggests that foods which may *loosen* stomal output include:

- foods containing fibre (e.g. raw fruit and vegetables, leafy green vegetables, wholemeal food, cereals, citrus fruits)
- some fluids (e.g. alcohol including beer, caffeinated drinks, citrus fruit juices)
- some food types (e.g. spicy foods, fried foods).

As patients readjust to their new bowel system they should be encouraged to introduce additional foods gradually, so their effects can be monitored. Any foods that are thought to have caused gastrointestinal upsets should not be eaten for a week or two. Patients can then try them again in order to establish whether the previous upset was caused by the particular food or was merely coincidental. Most patients can enjoy a varied diet. It is generally more helpful to encourage them to consider whether particular foods are sufficiently enjoyable to warrant occasional increases in effluent or flatulence rather than impose dietary embargoes on them.

Some foods have attributes that may be both helpful and unhelpful to patients. For example, prunes contain a specific laxative which increases stomal output (Thompson et al 1970) but they are also a good source of potassium (Iggulden 1999). It is also helpful to discuss with patients *how* and *when* they take foods. For example, alcohol, fizzy drinks and pure fruit juices taken on an empty stomach can overstimulate the gut, resulting in a watery stool and flatulence. However, they can be included within most people's normal diet.

Patients should also be given information about foods that can alleviate diarrhoea, odour and flatulence. Foods listed by Blackley (2004, p 179) and Meadows (1997, p 107) as *thickening* stool include bananas, rice, potatoes, pasta, cheese and bread. Eating marshmallows has also been reported as alleviating diarrhoea (Farbrother 1993). Eating natural yoghurt can help reduce odour and wind, and fennel tea or peppermint tea can help to ease flatulence.

Ileostomists should be made aware of foods that can swell in the gut and may therefore cause mechanical problems, stenosis or intestinal obstruction. These are generally foods that have a high fibre or cellulose content such as nuts, coconut, celery, sweetcorn and mushrooms (Blackley 2004, Meadows 1997). Other foods like oriental vegetables (e.g. in Chinese takeaways) can sometimes cause difficulties too. These foods should be eaten slowly, chewed well, and taken in moderation with ample fluids after, and not with, the meal.

If blockage does occur it is usually temporary, causing abdominal pain, and the stomal output will either cease or contain excessive amounts of watery fluid. Patients should be asked to describe their specific dietary intake of the preceding 24–48 hours in order to identify likely causes and appropriate treatment. Blackley (2004, p 182) suggests that if food blockage is suspected but the ileostomy is draining some stool, then oral fluids may be taken but solids should be avoided. However, if there is no effluent being passed nothing should be taken orally.

It is important to get a balance between giving patients sufficient information about possible problems to ensure they are well prepared for most eventualities and avoiding increasing anxiety. This can be achieved when written information such as that shown in Appendix 16.1 (Handout B) is used initially as a tool for discussion with individual patients, and only after discussion given to them to refer to later as necessary. It is inappropriate just to hand it to patients without ensuring they understand how that information relates to their situation as this can leave them with queries and increase anxiety.

Patients should be advised to seek help promptly from their doctor or stoma care nurse if there are significant changes in stomal output consistency, volume, or colour, and/or if they feel generally unwell with abdominal pain, distension, nausea or vomiting.

If bowel throughput is too speedy to allow maximum absorption of water and electrolytes from their remaining gut, ileostomists may benefit from decreasing this transit time by increasing intake of foods that thicken faeces and decreasing foods that make effluent more fluid or stimulate the bowel. Some patients may require medication to achieve similar effects (see Ch. 17). However, the need for medication should be reviewed at intervals as changing bowel absorption may mean individuals can reduce or do without medication.

INTERNAL BOWEL POUCHES

Residual bowel function following restorative proctocolectomy or Kock pouch formation is likely to be similar to that following conventional ileostomy diversion. Compensatory mechanisms to maintain normal body stores of water and salt which patients with ileostomies develop over time (see above) also develop in patients with these pouches, so dietary advice can be fairly similar.

Pearson (2002) suggests:

- patients with new stomas or ileo-anal pouches should follow a low fibre diet for 2–4 weeks after surgery before reintroducing small quantities of fibrous foods
- patients with a Kock pouch should introduce a pureed or soft low fibre diet for the first 2 weeks whilst the reservoir catheter is in situ; this can be followed by a low fibre diet for 4 weeks before gradually resuming a normal diet
- food must be chewed well
- high protein, high energy diets can help prevent weight loss
- small frequent meals, and commercial sip-feeds between meals if necessary, can help patients with poor appetites.

Some patients have been found to have reduced absorption following internal pouch surgery (Pearson 2002). Monitoring of fluid balance, weight, iron and vitamin B status, and any clinical signs of nutritional deficiency should be carried out during outpatient visits.

TRANSVERSE COLOSTOMY

This is often performed as an emergency procedure and patients are likely to be physically debilitated. Postoperative treatment will include correction of any electrolyte imbalance, but the patient's attitude and mental adjustment to their circumstances will also influence the type of food eaten. As time in which to mentally prepare for such surgery may have been minimal patients may require extra encouragement to resume meals as well as other activities.

Much of the above information relating to ileostomists will also be useful to patients with a transverse colostomy. However, they usually still have functioning ileum to enable some electrolyte absorption to occur. Generally, most colonic fluid reabsorption occurs in the proximal half of the large bowel. As these diversions lie fairly early on in the colonic pathway fluid absorption is reduced and effluent is usually initially fluid and then of a soft consistency which, in time, may get firmer. Fluids and then foods should be gradually reintroduced until a full diet is being eaten. Extra fluid may be needed if excess fluid is being eliminated, and advice on foods to thicken effluent and avoid overstimulating the gut should be given. Constipation is not usually a problem.

SIGMOID COLOSTOMY

Patients have often received substantial preoperative measures to empty their bowel, and may also have undergone major surgery such as abdominoperineal excision of rectum. Postoperatively bowel action may not occur for 4 or 5 days, and abdominal discomfort and flatulence are common in this early period. Once oral intake is resumed patients should first be encouraged to build up an adequate fluid intake, and then add foods that are light in fibre but with sufficient calories to aid healing and build up energy. Small amounts of fibre-containing foods should then be gradually added until patients are enjoying a balanced, high fibre diet taken as three meals a day. Pedder (1998) suggests that this includes five portions of fruit and vegetables daily, plenty of fluids, and that dietary advice should also take into consideration people's levels of activity.

If patients still have most of their colon in situ to fulfil its normal functions of absorbing water, sodium and potassium then, once they have resumed a varied diet, most of their nutritional needs will generally be met, and their effluent is likely to become more solid and be passed perhaps once or twice a day. Unless a specific diet is necessary because patients have another medical condition they do not have to restrict their diet.

Some patients report that if they eat excessive amounts of foods with a high fibre content or which are of the 'binding' type (e.g. eggs, boiled rice and tapioca) these can make their faeces too solid. This can cause a build-up which blocks the passage through the colostomy. Such substances do not have to be omitted from their diet, but should be taken in moderation coupled with an increased amount of fluids.

SOCIAL CONSIDERATIONS

Eating and drinking are social activities and therefore when patients are given information about the effects of their particular operation on their ability to eat, drink and digest food it is important to help them apply it to their particular circumstances and concerns. Generally it is helpful to first ask patients:

- *What they normally eat and drink.* This enables staff and patients to identify which elements of their normal diets can be continued, and where caution or adaptation might be desirable. This is much more helpful than just assuring patients vaguely that 'in time' they will be able to 'eat most things'.
- *Whether they were following particular modifications before their operation.* For example, a urostomist may have curtailed their fluid intake in an attempt to avoid incontinence, or an ileostomist may have curtailed fruit and vegetables to reduce bowel activity. Tactful questioning enables restrictive patterns that are no longer necessary to be identified. Some patients may just need general encouragement to try out a more varied diet, while others may need more specific help to plan how and when they could try out previously avoided foods, in small portions initially, so they can gain confidence in their ability to have a varied diet.

It is not uncommon for patients who have undergone stoma surgery to reject food because they feel unclean and antisocial when it results in stomal action. Any escape of odour from an unsealed appliance will exacerbate this problem. Encouragement to move towards eating regular meals and discreet monitoring of patients' food intake is advisable so help can be given with any difficulties at an early stage before a (new) curtailed pattern of eating or drinking becomes entrenched. Patients usually welcome written information to refer to and this is often available from their stoma care nurse or dietician (see examples in Appendix 16.1). The patient associations also produce literature which includes dietary advice (see Ch. 24). It is essential that any written advice, such as that shown in Appendix 16.1, is discussed with patients so they can relate the information to their own situation and have any questions answered.

CULTURAL DIETS

Individual patients may or may not follow religious or cultural eating patterns. It is always advisable to ask patients what they do, rather than make assumptions which can lead to inappropriate care (Downes 1999). However, it is also important that healthcare staff are aware of some of the main patterns so inappropriate advice or meals are not given: this can cause distress as well as reducing the credibility of any other information or advice that is subsequently given.

Asian diets

The three main religions are Islam (the religion of Muslims), Sikhism and Hinduism, and each have their own dietary restrictions (Henley & Schott 1999). Some of these may result in nutritional deficits (Barasi 1997, p 247–248), and this could be exacerbated if patients also have less small bowel with which to reabsorb nutriments. Henley & Schott (1999) provide a useful summary of foods that are likely to prove acceptable sources of nutriments to Asians.

Hindus will not eat any food that involves the taking of life and so are usually strict vegetarians. Some will not eat eggs. Even Hindus who are not strictly vegetarian will usually not eat beef (the cow is a sacred animal) or pork (considered unclean). They may not take substances made from animal-based gelatine such as jellies, marshmallows, and medication in capsule form such as Imodium (Black 2000).

Muslims will eat 'all wholesome foods which are lawful'. There are embargoes on particular foods, such as pork, and also requirements related to food preparation. For example, other meat can be eaten if it has been killed in the prescribed way (halal).

Sikhs may eat meat although few eat beef, and pork (considered unclean) and alcohol are forbidden.

Fasting

Hindus may fast one or two days a week, or on particular fast days, as may some Sikhs. Muslims may fast during the month of Ramadan. This entails abstaining from all food, liquid and tobacco between dawn and sunset, and meal times are rescheduled to take place outside these hours.

Jewish diet

Pork and all derivatives are prohibited but deer, sheep, goat and poultry are permitted. Orthodox Jews may require special (kosher) preparation of food, and may not combine meat and milk in the same meal or have both within a 2-hour timespan. It is advisable to ask patients if these are requirements they follow so that appropriate content and timing of meals and/or milk drinks may be achieved.

Chinese diet

Rice is the staple food and vegetables are always lightly cooked. Small amounts of meat, fish and poultry are often included in dishes.

DIETARY FIBRE

Dietary information given to patients should include discussion about the importance of including adequate dietary fibre in their daily diet. Recommended sources include vegetables, fruit, unrefined flour used in baking, cereals made from wheat, and unprocessed bran. As the lumen of ileum is smaller than colon it is important for ileostomists to get a balance between having sufficient fibre and not creating too much faecal bulk which could be more difficult to pass through their ileostomy. Most ileostomists can obtain sufficient fibre from meals without adding bran to them. Patients with transverse or sigmoid colostomies whose stool is liquid or very soft may find bran helps to firm up their stool and regulate stomal action.

Wheat or oat bran can be added to dishes, breakfast cereals, or sprinkled on beverages. Two or three teaspoonfuls of bran daily is usually sufficient when combined with other fibre-containing foods. Patients may need some encouragement to include sufficient fibre in their normal diet as, although it helps make effluent less liquid, it also increases the volume of stool passed and may increase the number of times pouches have to be changed.

FLATUS AND ODOUR

These create anxiety and problems in many patients with bowel stomas. Pringle & Swan (2001) found that more than 50% of colostomists in their study who survived to a year following surgery still had problems with flatus and around 37% reported bad odour. Such difficulties are likely to affect not only patients' willingness to eat a varied and nutritious diet but also their comfort in socialising and their sense of acceptability to themselves and others.

Patients can be helped by discussing with them both *how* flatus is produced and *what* activities and foods are likely to increase it, as well as appliance management (which is discussed in Ch. 4). Firstly, air can be *ingested*, particularly when talking when eating, chewing with an open mouth, smoking, chewing gum. Rushed eating, and eating and drinking at the same time are also likely to increase flatulence (Blackley 2004, p 179). Avoiding such habits can help reduce flatus derived from them.

Secondly, flatus is also *created by bacterial activity related to undigested carbohydrates including cellulose in the colon*, and is therefore related to what is eaten. Meadows (1997, p 106) cites Rideout (1987) as saying the average length of time from eating flatus-producing foods to passing flatus from the colon is 6 hours. Meadows (1997, p 107) suggests that foods which may cause flatus include beer, carbonated drinks, milk and milk products, onions, vegetables in the cabbage family (cabbage, broccoli, sprouts, sweetcorn). Blackley (2004, p 180) adds fresh and dried beans, radish and turnip, cauliflower, and wheat and bran products to this list. This does not mean patients should be advised to avoid such foods, but it is helpful to suggest they start with small portions, and do not eat several of these items in the same meal until their bowel has had some months to acclimatise itself after surgery. Many people find they can eat most of the above items without problems. Where items do cause discomfort people may like to try cooking/eating them in a different format. For example, onions in a casserole may not cause problems whereas raw onions may do so. Some foods may be more comfortably digested in soups than as whole items.

Odour is a common concern for patients and can have physical and psychological effects (Preston 1994). They may find it is helpful to consider this issue in two sections. Firstly, there is the reality that faeces does have an odour and that this will normally be contained within well-applied modern stomal equipment. Understandably, many patients experience their faecal odour as more noticeable than when it was rectally evacuated, as now it is being eliminated from a stoma that lies in a direct line below their nose, and faeces requires much more visible management than when it was evacuated straight into the toilet. Fears commonly expressed include that odour coming from their stomal action will be too offensive to be socially acceptable and/or that somehow the type of odour they can now smell will signal to everyone that they have a stoma if it works or if they have to change or empty equipment. Using a counselling style approach (as described in Chs 7 and 20) to help patients express any distress and come to realise the faecal odour is normal is generally a useful first step towards alleviating such fears. Patients then are usually more able to accept information about dietary and appliance management of odour. Many people report that as they become more competent and confident in managing their equipment so the odour seems less noticeable, and this information may help allay anxiety in new patients. Information and advice on appliance management and odour-containing products should be given (see Ch. 4).

Secondly, some foods may create more odour (see Appendix 16.1, Handout A) and patients may need to experiment with these foods and find combinations that are acceptable to them. For example, parsley can be included in fish and egg dishes or eaten after spicy foods. Patients may find they can have foods that create some odour but that it is inadvisable to couple them with foods which make their stoma more active or windy, as then the level of odour becomes more difficult to contain.

CONSTIPATION AND DIARRHOEA

It is always wise to ask patients what *they* mean by these terms, and obtain a detailed description of their situation and any factors that could be contributing to it, as described in Chapter 21. Generally patients may need help to deal with the immediate situation *and* to review whether they could prevent its recurrence by eating and drinking in a manner that results in softer or firmer bowel effluent. Foods that tend to loosen and thicken faeces have been discussed in the ileostomy section above, and are listed in Appendix 16.1 (Handout B). Medication to alleviate constipation and diarrhoea is discussed in Chapter 17. Means of alleviating constipation and temporary blockage of bowel (e.g. from a bolus of food) are also discussed in Chapter 21.

CONCLUSION

When providing dietary information and advice nurses must tailor it to patients' specific condition, type of surgery and resultant alterations in digesting and absorbing foods, and their individual needs and preferences. Such care helps patients understand and manage their situation more confidently. It therefore increases their likelihood of achieving a rehabilitated lifestyle which includes participating in occasions where eating and drinking take place.

APPENDIX 16.1

HANDOUT A: Information for patients following bowel stoma surgery

Like most people who have your type of operation you may have questions about what you can eat and drink. We hope that the information here will help you answer these questions. You may have additional questions about the things you like to eat and drink, or your individual situation and whether it affects what foods you can have. Do ask your healthcare team for any further information and help you want.

I. Staying well nourished and healthy

In *the first few months* after your operation your body will be adapting how it works to suit your shortened bowel, to enable you to gain the most benefit from your food. You can help this process by:

1. Drinking plenty of fluids (1500-2000 ml, i.e. 10–12 cups or 6–7 mugs daily). This can include water, fruit juice, tea, coffee, milk, alcohol (in moderation!). Remember alcohol and drinks containing caffeine (tea, coffee, cola) are dehydrating, so have other drinks as well.
2. Eating three regular meals a day, to help your bowel and stoma to settle down and work well.
3. Eating a balanced diet with carbohydrates, protein, fats, vitamins and minerals, but keeping the amount of fibre you eat low for the first couple of months only.
4. Checking with your nurse, doctor or dietician that what you normally eat and drink will give you the kind of balanced diet your body needs. Remember to tell them if you usually have a special diet or medication for a medical condition, as this may alter the advice you need now after your operation.
5. Some people are advised to include foods that are high in potassium and/or salt (sodium) for the first 6–8 weeks after surgery. Ask if you should do this. If the answer is 'yes' then the following foods can help you:
   - to increase *potassium*: fruit and vegetables (e.g. bananas, avocado, raw apple including the skin, prunes, dried apricots, raisins, tinned tomato, orange, prune juices), fish, chicken, Bovril, Marmite
   - to increase *sodium (salt)*: salt and salty foods, tinned meat, soups, and vegetables including tomato juice, cornflakes, Bovril, Marmite.

After the first couple of months:
- Continue to have a balanced diet with plenty of fluids.
- *Gradually* increase the amount of *fibre* you take in your diet, moving towards the five portions of fresh fruit or vegetables daily which are usually recommended. Other sources of fibre include cereals made from wheat, wholemeal bread (not just 'brown'), wholemeal pastas and rice.
- If you were originally advised to take extra salt or potassium in your diet this may no longer be necessary: ask your nurse, doctor or dietician.

1 of 2

II. Flatus (wind)

Flatus can collect in the bowel because of what we eat and how we eat, and is then relieved by 'burping' orally, or by it passing out via the stoma. Remember:

- eat slowly, taking in small amounts at a time and chew food well
- avoid eating and talking at the same time to cut down the amount of air you swallow
- avoid eating and drinking at the same time if this makes you swallow air: have your drink at the end of meals
- have regular meals – missed or irregular meals increase flatus
- smoking and chewing gum also increase the amount of air people swallow.

Flatus is mainly caused as the body acts on less digestible foods, usually in the large bowel (colon). People vary in which foods give them wind, and how much of a problem it is. Foods more commonly reported include:

- peas, beans, lentils, onions, cauliflower, sprouts, cabbage, broccoli
- carbonated drinks and beer
- high fibre foods including some wheat and bran products.

Take these in small amounts one at a time to begin with, so your body can more easily process them. If you do experience problems, try that food several times again, at about 2-weekly intervals, so you can identify whether it really does cause difficulties or was a chance coincidence. It can take about 6 hours from eating food to flatus being expelled from your stoma. If particular items are problematic but you enjoy them, experiment with the form in which you cook and eat them.

Foods said to reduce or relieve flatus include: plain yoghurt and buttermilk, fennel, peppermint, dill and aniseed (including liqueurs!).

III. Odour

Cheese, fish, eggs, spices and garlic may create a more noticeable odour in the faeces expelled from your stoma. However, the high quality of odour-containing materials used in modern appliances means that this is only likely to be noticed by you, for example when emptying or changing equipment. Foods said to reduce odour include parsley and spinach.

IV. Foods that are not digested

Some foods are indigestible and may pass through the stoma whole, especially in the early months after surgery. *These may include:* nuts, mushrooms, celery, sweetcorn, peppers, pineapple. You can still eat them unless they cause problems (see handout B), but start with small amounts and chew them well.

HANDOUT B: Dietary management of problems for stoma patients

This handout gives you some guidance on **problems** for which patients usually seek help. The basic information in handout A will also be useful to you. *Remember:*

- take regular meals: *do not* reduce or cut out meals or drinks in order to reduce your normal stomal output as this can cause flatus (wind), and could mean you don't take in the nourishment your body needs to function well
- ask your nurse or doctor for help if you need more specific advice, if your problems continue to occur, or if you have special dietary requirements.

I. Constipation

(a) *Increase* fluid intake (e.g. 2000 ml, which equals about 12 cups or 7 mugs a day). Drinks taken after meals (rather than with them) are less likely to cause flatus.

(b) *Increase* fibre-containing foods such as fresh fruit and vegetables, wholemeal bread, cereals, pasta, rice as these can help make faeces softer and more bulky and easier to pass when taken with a good fluid intake. If you are advised to also take wheat or oat bran: add 2–3 teaspoons daily to cereals, casseroles, or drinks.

(c) Eat regularly and in sufficient quantities to give your bowel a regular pattern of enough food to process and eliminate. This is important if you want to stop passing small amounts of hard faeces and have larger, softer, less frequent stomal actions.

(d) *Increase* the amount of exercise you take: this helps your bowel to work well.

(e) *Avoid* foods more likely to swell in the bowel (e.g. celery, nuts, coconut, sweetcorn, mushrooms). These sometimes cause blockage, or slow down the rate your food passes through the bowel, which makes faeces more solid. Also *avoid or reduce* 'binding' foods such as eggs, boiled rice, or tapioca.

II. Alternating diarrhoea and constipation

Seek help from your doctor or nurse so that the cause of this can be found and treated. It will help if you keep a record of what is happening so you can tell them:

- what you are eating and drinking, and at (about) what times
- what your bowel output is like (e.g. large/small amount; solid/soft/fluid consistency; lots/little flatus)
- about what time and/or how often your stoma acts
- whether your urinary output is more/less/the same as usual
- whether the appearance of your urine has changed (e.g. colour darker).

Remember, you should not delay seeking help if you do not have such information.

III. Diarrhoea

1. *Increase* fluids, especially those containing electrolytes so you replace those being lost in the diarrhoea, e.g. caffeine-free carbonated drinks, 'sports' and electrolyte drinks, weak tea with sugar, clear fruit juices.

2. Some food and drinks can make your bowel more active and/or output more fluid. Avoid foods and drinks which are:

1 of 2

- very acidic, e.g. stewed apple, fruit, more 'acid' fruit juices
- likely to have a laxative effect, e.g. prunes, chocolate
- flatus-producing, e.g. onions, greens, beans, peas, hot, spicy, or fatty foods.

3. *Reduce or avoid* alcohol, including beer, which can also increase bowel activity, and production of flatus as well as more liquid faeces.
4. Eat regular meals, with snacks in between if necessary, to give your bowel food to process, and help it slow down its level of activity.
5. *Include* foods which thicken faeces, such as bananas, potatoes, rice, pasta, bread and cheese. Marshmallows are also said to help!
6. Review what you have been eating and drinking which could be causing the diarrhoea. Omit such items until your bowel has settled, and then reintroduce them to meals in small amounts and one at a time to see if they do cause problems.
7. Seek advice from your nurse or doctor if the diarrhoea continues for more than 24 hours and/or if it might be caused by any medication you have been taking.

IV. Pain, discomfort, and possible food blockage

People with an *ileostomy* may experience more difficulty with certain foods because the small bowel is narrower than the large bowel (colon). High fibre foods and those which have indigestible cellulose/skins/pips are more likely to cause temporary 'pile-ups' before being evacuated, so should be taken in moderate amounts and chewed well. Examples include: nuts, potato skins, raw fruit and tomato skins, dried fruits, celery, sweetcorn, mushrooms, oriental vegetables.

Signs of partial blockage include: pain, abdominal distension, and reduction of normal ileostomy output or it may occur intermittently and perhaps more explosively, and be more watery and offensive. Generally, you should take one of these actions:

- *If you are not nauseated, and still have some stomal output:* continue to take fluids as this may dislodge the blocked items, but avoid food. Seek help from your doctor or stoma care nurse if this situation worsens, or is not resolved within 4-6 hours.
- *If nauseated, vomiting, and/or you have no stomal output:* contact your doctor or stoma care nurse promptly so further help can be given. Avoid food and drink.

2 of 2

References

Barasi M E 1997 Human nutrition: a health perspective. Arnold, London

Black P K 2000 Holistic stoma care. Baillière Tindall and RCN, Edinburgh

Blackley P 2004 Practical stoma wound and continence management, 2nd edn. Research publications, Vermont, Victoria, Australia

Bryan S, Cummings J A, McNeil N I 1982 Diet and health of people with an ileostomy. British Journal of Nutrition 47:399–406

Downes M 1999 False cultural assumptions: a bar to effective communication. Nursing Times 95(32):42–43

Farbrother M 1993 What can I eat? Nursing Times 89(14):63

Fillingham S, Douglas J 2004 Urological nursing, 3rd edn. Churchill Livingstone, Edinburgh

Hamilton H, Boorman J 1997 Nutrition. In: Bruce L, Finlay T M D (eds) Nursing in gastroenterology. Churchill Livingstone, New York, p 211–250

Henley A, Schott J 1999 Culture, religion and patient care in a multi-ethnic society. Age Concern England, London

Iggulden H 1999 Dehydration and electrolyte disturbance. Nursing Standard 13(19):48–56

Meadows C 1997 Stoma and fistula care. In: Bruce L, Finlay T M D (eds) Nursing in gastroenterology. Churchill Livingstone, New York, p 85–118

Nicholls R J 1996 Surgical procedures. In: Myers C (ed) Stoma care nursing. Arnold, London, p 90–122

Pearson M 2002 Dietary aspects of internal pouches. In: Williams J (ed) The essentials of pouch care nursing. Whurr, London, p 165–179

Pedder L 1998 Nursing's nutritional responsibilities. Nursing Standard 13(9):49–55

Preston J 1994 A perspective on the physical and psychological implications of odour for the ostomist. In: World Council of Enterostomal Therapists congress proceedings. Hollister, Libertyville, IL, p 245–247

Pringle W, Swan E 2001 Continuing care after discharge from hospital for stoma patients. British Journal of Nursing 10(19):1274–1288

Rideout B 1987 The patient with an ileostomy: nursing management and education. Nursing Clinics of North America 22:253

Stott C A 2000 Management of patients with urinary diversions In: World Council of Enterostomal Therapists congress proceedings. Hollister International, Libertyville, IL, p 22–26

Suvarna R, Pirmohamed M, Henderson L 2003 Possible interaction between warfarin and cranberry juice. British Medical Journal 327:1454

Thompson T J, Runcie J, Khan A 1970 The effects of diet on ileostomy function. Gut 11:482–485

Wood S 1996 Nutrition and the short bowel syndrome. In: Myers C (ed) Stoma care nursing. Arnold, London, p 79–89

Chapter 17

Medication and stoma care

Ann Richards

Clients with a stoma are just as likely as anyone else to suffer from other medical conditions needing treatment with drug therapy, sometimes on a long-term basis. As most medication is given orally and has to be absorbed into the bloodstream from the gastrointestinal tract, the presence of a stoma and the shortened length of the tract may influence the amount of drug available to the body. Drugs may also affect stomal action. Nurses looking after stoma patients should therefore have a good understanding of some of the basic pharmacological principles that underlie drug action.

DRUG ABSORPTION

Any medication given by mouth and swallowed has to be absorbed into the bloodstream before it can have a systemic action. The stomach plays only a minor role in absorbing drugs because gastric emptying is fast and the surface area available is small. For example, aspirin is acidic and more easily absorbed whilst in the stomach but even this drug is mostly absorbed in the small intestine where there is a much greater surface area available and a specially adapted epithelium.

Absorption of medication given orally may be delayed, reduced or even enhanced after food. Some drugs may bind temporarily to certain foods (Trounce 2004). If rapid action is required most drugs are better taken on an empty stomach – this is the case with some antibiotics – but if a drug is irritant to the gastrointestinal tract, it should be taken with food.

The amount of drug absorbed in the intestine is also affected by the 'transit time'. This is the time taken for nutrients to pass through the gastrointestinal tract. If there is a rapid transit time there is less absorption, and if the client has a slow transit time the drug is in the tract longer, so allowing more active ingredient to be absorbed. If a client has diarrhoea, very little of a medication may be absorbed. Some drugs (e.g. antimuscarinics such as atropine) may inhibit gastric motility and so cause slow or irregular absorption of other drugs. Drug absorption may be unpredictable in Crohn's disease due to inflammatory activity and this may contribute to the variable response to oral steroids seen in this condition (Howden & Brodie 1993).

Enteric coated tablets are protected from stomach acid and designed not to dissolve in the stomach, often because they are irritant to the mucosa. They are unsuitable for some patients, especially those with ileostomies, as tablets can pass through the gut unchanged. Aspirin and prednisolone are examples of medication that can be enteric coated.

Modified release preparations are designed to release their active component slowly. They may be unsuitable for some patients if their rapid transit time through the remaining bowel results in insufficient release of the active ingredient before (for example) ileostomy diversion.

Minor upsets in gastrointestinal function may be well tolerated by the majority of the population. However, in stoma patients minor disturbances may have more major repercussions. Any sudden change in stomal action is likely to cause problems and drugs causing irritation may mean that the stool becomes too liquid to be contained by the client's normal stomal equipment. People with bowel stomas are usually more aware of the consistency of their stool than the general population. As practically any drug may alter bowel activity it may be advisable to warn stoma patients of this possibility. Having said this, the majority of side effects caused by drugs are no more likely to affect stoma patients than any other people. This should also be emphasised as patients may be afraid to take medication for other disorders in case stomal action is disturbed. Some patients have been known to be afraid of taking even two paracetamol for a headache in case the stomal action is upset.

In this chapter drugs will be looked at in four categories:

1. drugs given to affect stomal action
2. drugs prescribed for other reasons but having an incidental effect on stomal action
3. drugs with a direct action on the gut
4. other drugs relevant to stoma care.

DRUGS GIVEN FOR THEIR EFFECTS ON STOMAL ACTION

Both prescribers of medication and nurses administering it should think carefully before giving the medication to any client but when this client has a stoma this brings yet another factor for consideration into the equation. The mode of action of the drug needs to be considered and whether the stoma will adversely affect this. For example, clients with a double-barrelled stoma may require the distal loop to be cleared. An oral laxative will not be suitable for this role, although it may be used to clear the proximal loop before stoma closure. Some stimulant laxatives may have an effect on the distal loop as they increase intestinal motility, but this is insufficient to push debris through the loop. In these instances washouts of the distal loop are necessary (see Ch. 4).

Expecting patients to retain suppositories when they no longer have sphincter muscles and therefore no voluntary muscular control over bowel evacuation is inappropriate. Instilling olive oil into the stoma via a Foley catheter to lubricate the faeces may sometimes relieve constipation. The balloon is blown up slightly to temporarily stop the oil coming back out. This procedure is discussed in Chapter 21.

TREATING CONSTIPATION

Colostomists may suffer from constipation and whenever possible this should be treated by increasing fluid intake or dietary fibre. The latter will increase the bulk of the stool and soften it, thus helping to prevent constipation. In diarrhoea, fibre may also help by absorbing water and thickening the stool (see Ch. 16). When there is a disturbance in bowel function, dietary causes should always be investigated first – has the client eaten anything unusual? Have they changed their usual diet at all?

Colostomists with cancer may be given opioid analgesia, which will cause constipation and thus may require a laxative. Diet alone is not usually sufficient to solve this problem.

Laxatives

These are drugs which accelerate the passage of food through the intestine. In the general population, they are among the most abused drugs (Galbraith et al 1999).

Action may be by:

- increasing the volume of non-absorbable solid residue with bulk laxatives
- increasing motility and secretion with stimulant laxatives
- increasing the water content with osmotic laxatives
- softening the consistency of the faeces with faecal softeners.

Bulk-forming laxatives

These agents have two modes of action dependent on the amount of fluid that is taken with them. They work by the absorption of fluid from the gut. If given with a lot of fluid they will increase the size of the faecal mass and lessen the viscosity ('stickiness'), thus making small, hard stools larger, softer and bulkier. If given with no fluid or minimal fluid in cases where the stool is very runny, they will absorb water and so increase the viscosity of the stool, decreasing its fluidity. It is important when advising clients to explain the possible dual role of these agents and also the dangers of too little fluid intake when there is not a fluid stool. This may actually cause an obstruction of the colon.

These agents are especially useful when stools are small and hard. They help to relieve constipation by increasing the faecal mass, which then stimulates peristalsis. However, the most common cause of constipation is a dietary one and it is important to discuss their diet with clients, giving advice as to any improvements that may be made (see Ch. 16).

Patients may complain that, although the stoma is working several times a day, only a small amount of stool is being passed each time. Once mechanical causes such as stenosis have been eliminated a bulking agent should be tried, which will increase the fluid volume and lower the viscosity of the intestinal contents, thus also softening the stool. It is essential that adequate fluid intake is maintained to prevent the possibility of obstruction and these preparations should not be taken immediately before going to bed. Flatulence and abdominal distension are side effects. Unprocessed wheat bran, taken with food, is most effective, but other examples include methylcellulose (Celevac), ispaghula (Fybogel, Isogel) and sterculia (Normacol). Flax seed is a natural food high in fibre, lignin and omega-3 essential fatty acids and is sometimes used for constipation.

Agents such as methylcellulose may be given to increase the viscosity of a very runny stool. If used for this purpose the manufacturer recommends they should be taken with the minimum required liquid and fluids withheld for 30 minutes before and after each dose. Granules are difficult to take dry but may be added to jam or marmalade to help them slip down readily with a small amount of fluid.

Stimulant laxatives

These are used much less than used to be the case but anthraquinones such as senna (Senokot) may be used if increased fibre and bulk-forming laxatives are not tolerated. This group also includes rhubarb. Anthraquinones change the colour of the urine to brown if it is acid, or red if it is alkaline and clients should be warned that such changes occur. Docusate sodium is sometimes used and this is both a stimulant and a softening agent. Any stimulant laxative causes increased intestinal motility and may cause abdominal cramp.

Osmotic laxatives

These act by retaining fluid in the bowel by osmosis.

Lactulose is a semi-synthetic disaccharide, which is not absorbed from the gastrointestinal tract and holds water osmotically. As it also discourages ammonia-producing microorganisms it is useful in liver failure. Magnesium salts are also in this category but should not be used as they are contraindicated in any conditions of the gastrointestinal tract.

Faecal softeners

This type of laxative is most useful in haemorrhoids and anal fissure. Liquid paraffin is the best known but its prolonged use can interfere with the absorption of fat-soluble vitamins and also may cause a granulomatous reaction that could be related to the development of carcinoma of the colon. For these reasons it is probably best avoided by stoma patients.

TREATING DIARRHOEA

Anti-diarrhoeals

Any ostomist may suffer from diarrhoea. However, some patients who have had resection of the ileum or ileocaecal area may have a persistently high output, fluid stool due to loss of special transport functions (see Ch. 2). They may need a regular dose of a constipating agent.

Fibre and bulk-forming drugs may be tried but it is often difficult to adjust the dose appropriately. Some ileostomists find they cannot use high levels of fibre as the smaller lumen of the ileum, compared to the colon, means that the fibre collects in a bolus that may be difficult to pass. Anti-motility agents (described below) may be more effective for recurrent diarrhoea.

Octreotide is a somatostatin analogue, which reduces intestinal output and may be useful in ileostomy diarrhoea. It may be used in those with high output jejunostomies or ileostomies.

Fluid and electrolyte balance may need to be addressed in clients with a high output stoma, and oral rehydration solutions such as Dioralyte may be needed together with an anti-diarrhoeal agent such as loperamide (Meadows 1997). Clients with diarrhoea may also need to consider different appliances and skin care aids (see Ch. 21).

Anti-motility drugs

These drugs are especially useful when the problem is a rapid transit time as they slow down the motility of the gut. Where the stool is too fluid, a bulk-forming agent may be tried (see above) but there is often difficulty in adjusting the dose appropriately. Following any bowel shortening surgery there is a period of time, before adaptation can occur, when transit time is shorter and these drugs are useful. They increase the length of time the chyme is in contact with the mucosa and thus allow more absorption to occur per unit surface area.

Codeine phosphate activates opioid receptors on the smooth muscle of the bowel, which reduces peristalsis and increases segmentation contractions so that passage of contents is delayed and more water is absorbed. Tolerance may develop with prolonged use and occasionally dependence has been known (Laurence et al 1997). If the client is also in pain then this drug may be useful as a dual-purpose preparation.

Co-phenotrope (Lomotil) is a mixture of diphenoxylate hydrochloride and atropine sulphate. The former is a drug similar in structure to pethidine that has a similar effect on the bowel to morphine. The amount of atropine added is very small and is there partly to discourage abuse (Laurence et al 1997). Side effects include nausea, vomiting and abdominal cramps. In overdose, respiratory depression may occur.

Loperamide impairs propulsion in the gut by an action on the longitudinal and circular muscles which is not fully understood but is at least partly due to its action on the opioid receptors. In structure it is similar to diphenoxylate. Possible side effects include nausea, vomiting and abdominal cramps. Anti-diarrhoeal medication is best taken an hour before eating for maximum effect (Meadows 1997). People who eat a vegan diet (including many followers of the Hindu religion) may be unwilling to take gelatinous capsules which might contain animal products. They should be offered loperamide syrup instead of capsules (Black 2000).

The action of all three of these anti-motility drugs can be reversed by naloxone, which is the antidote to all opioid drugs. There are receptors for opioids on body cells and the drug actions occur when the opioid enters these receptors. Naloxone has a similar chemical structure to morphine, but none of its actions. It also fits the opioid receptors and will push the opioids out of the receptors to sit there itself. Naloxone, however, does not have any action on the cells and so the effects of the opioid are reversed. This means that naloxone antagonises all the effects of these drugs including respiratory depression and analgesia.

In clients with short bowel syndrome where diarrhoea may be being induced by bile acids, colestyramine may be used to bind the bile acids and prevent their effect on the colon. Although it may lessen diarrhoea, it may increase steatorrhoea due to further depleting of the bile acid pool. In some clients with very poor fat absorption, pancreatic enzymes (pancreatin) may be given to improve this.

If acid hypersecretion is a problem there are drugs available to decrease gastric acid secretion, for example, ranitidine and omeprazole.

DRUGS HAVING AN INCIDENTAL EFFECT ON STOMAL ACTION

ANTACIDS

These drugs reduce gastric acidity. They are usually taken for dyspepsia, in the presence of an ulcer or not, or reflux oesophagitis. Mostly they are magnesium or aluminium salts. All magnesium salts (e.g. magnesium hydroxide or trisilicate) can cause diarrhoea. Aluminium salts (e.g. aluminium hydroxide) tend to cause constipation. These bowel effects may be increased in stoma patients, and should be borne in mind when the agents are used.

All aluminium and magnesium containing antacids can interfere with the absorption of other drugs especially iron, digoxin, warfarin and some non-steroidal anti-inflammatories and so are better not taken with other oral medications. They may also damage enteric coatings designed to prevent dissolution in the stomach.

DRUGS THAT AFFECT THE STOMA BY THEIR ACTION ON THE AUTONOMIC NERVOUS SYSTEM

The autonomic nervous system consists of two parts, the sympathetic and the parasympathetic (see Ch. 2), and controls the activity of the gastrointestinal tract. Parasympathetic stimulation increases gut motility and activity, whereas sympathetic stimulation causes inhibition and slowing of gastrointestinal activity. Normally there is a balance between the two. If a drug increases the activity of the parasympathetic nervous system or decreases the activity of the sympathetic nervous system (rather like removing the brakes), it is likely to increase peristalsis and thus may cause diarrhoea. A drug that increases sympathetic activity, or decreases parasympathetic activity, is likely to cause constipation by decreasing peristalsis (Table 17.1).

Drugs increasing parasympathetic activity

Stimulation of the parasympathetic branch increases the release of the chemical acetylcholine where the nerve endings meet the smooth muscle of the gut.

The gut muscle is stimulated to contract by acetylcholine and thus the motility of the gut is increased. When acetylcholine is released in the body a cholinesterase enzyme rapidly destroys it. If the activity of this enzyme is decreased by drugs, this will prolong the action of acetylcholine in the body. Such drugs include neostigmine and pyridostigmine, which are used in the treatment of myasthenia gravis where there is reduced response to acetylcholine at the neuromuscular junction. This leads to weakness of skeletal muscle contraction. These drugs enhance neuromuscular activity by delaying the breakdown of acetylcholine in the body and thus prolonging its action. This means that the person has better skeletal muscle contraction but side effects of the acetylcholine on the autonomic nervous system include increased salivation, increased gastrointestinal secretions and increased motility.

Anti-dopaminergic agents such as metoclopramide and domperidone, which are used as antiemetics, also accelerate gastric emptying. This may affect other drugs administered orally and cause an earlier and higher peak concentration. Metoclopramide has been extensively studied and has been shown to accelerate the absorption of paracetamol, levodopa, ethanol and some antibiotics from the upper small intestine (Howden 1990).

Distigmine (Ubretid) is sometimes used in the treatment of a neurogenic bladder and because it delays the breakdown of acetylcholine it may also cause diarrhoea.

Bethanechol stimulates the parasympathetic nervous system and causes contraction of the detrusor muscle in the bladder. It used to be used in urinary retention, especially postoperatively, but it has now

Table 17.1 Gastrointestinal effects of drugs that affect the autonomous nervous system

Effect of drug on the autonomic nervous system	Effect on gastrointestinal motility and secretions	Result for the client
Increases parasympathetic activity	Increases peristalsis Increases secretions Relaxes sphincters	Possible diarrhoea
Decreases parasympathetic activity	Decreases peristalsis Decreases secretions	Possible constipating effect
Increases sympathetic activity	Decreases peristalsis Contracts sphincters	Possible constipating effect
Decreases sympathetic activity	Increases peristalsis Relaxes sphincters	Possible diarrhoea

been superseded by catheterisation. One of the side effects of the drug is that it enhances parasympathetic activity in the gut and thus increases intestinal motility, which may cause abdominal cramps and diarrhoea.

Drugs decreasing parasympathetic activity

Any drug that prevents the action of acetylcholine will cause relaxation of the smooth muscle in the gut, a loss of muscle tone and peristalsis and thus perhaps constipation. Such drugs are called antimuscarinics and include belladonna and the alkaloid atropine which is obtained from it. Atropine competes for the same receptors as acetylcholine and by occupying the acetylcholine receptors it renders the acetylcholine ineffective. This means that peristalsis is reduced and thus spasm reduced and colic helped. Hyoscine butylbromide (Buscopan) is also such a drug. It relaxes smooth muscle in the gastrointestinal tract and acts as an antispasmodic.

Synthetic antimuscarinic drugs such as dicycloverine (Merbentyl) may be used to reduce abnormal activity of the gut in irritable bowel syndrome and may help to reduce colic and pain. Propantheline (Pro-Banthine) used to be used to reduce acid secretion in the stomach and may be used to reduce muscle spasm and for urinary frequency. These drugs have a variety of side effects due to their effect on the parasympathetic nervous system. These include a dry mouth, dilation of the pupil, urinary hesitancy and of course constipation.

Other drugs with antimuscarinic action include some of the anti-parkinsonian drugs such as orphenadrine (Disipal) and trihexphenidyl, previously benzhexol (Artane), which correct the relative excess of acetylcholine in the central nervous system in Parkinson's disease. As a side effect they will reduce gastric motility and cause constipation.

Drugs increasing sympathetic activity

Increased activity of the sympathetic nervous system causes a reduction in gastric motility and thus constipation. The rate of gastric emptying may also be slowed and this may modify the concentration-profile of a single dose of a number of drugs, producing delayed and attenuated peak concentrations but usually not altering the total amount of drug absorbed. This is most important when an early high peak concentration is needed as in antibiotic or analgesic administration. Tricyclic antidepressants such as amitriptyline and imipramine are examples.

Drugs decreasing sympathetic activity

These drugs may reduce the amount of noradrenaline released and so reduce sympathetic activity, resulting in diarrhoea. Methyldopa used to be a very common drug used to control blood pressure but with the advent of modern drugs such as ACE inhibitors, e.g. ramipril, its use has declined. It is often used in pregnancy, however, because it is known to be safe.

DRUGS WITH A DIRECT ACTION ON THE GUT

Mebeverine (Colofac) has a direct effect on colonic hypermotility and may be used to relieve the spasm of intestinal muscle in irritable bowel syndrome. It is not an antimuscarinic and so does not have troublesome side effects such as a dry mouth.

Peppermint oil is believed to have a direct muscle relaxing activity. It is administered as Colpermin or Mintec and helps to relieve symptoms of pain and bloating due to intestinal spasm in irritable bowel disease or other gastrointestinal disorders. Capsules should be swallowed whole with a glass of water, 30–60 minutes before meals. The capsules must not be broken or chewed, as this would release peppermint oil and cause local irritation of the mouth or oesophagus. Heartburn is the most common side effect but occasionally allergic reactions may occur including bradycardia, headache, muscle tremor, ataxia (difficulty in coordinating movements) and a reddish skin rash. Peppermint oil should not be given to those who have a sensitivity to menthol.

Calcium channel blockers such as nifedipine and benzodiazepines such as diazepam may constipate to varying degrees. This is because impaired propulsion allows more water to be absorbed from the gut and thus the gut contents become more solid.

Opioid analgesics were mentioned earlier and when needed for intractable pain the associated constipation should be anticipated and a laxative considered. The action of morphine on the gut is complex. It increases tone and rhythmic contractions of the intestine but diminishes propulsive activity (Rang et al 2003). This means its overall effect is constipating. The effects of pethidine are similar to those of morphine and in equianalgesic doses it causes the same amount of constipation.

Non-steroidal anti-inflammatory drugs (NSAIDs) such as nefopam and ibuprofen are much less likely to cause constipation but these drugs may all reduce the thickness of the mucus lining of the stomach and intestines and lead to an increased risk of peptic ulcer formation. Ibuprofen appears to have the lowest risk. NSAIDs have been heavily implicated in causing damage to the small intestine and there are a number of reports of small intestine ulceration or perforation attributed to NSAIDs (Howden & Brodie 1993). A case-control study of 268 patients admitted with small or large bowel bleeding or perforation showed a positive association with NSAID ingestion - patients were more than twice as likely to have taken NSAIDs than controls (Langham et al 1985). It must also be noted that in asthma these drugs can lead to a worsening of the condition.

OTHER DRUGS RELEVANT TO STOMA CARE

Diuretics should be used with caution for patients with ileostomies as they may cause dehydration. Potassium depletion may occur and so it is usually advisable to use a potassium-sparing diuretic in these clients (British National Formulary 2004).

Hypokalaemia may occur in some ileostomists and this may mean patients are more sensitive to digoxin. Stoma patients who are taking digoxin may need potassium supplements or a potassium-sparing diuretic. If potassium is to be used modified release formulations of potassium are unsuitable and liquid formulations may be preferred. Patients with strictures should not be prescribed slow release formulations of potassium salts, as there is a danger of small bowel ulceration and perforation (Howden & Brodie 1993).

Iron preparations may cause loose stools and may also contribute to sore skin in these clients. It may be necessary to use an intramuscular preparation if iron is really needed. Again, modified release formulations should be avoided.

HORMONAL CONTRACEPTION

Detailed discussion of oral contraception is not possible in this chapter: readers should consult specialist texts. Most hormonal contraception is a combination of the synthetic hormones ethinyloestradiol and progestogens. These are both well absorbed from the upper small intestine when taken orally. They are transported to the liver where they are metabolised and then returned to the large bowel in the bile. Progestogen is excreted but oestrogen is reabsorbed from the large bowel as the bacteria there hydrolyse it into a reabsorbable form (this is the enterohepatic circulation). This process may be interrupted by the use of some broad spectrum antibiotics (e.g. ampicillin and tetracycline) and a small number of pregnancies have been linked with antibiotic use (Kovacs et al 1989). There is, however, still a lack of evidence regarding the use of antibiotics and combined oral contraceptive efficacy (Weaver & Glasier 1999). Rifampicin increases the metabolism of the hormones and its use reduces contraceptive efficacy for up to a month (Orme & Back 1991). St John's wort is a herbal remedy that can potentially reduce the efficacy of oral contraception due to its effect on liver enzymes (Chief Medical Officer 2000).

In clients with an ileostomy there is no enterohepatic circulation (from the large bowel back into the circulation) but the half-life elimination of 5–8 hours for oestrogens is not significantly changed and Grimmer et al (1986) note that there does not appear to be an altered hormone level in the blood in women following a total colectomy with ileostomy. The recommendation from the faculty of Family Planning and Reproductive Health Care Clinical Effectiveness Unit (FFPRHC) made in 2003 is that women should be advised that the efficacy of oral contraception is unlikely to be reduced by large bowel disease but may be potentially reduced in women with Crohn's disease who have small bowel disease and malabsorption. They also recommend that women with irritable bowel disease should stop combined oral contraception at least 4 weeks prior to major elective surgery because of the risk of venous thromboembolism.

NATURAL PRODUCTS

Many natural products are taken in an attempt to enhance health and some can actually interfere with either the absorption or metabolism of certain drugs.

Cranberry juice

This is taken in cystitis and urinary tract infections both as a treatment and preventative measure. It is also recommended following urinary diversion as it helps to break up mucus (Stott 2000). Leaver (1996) states it may be useful for its urinary antiseptic properties for people with ileal conduits.

Patients with bowel disease, especially those who have had resection of part of their gastrointestinal tract, have an increased incidence of kidney stones (Worcester 2002). Calcium oxalate stones and uric acid stones both have increased incidence partly explained by a decreased urinary volume due to loss of water and salts in the stool. Loss of bicarbonate in an ileostomy leads to an acid urine which encourages the formation of uric acid stones. Treatment with alkalinisation agents to raise the pH of the urine to about 6.5 may be needed. Cranberry helps to acidify the urine so in this instance would not be linked to prevention of kidney stones and although an alkaline urine may be linked to the formation of some types of urinary calculi, these are rare. Cranberries are high in oxalate compounds and these may actually promote the formation of kidney stones. One study (Terris et al 2001) reported significantly higher levels of oxalate in the urine of patients taking cranberry supplements and concluded that patients should be warned of the possible risk of kidney stones that may be associated with cranberry supplements. Recent evidence from medical practice has highlighted a possible interaction between warfarin and cranberry juice (Suvarna et al 2003). Cranberry juice contains antioxidants, including flavonoids, and these inhibit some of the drug metabolising enzymes in the liver. This may interfere with the metabolism of warfarin in the body, leading to dangers of haemorrhage in some patients. For this reason the Committee on Safety of Medicines has recommended (2003) that patients taking warfarin should be advised to avoid cranberry juice.

St John's wort

This herbal remedy appears to be effective in mild to moderate depression and, taken on its own, has an encouraging safety profile (Izzo 2004). However, it lowers the concentration of several drugs including warfarin and oral contraceptives. It may also interact with certain antidepressants with serious consequences. Patients considering this supplement need to be warned about this.

CONCLUSION

Although there are many drugs that may affect bowel function, and rapid transit time may present a problem on occasions, patients with a stoma can take most drugs without suffering any more side effects than other people. Drug absorption may sometimes be unpredictable, as in Crohn's disease due to malabsorption and inflammatory activity or complications of the disease such as enteroenteric fistula, stricture formation or secondary bacterial overgrowth. Each client needs to be considered as an individual and a careful history, including diet, needs to be taken before any drug therapy is commenced. A system for monitoring the effects of any drug therapy should be set up for patients who might not otherwise be in regular contact with a doctor or nurse.

References

Black P K 2000 Holistic stoma care. Baillière Tindall & RCN, Edinburgh

British National Formulary March 2004 No. 47. British Medical Association and the Royal Pharmaceutical Society of Great Britain, London 2003 (www.BNF.org)

Chief Medical Officer (CM) 2000 Important interactions between St John's Wort preparations and prescribed medication (4). Department of Health, London

Committee on Safety of Medicines 2003 Possible interaction between warfarin and cranberry juice. Current problems in Pharmacovigilance 327:1454

Family Planning and Reproductive Health Care Clinical Effectiveness Unit (FFPRHC) 2003 Contraceptive choices for women with inflammatory bowel disease. Journal of Family Planning and Reproductive Health Care 29(3):127–135

Galbraith A, Bullock S, Manias E et al 1999. Fundamentals of pharmacology. Addison Wesley, Harlow.

Grimmer S F M, Back D J, Orme M et al 1986 The bioavailability of ethinyloestradiol and levonorgestrel in patients with an ileostomy. Contraception 33:51–59

Howden C W 1990 Drug interactions and the gastroenterologist. GI Futures and Clinical Practice

Howden C W, Brodie M J 1993 Drug absorption and bioavailability. In: Bouchier A D, Allen R N, Hodgson H J F, Keighley M R B Gastroenterology Volume 1, 2nd edn. W B Saunders, London, p 710–718

Izzo A A 2004 Drug interactions with St John's Wort: a review of the clinical evidence. International Journal of Clinical Pharmacology and Therapeutics 42(3):139–148

Kovacs G T, Riddoch G, Duncombe P et al 1989 Inadvertent pregnancies in oral contraceptive users. Medical Journal of Australia 150:549–551

Langham M J S, Morgan L, Worrall A 1985 Use of anti-inflammatory drugs by patients admitted with small or large bowel perforations and haemorrhage. British Medical Journal 290:347–349

Laurence D R, Bennett P N, Brown M J 1997 Clinical Pharmacology, 8th edn. Churchill Livingstone, London

Leaver R 1996 Cranberry juice. Professional Nurse 11(8):525–526

Meadows C 1997 Stoma and fistula care. In: Bruce L, Finlay T M D (eds) Nursing in gastroenterology. Churchill Livingstone, London, p 85–118

Orme M, Back D J 1991 Oral contraceptive steroids – pharmacological issues of interest to the prescribing physician. Advances in Contraception 7:376-380

Rang H P, Dale M M, Ritter J M, Moore P 2003 Pharmacology. Churchill Livingstone, London

Stott C A 2000 Management of patients with urinary diversions In: World Council of Enterostomal Therapists congress proceedings. Hollister International, Libertyville, IL, p 22–26

Suvarna R, Pirmohamed M, Henderson L 2003 Possible interaction between warfarin and cranberry juice. British Medical Journal 327:1454

Terris M K, Issa M M, Tacker J R 2001 Dietary supplementation with cranberry concentrate tablets may increase the risk of nephrolithiasis. Urology 57(1):26–29

Trounce J 2004 Clinical pharmacology for nurses. Churchill Livingstone, London

Weaver K, Glasier A 1999 Interaction between broad spectrum antibiotics and the combined oral contraceptive pill. Contraception 59:71–78

Worcester E M 2002 Stones from bowel disease. Endocrinology and Metabolism Clinics of North America 31(4):979–999

Chapter 18

Care of patients receiving antitumour chemotherapy or radiotherapy

Brigid Breckman

Treatment of bowel and bladder cancers includes various combinations of surgery, chemotherapy and radiotherapy. Overviews of such treatments are provided by various authors (e.g. Fenwick 2004, Northover et al 2002, Tobias & Souhami 2003). The combination of regimes differs between countries as can the timing of when patients are offered treatment. In some countries treatment differs between centres. In other countries national cancer treatment regimes are reviewed and recommended by particular organisations. In the UK the National Institute for Clinical Excellence (NICE) provides such guidance. Guidelines are also provided by some professional groups (e.g. Association of Coloproctology of Great Britain and Ireland 2001).

In addition, patients' treatment can differ from conventional regimes because they are taking part in a trial of new forms or combinations of antitumour therapy. Updating information about treatments and trials must therefore become regular practice. Information can be downloaded from various websites by professionals and patients (e.g. NICE 2002a, 2002b, 2003; see Ch. 24).

Multidisciplinary approaches to cancer management have increased patients' awareness that they may receive more than one mode of treatment. Internet access is increasing people's awareness that different treatment regimes exist. They are therefore more likely to ask what these treatments entail, and what benefits and side effects they might experience from them.

In this chapter principles underlying chemotherapy and radiotherapy are discussed, focusing on aspects to consider when patients have a stoma and management of more common side effects.

Currently, in the UK, patients are more likely to have chemotherapy than radiotherapy after they have acquired a stoma for several reasons:

1. Radiotherapy may not now be considered the best treatment. Midgley & Kerr (2001) suggest it provides no benefit for *colonic* cancer. Keane et al (2001) describe cystectomy and chemotherapy as the treatments for invasive bladder tumours.
2. Radiotherapy may be given preoperatively. Midgley & Kerr (2001) suggest radiotherapy for *rectal* cancer is beneficial, and may be more effective and reduce toxicity when given before rather than after surgery.
3. Fewer patients may require stomas. Downing (2001) suggests sphincter-preserving surgery is now performed in over 50% of surgically resectable colorectal tumours. Concurrent chemoradiotherapy is now usually the primary treatment for anal cancers (NICE 2004).

Both chemotherapy and radiotherapy act on cells' reproductive cycle. Stoma patients usually receive chemotherapy systemically so it can potentially act on cells throughout their body. However, radiotherapy is localised to acting on cells within the fields of the radiation beam(s).

THE CELL CYCLE

Both normal and cancer cells go through several phases in order to grow and replicate themselves. The phases of the cell cycle are:

G1: *the first gap or growth phase, also called the intermitotic* phase. Cells produce ribonucleic acid (RNA) and protein in preparation for deoxyribonucleic acid (DNA) synthesis.

S: *the synthesis phase.* Cells double their DNA content so that the normal amount will be available for each new cell when the original cell divides in two.

G2: *the second gap or growth phase,* also called the *premitotic* phase. Synthesis of RNA and proteins continues.

M: *mitotic phase.* Cell division (*mitosis*) takes place. Each daughter cell has the same number and type of chromosomes as the parent cell.

Following mitosis cells either start the cell cycle again or may enter a resting phase:

G0: *the resting phase,* when cells may also be described as 'out of cycle'. This phase can be considered a sub-phase of G1.

Cells that are out of the reproductive cycle may:

- remain out of cycle and eventually die, or
- remain alive and begin cycling again.

Different types of cell take different lengths of time to divide. Normal cells divide in order to replace lost cells. This process maintains a constant normal cell population.

Tumour cells appear to have lost control mechanisms which prevent cells from growing until replacement is required. Human tumour cells are thought to have an average cycle time of 48 hours. This is not more rapid than the cycle of most normal cells. The reason tumours become larger is because their cell division creates additional cells rather than replacements (Dougherty & Bailey 2001). The rate of tumour growth can be expressed as the time it takes for a particular population of cancer cells to double in size. This *doubling time* is dependent on the tumour's:

- histological type
- age
- primary or metastatic status.

The histological type of a tumour affects the length of time it takes to complete a cell cycle. This in turn affects the length of time it takes a specific type of tumour to double in size. Adenocarcinomas of the bowel have doubling times in excess of 70 days (Dougherty & Bailey 2001). The growth of a cancer is only detectable and observable during the last 10–14 of its 35–40 doubling times, so most tumours are only detected at later stages of development.

The *growth fraction* is the proportion of viable tumour cells that are in the active division cycle at any one time. In early stages of tumour development the growth fraction is high. As tumour volume/size increases, its blood supply is likely to become poorer, leading to lower supplies of oxygen and nutrients. The growth fraction reduces, with more tumour cells being in a slowly dividing or resting (G0) mode. The rate of tumour growth slows.

CHEMOTHERAPY

Chemotherapy agents/cytotoxic drugs are generally most effective against rapidly dividing cells. However, tumours may not be detected until they have passed their most prolific stage. This can mean that chemotherapy is commenced at a point where its potential effectiveness may be reduced because tumour cell division has lessened.

Some cytotoxic agents are most effective against cells that are in a particular phase of the cell cycle. This *phase-specific* function means that when tumour cells enter other phases (including the resting (G0) phase) this reduces the opportunity drugs have to act on them.

Surgery, radiotherapy, and non-cycle-specific chemotherapy can reduce the volume of tumour cells. An increase in tumour cell division and/or resting tumour cells re-entering the cell cycle can then occur. In these circumstances the opportunity for phase-specific chemotherapy to be effective can increase. For example, patients whose overall amount of primary and secondary tumour is reduced by surgical resection of their colorectal primary may then be in a better position to benefit from fluorouracil (5FU), which is an S-phase-specific agent.

FREQUENCY OF TREATMENT MODULES

Cytotoxic drugs act on both normal and cancer cells. Since they are most effective in inhibiting rapidly dividing cells they affect tissues where cell repair and division activities are high. These include:

- stem cells and mature cells in the bone marrow
- the mucosal epithelium lining of the gastrointestinal tract
- hair follicles
- the germinal epithelium of the seminiferous tubules of the male testicles.

Normal cells have a greater ability to repair minor damage and remain viable than do cancer cells. This difference is used to create chemotherapy regimes that inhibit tumour growth while inflicting less damage on normal cells, enabling them to recover between each treatment.

Each regime has a length of time allocated between modules that is thought likely to be sufficient to allow normal cell recovery but not cancer cells. However, such recovery cannot be assumed to occur. Assessment of patients' fitness to undergo chemotherapy must take place before each treatment module. Blood counts are checked because they are likely to be affected by cytotoxic drugs (see below). The ability of the patient's body to eliminate their specific cytotoxic agents must also be monitored.

Impaired liver or kidney function could lead to the drug(s) staying in the body for longer than planned. When this occurs the level of damage to normal cells may be too high to enable adequate recovery of function in the normal timespan between treatment modules.

OVERALL LENGTH OF TREATMENT

The concept of *fractional cell kill* is used to aid programming of treatment (Tobias & Souhami 2003, p 71–72). It has been established that certain cytotoxic drugs, when given to treat specific histological types of tumour, are likely to kill a fixed fraction or proportion of tumour cells regardless of the size of the tumour. While the bulk of a tumour may be fairly easily eradicated the small amount remaining must be treated regularly, to reduce it by the same fraction each treatment, until all the malignant cells have been eradicated. This includes cells that have remained alive but out of cycle as they can begin cycling again. However, treating cancers is not always such an orderly process. Tumours may not be uniformly exposed to the drugs (e.g. solid tumours with poor vascularisation). Tumour cells can become resistant to chemotherapeutic agents, or their rate of regrowth can alter. It is preferable to treat cancers when they are small and there is less tumour to destroy.

The best timespan for chemotherapy treatment for patients with advanced colorectal disease, where chemotherapy is often palliative, is being tested in trials. Currently, patients are typically treated for 6 months or until tumour progression occurs (NICE 2002a).

MODE OF DELIVERY

Both the timespan and mode used when cytotoxic drugs are given affects the degree to which specific drugs act on cycling cells. Drugs given to treat a specific histological type of tumour need to act in the body for sufficient time to enable disruption of that tumour cell cycle to occur. Non-phase-specific drugs can be effective throughout tumour and normal cell cycles. Phase-specific drugs are generally only effective during that specific phase of the cell cycle. Each cytotoxic drug has its own half-life. This affects the levels of toxicity occurring during and after its delivery to patients, and how long these continue. These factors influence:

- the modes of delivery for which the drug is pharmacologically suitable
- the degree to which that drug is likely to be acting for enough time to cover the period of a tumour cell cycle
- the differences in levels of cell disruption likely to occur when the drug is given via different modalities (e.g. by continuous infusion or intermittent bolus injection)
- pharmacological effects which will occur when an agent is given singly or in combination with others
- whether the effects of particular regimes on patients' cancer and quality of life are of a level to warrant them being offered as treatment.

CHOICE OF CHEMOTHERAPY REGIME

Our knowledge of how cancers function, and the benefits and side effects of the various chemotherapy regimes, particularly for colorectal cancer, is increasing (NICE 2003, 2004). Media coverage of cancer treatment is greater, as is internet access to information about cancer treatments and trials. Increasingly, patients expect to discuss aspects of treatment in more depth. This may include the degree to which particular regimes could increase life expectancy, decrease disease progression and symptoms from residual tumour, and affect the quality of their lives. Such discussions should primarily be with the cancer specialist who (with other members of the multidisciplinary team) is assessing whether chemotherapy is advisable for the particular patient and, if so, which standard or trial regime(s) could be given. Information regarding potential disruption of fertility, the possibility of banking sperm or ova, and the need for contraception should be included as appropriate (Quinn 2003). Patients and their families are also likely to ask nurses to support them as they clarify their understanding of their situation, any treatment being offered, and the implications for their current and future wellbeing. Such factors need to be adequately understood if patients are to give informed consent to treatment (Foster 2002).

The timespan between when patients undergo surgery and when they discuss whether chemotherapy options are advisable is short nowadays. As more conventional and trial regimes are developed the choice of drugs, modes of delivery, and side effects which patients could experience from them are liable to differ. Systematic updating is essential so current information is easily usable with patients undergoing a variety of regimes. Background knowledge of common side effects, including those most likely to affect stomal action, must be gained. When a specific regime is prescribed we can then ascertain which of those side effects are most likely to occur and plan and provide care that is tailored to each patient's particular situation.

Cytotoxic drugs, their potential side effects, and measures that can be taken to recognise and alleviate them are described by several authors (e.g. Bridgewater & Gore 2001, Dougherty & Bailey 2001). Side effects more relevant to the care of patients with stomas are outlined here, rather than a comprehensive description of all side effects from cytotoxic drugs.

GENERAL SIDE EFFECTS

Bone marrow suppression

The shorter a cell's cycle is the more frequently cytotoxic agents (particularly phase-specific ones) have the opportunity to disrupt its system of creating replacement cells. The results of this can be seen in the bone marrow, where stem cells divide rapidly to replicate blood cells and ensure their levels are maintained in the blood:

- white blood cells divide every 6-8 hours
- platelets divide every 7-10 days
- red blood cells divide approximately every 120 days.

These cycle timings mean that, when chemotherapy is given, reduction of white blood cells (neutropenia) occurs sooner than reduction of platelet levels (thrombocytopenia). Neutropenia is also generally more severe. Anaemia, arising from reduction in red blood cell levels, occurs later (Dougherty & Bailey 2001).

Peripheral blood counts are usually at their lowest 7–10 days after chemotherapy has been given. These can result in increased susceptibility to infection and patients may find their stoma bleeds more readily when being cleaned. In more severe anaemia the stoma itself may look more pallid. Patients should be encouraged to note and report such symptoms, and any signs of infection or skin damage, to their doctor in case further investigations such as a blood count or sending swabs for culture and sensitivity might be required. Gentle handling of the stoma and removal of stomal equipment should be encouraged.

Alopecia

Patients should be informed, before treatment commences, if the drugs to be used may cause hair loss. Dougherty & Bailey (2001) state that 60–90% of hair follicles are actively dividing at any one time, and that cytotoxic drugs can damage their epithelial cells. Stem cells at the base of the shaft may atrophy; hairs become thinner, more fragile, and can break off or fall away. Patients may experience considerable physical discomfort and psychological distress from losing some or all of their hair. Patients who are still coming to terms with changes in their body image due to surgery can find it extra difficult to cope with the additional changes in self-image resulting from their hair loss (Dryden 2003).

If cytotoxic regimes are likely to cause hair loss, patients should be measured for a wig before treatment starts. This enables them to match their hair colour and style more easily than later, when hair may be sparse. Knowing that their wig will be available whenever they need it can be comforting. Discussion about hair care and alternative head coverings such as hats and scarves encourages patients to believe they can still make themselves look and feel attractive. Drum (1996) suggests that use of a soft brush and wide-toothed comb, a mild shampoo, conditioner for fine or limp hair, and patting hair dry, or using the lowest hairdryer setting can be helpful. Patients can be reassured that their hair will grow again at the end of their treatment, and may even have started to grow before treatment is completed. The process of scalp hypothermia, or scalp cooling, can be used to reduce hair loss for some patients but its effectiveness is significantly reduced if they have abnormal liver function (Dougherty 1996).

Cystitis

Some cytotoxic agents are excreted through the urinary system and a chemical cystitis may develop, caused by the proximity of the drugs to the bladder mucosa. Drugs that may produce cystitis should be given early in the day, when the patient is awake and can be encouraged to maintain a high fluid intake, and empty their bladder frequently. Patients should be encouraged to report burning, pain, or frequency of micturition and any signs of blood in the urine. Colouration of urine after administration of some drugs can occur (e.g. red-orange after doxorubicin).

Cystitis can be very painful. It is important that patients are given information which is sufficiently specific to help them maintain adequate hydration. Generally, increased fluids should be taken during treatment and for 48–72 hours after its completion. Establishing each patient's normal intake and then relating advice to it, such as suggesting they double it during the relevant period, helps patients know what they should aim to achieve. Antiemetics and intravenous fluids may be needed by some patients if they are nauseated and unable to maintain an adequate oral fluid intake.

Peripheral neuritis

As a result of some cytotoxic drugs, patients may report a tingling in the fingers or less ability to manage fine hand movements, for example when carrying out stoma care. This must be reported promptly to the medical staff as the condition can be progressive if it is not treated at an early stage. Management of stoma care may have to be simplified. Occupational therapists can also provide helpful advice and aids to make a range of activities easier.

Palmar plantar erythrodysaesthesia (hand foot syndrome)

Prolonged treatment with fluorouracil (5FU) can produce painful blistering of the hands and feet. This often improves with pyridoxine (Young & Rea 2001). Patients should be encouraged to report symptoms promptly so that they can be alleviated and any interference with their ability to manage their stoma care minimised.

SIDE EFFECTS WHICH MAY AFFECT STOMAL ACTION

Altered stomal action may indicate that problems could occur, or are beginning to do so. In this next section side effects of chemotherapy which affect stomal action are first outlined separately in order to clarify why they occur and how they can be individually treated. However, they also have a combined effect on patients' ability to eat, drink, and maintain adequate nourishment. Ways of managing these combined effects are discussed in the nursing care section.

Stomatitis

Several cytotoxic drugs can cause inflammation of the oral and oesophageal mucous membranes. The squamous epithelial mucosal lining of the mouth regenerates every 10–14 days (Dougherty & Bailey 2001). The first symptoms of stomatitis (e.g. pale dry mucous membranes) can arise 3 days following chemotherapy, while diffuse ulceration may occur up to 7 days after treatment. Difficulties can be compounded by low blood counts increasing the risk of infection and bleeding.

Patients should be warned if stomatitis could occur with their particular regime. If possible, dental and oral problems should be dealt with before chemotherapy begins. Adequate oral hygiene routines should be established. A soft toothbrush and use of antibacterial mouthwashes and emollients to keep lips moist are helpful. Antifungal and antibacterial suspensions can be useful if problems do arise (Dougherty & Bailey 2001, Young & Rea 2001). Patients receiving 5FU may find sucking ice chips 5 minutes before chemotherapy is given, and continuing this for 30 minutes afterwards, aids prevention of stomatitis (Dougherty & Bailey 2001).

Anorexia, nausea and vomiting

These side effects occur with many antitumour drugs. They may be the result of drugs acting as an irritant on the stomach or duodenum, or the drugs may stimulate the vomiting centre of the brain. The presence and severity of these side effects depends on the drug(s) used, dosage, frequency and method of administration, extent of the disease, and personal factors such as the patient's tendency to experience travel sickness. Symptoms may be classified according to their time of occurrence:

- anticipatory: before treatment begins
- acute: within 2–24 hours of treatment
- delayed: lasting 3–5 days following treatment.

Patients may be unable to tolerate their normal diet for quite an extended period, experiencing difficulty in maintaining adequate nutrition and hydration as well as having to cope with the distress and fatigue that occur with these side effects (Krishnasamy 2001a). Antiemetics should be given before cytotoxic regimes which usually cause nausea or vomiting as well as during treatment if symptoms occur. Some antiemetics can increase gut motility (e.g. metoclopramide) and may be less suitable for patients following bowel resection (Taylor 1997). The choice of antiemetic will depend on:

- the purpose for which it is being given
- where and how it will act in the body

- the time when symptoms are likely to be, or are occurring and thus need relieving
- the route of administration best suited to the patient and their situation (Taylor 1997).

5-Hydroxytryptamine (5-HT3) antagonists such as odansetron have been found helpful in preventing and controlling acute nausea and vomiting but appear to be less successful with delayed nausea and vomiting (Dougherty & Bailey 2001).

Patients who experience anticipatory nausea may benefit from taking a mild tranquilliser before coming for treatment, but should then be accompanied on their journey to and from the hospital. Some antiemetics, such as lorazepam, not only have a sedative effect but can also cause temporary short-acting amnesia, particularly if given intravenously. This is beneficial in that it can help patients blur their recall of symptoms they experienced during their treatment. However, this combination of sedation and forgetfulness has been known to cause distress to patients if they then forget to perform normal functions such as emptying their bladder. Patients may need reminding to attend to their stoma care, and both they and their families should be alerted to this possible need.

Non-invasive techniques can also help alleviate these side effects. Research into acupressure, acupuncture, progressive relaxation and hypnosis is indicating these approaches are beneficial for some patients (Dougherty & Bailey 2001, Eckert 2001). Acupressure armbands to reduce nausea are available from many chemists.

Altered bowel output

Changed dietary intake is likely to result in altered bowel output and this may also occur if the patient's regime contains cytotoxic drugs that directly affect bowel function. It is advisable to establish what patients mean when they report diarrhoea or constipation, and encourage prompt reporting of symptoms to the medical staff.

Diarrhoea

Epithelial cells lining the bowel are replaced frequently. If their cell cycle is affected by cytotoxic drugs (e.g. 5FU) this may cause the bowel to become inflamed and oedematous (Dougherty & Bailey 2001). Villi and microvilli become flattened and the overall size of the absorptive surface of the bowel becomes smaller. This can result in food passing more rapidly through the gut, reducing absorption of nutrients and increasing the frequency and fluidity of bowel actions. Such changes can result in patients having to change their stomal equipment to accommodate the altered bowel effluent as well as revise their diet.

Constipation

This may occur if cytotoxic agents interfere with the function of the autonomic nervous system supplying portions of the gut, resulting in less peristalsis and, in severe cases, faecal impaction leading to paralytic ileus. The constipation normally arises in the upper part of the colon and may not be felt on digital examination of a sigmoid colostomy.

Patients who are constipated are usually advised to increase their fluid intake and the amount of roughage in their diet. This may not be realistic if the patient is also nauseated. It may be more helpful to use stool softeners or mild laxatives prophylactically, and an oil retention enema to aid clearance of hard faeces if necessary (see Ch. 21).

NURSING CARE

As a prelude to caring for patients undergoing chemotherapy we should establish what each individual's situation is likely to be. The following questions are useful for structuring information gathering:

(a) What alterations in the normal gastrointestinal or urinary pathway have already occurred due to this patient's disease, surgery, and any previous radiotherapy?
(b) What chemotherapy regime will this patient now have?
(c) What side effects are known to be likely when the drug(s) are given in the format, dosage and frequency being prescribed?
(d) How can these (and any other) side effects best be recognised, monitored and minimised?
(e) Are there additional implications regarding this particular treatment, its effects, and its management because of the surgery this patient has had and/or because the patient has this type of stoma?

The increased understanding gained from answers to these questions helps us tailor information to each patient's needs. It will also increase our ability to recognise the implications of information patients give us, and the actions we should take in response.

Generally, when people undergoing chemotherapy are asked if they have problems, they compare how they are at that time with how they normally function. If the period of time between surgery and chemotherapy is short, stoma patients may not have developed a clear sense of how their new elimination system works, or what their peristomal skin is normally like. They may still be psychologically working through what is happening to them. Their emotions and sense of wellbeing may fluctuate considerably. They may not have a sense of what is 'normal' to use for comparisons. It is therefore particularly important to assess patients before they start treatment so that baseline information is obtained and problems are addressed. Use of chemotherapy symptom assessment scales (e.g. C-SAS) by patients after each treatment enables their experience, problems, and the effects of measures to resolve them to be better understood (Brown et al 2001, Dikken 2003). Indication of how bothersome patients find their symptoms is important. Staff may underestimate this, or attribute different levels of importance to symptoms compared with patients (Tanghe et al 1998).

Strategies to help patients deal with problems should combine four approaches. These are:

- management of food and fluids so they are provided in a form and at times when patients can best enjoy or tolerate them
- reduction of symptoms through medication that is of a type and frequency appropriate for the individual's needs
- management of patients' external experience and environment; for example, provision of a comfortable place in which to receive treatment, an absence of food or unpleasant smells, provision of suitable stomal equipment and help with stoma care when required
- promotion of patients' internal wellbeing; for example, helping them use relaxation, distraction or guided imagery before and during treatment (Krishnasamy 2001a, Drum 1996), or engaging in measures that help them feel they have some control over their situation (Wells 2001).

Managing dietary intake

Patients can feel bewildered and overwhelmed by the various changes in their ability to eat and drink normally. Many patients benefit from being given an outline of the cell cycle and how chemotherapy interrupts that cycle in order to destroy tumour cells. Having then explained that chemotherapy is timed to allow normal cells to recover to a greater extent than tumour cells, it is possible to identify symptoms that patients may experience because the cells making up particular tissues have frequent reproductive cycles. Such explanations help patients realise their symptoms may be undesirable but there are reasons why they occur, and they can trust assurances the symptoms will resolve after chemotherapy has ended.

For example, patients may experience changes in their perception of taste. This is thought to arise from the effects of chemotherapy on the tongue's taste buds, which are replaced every 3–5 days (Dougherty & Bailey 2001). Patients with a general decrease in taste sensation can be encouraged to try adding different herbs and flavourings to food to make it less bland. If meat tastes bitter, alternatives such as cheese, eggs, fish or pulses may be more acceptable (Stubbs 1989). Tea, coffee and alcohol may also taste different (Ream et al 1997).

Patients and their families can be distressed to find carefully prepared or favourite meals are now distasteful. Generally, it is helpful to first establish with patients which symptoms they are experiencing, and make a list of the qualities their food probably should have as a result of their combination of symptoms. Patients who have the symptoms outlined earlier may require food and drink that:

- is given in conjunction with antiemetic medication
- does not trigger nausea and vomiting
- is of a consistency that can be swallowed even if they have a sore mouth
- is palatable to their altered sense of taste
- is tempting when they may not feel like eating
- is sufficiently nutritious and digestible to enable adequate absorption as food passes through the bowel (which may have less absorptive capacity than usual, and be passing food through it more rapidly)
- enables adequate hydration to be maintained
- helps maintain normal urinary and faecal output.

These criteria can generally be fulfilled when patients have a diet that is:

- high calorie
- high protein
- soft
- bland or non-irritant
- easily digestible
- low residue

- low in milk or milk products (which can cause diarrhoea)
- adequate in fluid intake.

This includes chicken, fish, pasta, boiled or steamed vegetables (Dougherty & Bailey 2001). Items that lengthen the time taken for foods to pass through the bowel can be useful if diarrhoea occurs (e.g. bananas, eggs). Effervescent drinks such as soda water (Topping 1991) or ginger beer (Taylor 1997) can reduce nausea and aid fluid intake. Having small sized meals and sipping drinks over time can make it easier for patients to take in adequate daily nutriments.

It is important that patients understand the need for this kind of diet while undergoing chemotherapy. It is different to that generally recommended to stoma patients, particularly relating to fibre intake and its use to manage bowel effluent consistency (see Ch. 16). Helping patients link foods they enjoy to the two lists of criteria above will enable them to understand how they can minimise symptoms and promote adequate nutrition. Further discussion after chemotherapy is completed can help patients revert to a more extensive higher fibre diet.

Use of medication

Medication may also be needed to slow down gut motility, thus aiding absorption of nutrients and fluids and reduction of diarrhoea. It is important that the medication prescribed is suitable for resolving the problem and can actually be taken and retained by the patient. Symptoms such as nausea and stomatitis may reduce their ability to use bulky tablets or granules.

Managing altered stomal output

Patients may require additional care because they have a stoma. They should be reminded to report any changes in the appearance of their stoma as some cytotoxic drugs can cause mucosal ulceration of the stoma (Topping 1991). Blackley (2004) suggests that bathing the stoma with a cool saline solution, and application of gelatin/pectin compound powder when the bag is changed will help control bleeding and heal ulceration.

Some patients find their stoma becomes swollen and tender for several days following chemotherapy (Black 2000). They should be taught how to assess whether the gasket size of their equipment requires alteration, and given larger sized equipment for use at these times if appropriate. If these symptoms do occur patients who irrigate should be advised to wear a bag instead, and taught how to manage it, as the irrigation procedure could cause additional trauma to bowel in this condition. They may also need to discontinue irrigation if their chemotherapy causes diarrhoea. Some patients have reported their continent colostomy plugs were less effective during chemotherapy and that change to a bag was necessary.

Patients who normally use a closed colostomy bag may prefer to use a drainable appliance during treatment with the larger capacity, greater adhesion, and ease of management of more fluid faeces that these bags generally provide. Extra skin protection may also be required if the bag adhesive does not incorporate a peristomal wafer.

Patients whose chemotherapy is given by intravenous infusion will require help emptying or changing their bags while the infusion is in progress as well as before and after treatment if they are nauseated or drowsy from sedatives. If they have had medication which could have amnesic effects they may also need tactful reminders to check whether their equipment needs attention. Changes in appliance needs while chemotherapy is being given must be discussed with each patient, and agreement reached over how those needs are best met, rather than staff insisting that patients change from a familiar appliance to an unfamiliar one when they may already be stressed.

Psychological care

Patients with cancer require psychological support in addition to physical treatment (Deeny & McGuigan 1999, Wells 2001). Relatives also need opportunities to express their concerns and receive support (Plant 2001). Informational and psychological strategies described in other chapters (7–9, 22) can help patients receiving chemotherapy. Some patients find it increasingly difficult to come for each treatment, particularly if they are having unpleasant side effects or have developed a needle phobia. Counselling skills can be used to help patients describe their experiences, fears, feelings and needs. Empathic understanding of these by staff can help patients feel more able to cope with their situation (Lanceley 2001). Patients may feel chemotherapy takes over their lives if they have barely recovered from side effects from one course before the next is due. Discussions between the patient, family and staff

can lead to a reduction in problems and the patient and their family feeling more in control of their situation (Rushworth 1994, Wells 2001). Some patients find keeping diaries of their experiences is beneficial. It gives them an outlet for expressing thoughts and feelings, and a record they can use, if they wish, to discuss their situation with staff.

Stoma patients will already have had to contend with changes in how they look, eliminate urine or faeces and, for some, how they can function sexually after their surgery. Both chemotherapy and radiotherapy can bring further changes in appearance, elimination, and sexual function (Dryden 2003, Quinn 2003, White & Faithfull 2003). Where stoma surgery was palliative, or when chemotherapy is being given as an adjuvant to surgery, there may have been little time for patients to come to terms with their surgically changed body image before chemotherapy commences, bringing further changes. This can result in patients taking longer and needing more specific help to come to terms with their stoma and the effects of chemotherapy. Where chemotherapy is being provided as treatment for recurrent disease some patients may experience even greater psychological disturbance than at the time of the original diagnosis of cancer (Wells 2001). Ways of helping people experiencing loss and change are discussed in Chapters 20 and 22.

RADIOTHERAPY

Patients who have a stoma while undergoing radiotherapy include those:

- whose previous treatment of non-cancerous conditions included stoma formation, and who now require radiotherapy for cancer
- whose pelvis made adequate resection of bowel or bladder tumour difficult, and who now require radiotherapy to localised tumour to aid symptom control (Young & Rea 2001).

Radiotherapy is a process of using ionising, or high-energy, radiation to penetrate body tissues and cause damage to cells by affecting their biochemical and molecular structure. Faithfull & Wells (2003) provide a detailed account of the principles of radiotherapy, the different sources of radiation, and the nursing care of patients receiving treatment via these various sources. Most stoma patients receive external beam or teletherapy, the type of radiotherapy discussed here. Parts of the body which lie within the pathway of the beam of radiation can be affected by it.

Principles guiding treatment:

1. The treatment field(s) selected and the total amount of radiation given should enable maximum tumour damage to occur with minimal damage to normal tissues.
2. The nature of the cell damage or reaction which could be caused by the radiation must be considered. Radiotherapy can cause two types of tissue reaction. These are described as early and usually acute reactions, or later, chronic reactions.

   Early reactions occur in cells that have rapid mitotic rates because radiation creates most damage when cells are undergoing mitosis. This means that if a tumour lies in close proximity to the bowel (for example) the potential damage to gastrointestinal epithelium with its frequent mitosis has to be considered as well as the potential effect radiation could have on the cancer cells. Although radiotherapy is most effective in destroying or damaging the reproductive abilities of cells with a frequent mitotic rate, these cells also tend to be able to repair or reproduce themselves fairly easily. Since normal cells recover more readily than cancer cells it is generally possible for the body to recover from early acute reactions as long as the level of radiation to normal tissue is kept sufficiently low, and the frequency with which each dose is given enables some tissue repair to take place between treatments.

   Late reactions occur in cells that have a low capacity to reproduce or repair themselves (e.g. the brain, spinal cord, lung and kidney). Such cells have a low rate of reproduction. The effects of radiation on them does not show up until they seek to divide and the damage to the DNA becomes apparent, which may be months or years after treatment. Since this damage may be permanent it is the potential for this kind of damage (created by the presence of tissues that have a low reproduction/proliferation rate in the treatment field) which is critical in deciding the radiation dose that can be safely given to a patient (Tobias & Souhami 2003).
3. A suitable source of radiation must be used. High energy radiation produced by a linear accelerator enables penetration of the beam accurately to the depth required to achieve maximum tumour damage and minimal damage to normal surrounding tissues.

4. The total dosage of radiation required must be identified, based on the histological type of the tumour and thus its potential reactions, whether the cancer is a primary or metastatic tumour, whether the goal is curative or palliative treatment, and the probable capacity of the normal tissues within the treatment field to repair or reproduce themselves.
5. This total dose is divided into fractions or smaller doses which will be given at each treatment. This allows recovery of tumour cells as well as normal cells between treatments, so a larger dose of radiation must be given. Since the recovery rate of normal tissue is quicker than that of malignant tissue this strategy enables normal tissue damage to be minimised.

PREPARATION FOR TREATMENT

Investigations that will be carried out before radiotherapy is given include scans, X-rays and blood tests. They are used to establish a full picture of the patient's disease: its location, extent, and any metastases. This is important as spread of the disease may mean altering the field of radiotherapy or considering alternative treatment. Adequate explanations of what these preparations entail (particularly the use of the simulator, described below), time for patients to ask questions and express concerns, and appropriate support for each patient and their family should be given before and during this period of preparation for treatment (Wells 2003).

Sometimes patients' willingness to consider longer-term side effects is limited, perhaps because their prime focus is on getting their cancer treated or managing their situation daily. In such circumstances they should be informed that side effects could occur, then asked when they might like to discuss these. For example, White & Faithfull (2003) describe various effects on sexual function which arise from pelvic irradiation. However, discussion before radiotherapy sometimes focuses narrowly on whether patients' fertility could be affected by their treatment fields. This enables banking of sperm or ova before radiotherapy begins (Quinn 2003). But unless we state that wider information is available, patients may not realise they can obtain it, then or later, or know who has sufficient knowledge of the effects of all their treatments to provide it.

Identification of the exact area to be treated will be carried out using a simulator. This establishes the length, width and depth of the tumour. It relates the tumour to reference marks on the patient's body and can reproduce the field sizes of the therapy unit. CT scans may also be used to identify what the effects of different treatment programmes on tumour and normal tissues would be, and thus aid choice of the most suitable treatment plan. This treatment plan shows the tumour and also vital areas which must receive as low a dose of radiation as possible, plus the number of fields to be used, their size and angulation. The treatment plan is then transferred to the patient's body by use of tattoo marks or skin marks with indelible ink, and a check film is taken of all the treatment fields with the patient lying in the treatment position. In this way precisely the right dose to the correct area can be achieved at each treatment.

Side effects from radiotherapy vary depending on the area treated, the dose given, the frequency of treatment, and the degree of involvement of normal tissues. Conformal modes of radiotherapy are reducing the amount of normal tissues lying within treatment fields and thus the side effects that arise. Side effects that stoma patients are more likely to experience are discussed here.

GENERAL SIDE EFFECTS

Bone marrow depression

This can be caused by radiation if large areas of bone, such as the spine or iliac crest, lie within the treatment area. Regular blood counts are necessary so that early warning of possible anaemia, leucopenia or thrombocytopenia is obtained. Patients may experience symptoms of a low-grade anaemia for some months after they have completed treatment.

General fatigue and malaise

Many patients experience weariness and less ability to concentrate on or carry out normal activities during the treatment period and for some time afterwards (Faithfull 2003a, Heggie et al 1997). These side effects may be due to physiological processes, such as the breakdown of the cancer or the effects of bone marrow irradiation. They may also be the result of the patient's psychological and social situation. Most patients continue to live at home and travel to their treatment centre daily for up to 5 days each week. This can be very tiring. Patients should be encouraged to review their situation,

involving family and friends as appropriate, so that realistic expectations of what the patient could do and/or is likely to need help with are developed. Plans for practical and emotional support can then be made and acted upon.

Fatigue and other side effects can leave patients with diminished interest in sex during and after radiotherapy (Faithfull 2001). Some patients (incorrectly) fear sexual contact can irradiate their partners. Being cuddled, held or massaged can raise patients' self-esteem and help couples feel closer. However, they may need to clarify the differences between activities which feel beneficial and those which feel 'too much'. Mentioning sexual as well as other activities when discussing how patients can pace their use of limited energy invites them to discuss them further if they wish (see also Ch. 5; Krishnasamy 2001b, White & Faithfull 2003).

Patients receiving radiotherapy may also be seeking to come to terms with newly gained knowledge that they have cancer, or recurrent cancer. The feelings and concerns thus raised may leave them feeling drained of energy, perhaps due to anxiety and less ability to relax or sleep well. Opportunities for patients and their families to voice fears, feelings and needs should be an integral part of the care that is offered by staff, so that relevant information, care and support can be provided and its usefulness evaluated (Deeny & McGuigan 1999).

SIDE EFFECTS AFFECTING THE STOMA OR STOMAL ACTION

Gastrointestinal symptoms from abdominal and pelvic irradiation often occur in clusters rather than singly. Their cumulative effects can impair patients' quality of life considerably. Faithfull (2003b) provides a more comprehensive overview of gastrointestinal effects of radiotherapy and their treatment than is possible here.

Nausea, vomiting and anorexia

Although these side effects do not occur with all patients receiving radiotherapy, when they do occur the resultant distress is sometimes underestimated by staff.

Nausea may be the result of raised uric acid levels caused by rapid tumour breakdown or other biochemical imbalances in the blood. The position of the tumour itself or unavoidable involvement of the gastrointestinal tract in the treatment areas of the mediastinum, abdomen and pelvis can all cause patients to feel nauseated and may also produce abdominal discomfort.

Gastrointestinal alterations

If the stoma lies within the treatment area it will be protected by a lead shield during treatment. However, Topping (1991, p 304) reports that stomal ulceration can occur. She describes a sequence of events where, initially, the stoma appears oedematous; then superficial ulceration occurs, and the stoma may later secrete exudate which coagulates as a whitish membrane. Observation of the stoma and use of an appliance with a larger gasket size when appropriate is advocated, and radiotherapy may have to be temporarily postponed in severe cases to enable these effects to subside. Bathing the stoma with a cool saline solution when the bag is changed and applying gelatin/pectin powder to it can aid healing (Blackley 2004, p 221).

Patients with a mucous fistula may find this produces more mucus. Extra skin protection may be needed around the fistula, and if the discharge is sizeable or malodorous patients may prefer to wear a small stomal appliance to contain both the mucus and odour.

Since gastrointestinal mucosa has a high rate of mitosis damage can occur to any bowel lying within the treatment field. Heggie et al (1997) report that increased flatus can occur. Faithfull (2001, p 243–245) suggests diarrhoea could arise from several causes:

- Damage to stem cells in the small intestine, resulting in shortened villi and reduced tissue surface for absorption.
- Reduction of bile salts absorption (normally thought to take place in the small intestine). Unabsorbed bile salts inhibit water resorption and stimulate peristalsis distally in the colon, increasing the likelihood of diarrhoea.
- Reduction of carbohydrate absorption, which can raise osmolarity and thus increase peristalsis. Bacterial fomentation of carbohydrates in the colon produces gas and results in diarrhoea and discomfort.
- Release of prostaglandins in response to radiation cell damage. These are known to stimulate smooth muscle, causing diarrhoea in animal studies.

Management of bowel problems and skin care are discussed in the nursing section.

NURSING CARE

Nurses must work closely with radiotherapy and medical colleagues to ensure patients are well prepared for undergoing radiotherapy. They need adequate time in which to gain information and discuss concerns about their radiotherapy *before* it actually takes place. Strategies used to prepare patients for surgery (see Ch. 7) can also be used to identify with patients the information and physical and psychological care which they will need before, during and after their radiotherapy.

It is important to start by asking patients what 'having radiotherapy' means to them, because there are many misconceptions about this form of treatment. Such beliefs include that it is given because surgery was unsuccessful, that it causes burns, scars and pain, and that it makes patients radioactive (Faithfull 2001). When people's concepts of radiotherapy are identified before information is given we can then make sure that the information they are given is accurate and specific enough to help patients gain a concept of radiotherapy that is factually correct.

Patients can find the equipment and processes used to deliver radiotherapy quite alarming unless they are well prepared. They should be told that staff will leave the room while their treatment is given. It is important to stress that, while their individual radiation doses are beneficial for them, staff leave the room to avoid getting a succession of small doses of radiation each time a patient is treated, as these amounts could add up over time to inappropriate levels. Patients should also be told that staff will be monitoring them as they receive their treatment and, as they can see and hear patients from outside the room, patients can communicate with them and receive help promptly. Even with such preparation patients do report that the experience of staff vanishing from the room leaving them to be given treatment they cannot see, hear or feel can be daunting.

Patients' overall situation needs to be regularly assessed throughout the treatment period, and they should also be encouraged to report problems or concerns at an early stage. Staff who are aware of potential side effects can discreetly enquire about problems without alarming patients, and correct misunderstandings about why they are occurring. Heggie et al (1997) reported that 48% of their stoma patients receiving radiotherapy experienced tiredness. This was deemed normal by radiation therapists.

However, patients may experience such tiredness as similar to the fatigue and general malaise they had when their cancer was originally diagnosed, and can assume that this means their disease is spreading. Reassurance that this is not the case is more likely to be believed if it is linked to a simple explanation of why these side effects may occur. Patients and their families usually benefit from discussing how they can pace activities (see *example* of Nurse Beech's work with Mr and Mrs Earl in Ch. 8 (Patient scenario 8.5); use of 'just do's' and contracts in Ch. 9).

Ireland & Wells (2003) provide a useful account of the effects of radiotherapy on nutritional status. Alterations in food intake and bowel activity often go together, coinciding with growing fatigue.

Patients in these circumstances often require help to achieve:

- elimination or reduction of nausea
- an intake of foods and fluids which they can enjoy (or at least tolerate) and which will aid tissue repair, fulfil nutritional needs generally, and minimise production of flatus
- a regime of analgesics (if required) of a type and frequency to control their pain effectively
- a regime of medication which reduces or resolves problems in bowel action
- use of easily managed stomal equipment suitable for their current bowel activity and skin protection needs
- a pattern of daily activities which enables them to gain sufficient rest and continue with at least some of their chosen activities
- adequate help for the patient from family, friends and/or healthcare agencies.

Once such goals have been identified then strategies to achieve them can be chosen. Patients who are having radiotherapy to relieve pain should be told that this is unlikely to be achieved immediately treatment commences. Their situation should be regularly monitored so analgesics can be revised as radiotherapy takes effect.

Prophylactic use of antiemetics appears to be low, unlike their systematic use with chemotherapy. 5-HT3 antagonists are usually prescribed when symptoms occur, with effective results when given in adequate dosage and frequency (Faithfull 2003b). Patients who keep a record of symptoms and when they occur can help pinpoint times when they feel most and least nauseous, and adjust their antiemetics and meals accordingly.

The basis for managing radiation-induced diarrhoea varies between advisers. Traditionally, patients receiving pelvic irradiation have been recommended to reduce the amount of faecal output through low fibre diets (Faithfull 2001). Faithfull suggests there is little evidence that this approach was effective, but growing evidence that elemental and low fat diets do reduce diarrhoea. Ireland & Wells (2003) suggest that, because bile acid absorption is impaired with pelvic irradiation, low fat diets tend to be better tolerated by gut mucosa. They list foods to be recommended and avoided. However, patients may associate '40 g fat diets' with weight loss programmes and be concerned that reduction in diarrhoea could be accompanied by unwanted weight loss.

Medication may also combine benefits with problems. Taking bile acid sequestrants to bind bile salts in the intestine reduces diarrhoea but patients may find they are unpalatable and nauseous. Medications that reduce gut motility (e.g. loperamide, codeine phosphate) may result in constipation, dizziness, and only short-term relief. There is some evidence that sucralfate reduces diarrhoea and late bowel disturbances in patients receiving radiotherapy for prostate and bladder cancer (Faithfull 2003b). Patients who have had small bowel resection before requiring radiotherapy, or who have other bowel conditions as well as cancer, may require specialist advice.

Patients whose bowel stomal actions increase or become more fluid may need to use drainable bags. Their larger capacity and ability to be emptied enables faeces and flatus to be disposed of without numerous bag changes. When appliances lie within the radiotherapy area their use needs to be compatible with:

- containment of stomal effluent
- radiotherapy delivery to target areas
- avoidance or management of radiation-induced skin problems.

Management of alterations to radiotherapy delivery and skin integrity

Radiotherapy departments generally give skin care guidance to all patients. Wells & MacBride (2003) provide more detailed descriptions of preventative measures for maintaining skin integrity, and management of radiation skin reactions. Patients whose stomal equipment lies outside the radiotherapy area should follow the same guidance as patients without stomas. Factors that require consideration when equipment lies within the radiotherapy area are outlined here.

Normally, as superficial cells from the epidermis are shed they are replaced by new cells created by mitosis in the basal layer of the skin. Radiotherapy affects basal cell mitosis within the treatment area, thereby reducing replacement of epidermis. Skin and hair can be affected at entry and exit sites of radiation beams. As epidermal renewal time is 2–3 weeks reactions generally start to appear when patients have had this length of radiotherapy and continue until about 3 weeks after treatment completion.

In order to minimise skin damage modern radiotherapy systems enable the maximum radiation dosage to occur below the skin surface between 0.5 5 cm (Jansson 1992). This is known as *the skin sparing technique*. Skin reactions can occur to some degree, but are further minimised when moisturising or aqueous cream is applied to beam entry and exit points from commencement of radiotherapy (Campbell & Lane 1996).

Where stomal equipment lies within the radiotherapy area there are two issues to be resolved. Firstly, any metal in equipment (including skin protectives) can alter the radiation beam and thus the skin sparing process. Secondly, the thickness of the equipment can alter the skin sparing process. Instead of radiotherapy being delivered at the specified distance below the skin it will be delivered that distance below the appliance. Irradiation could begin at the skin surface rather than beneath it (Figs 18.1 and 18.2).

Blackley (2004, p 221) suggests that, although stomal equipment can remain in situ within the treatment area when photon beams are used, it will have to be removed when electron beams are used in order to ensure correct delivery of radiation dosage to target tissues is achieved, combined with skin sparing. However, daily removal of stomal equipment can cause skin damage, as can eruption of urine or faeces onto the skin during treatment when patients are expected to lie still and cannot contain this effluent. Discussion about patients' actual equipment and how their radiotherapy sessions can best be managed should take place before radiotherapy is commenced. Modern appliances and skin care aids are usually slim and non-metallic. A compromise over their presence may need to be reached, particularly if substantial amounts of effluent are being passed or patients are distressed by stomal activity during radiotherapy.

During and after the period when radiotherapy is being given it is important to recognise types of

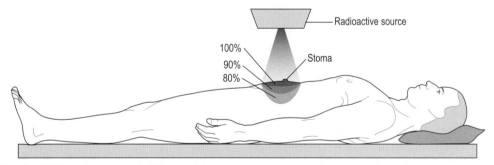

Figure 18.1 Depth below skin at which radiotherapy acts.

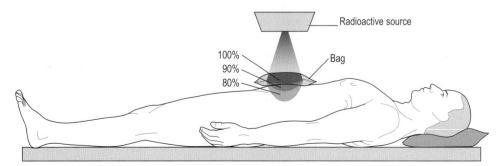

Figure 18.2 Stomal equipment containing metal applied to the skin results in radiation of tissue at less depth than planned.

skin reaction which may occur so appropriate treatment can be given promptly. Faithfull (2001) describes four *skin reactions*:

1. *Erythema*, which is a reddening of the skin. There may also be slight inflammation.
2. *Dry desquamation* where the skin becomes dry and scaly, with flaking of superficial layers of the skin. The area is slightly inflamed and may itch and burn.
3. *Moist desquamation*, which occurs as a result of blistering and sloughing of the epidermis, leaving a painful area of dermis which may exude serum. Radiotherapy generally has to be postponed for a while to enable healing to take place.
4. *Necrosis*, which occurs infrequently, caused by a combination of ischaemia and vascular occlusion resulting in cell death.

Stoma patients may need to manage skin which lies:

- directly under the appliance adhesive
- under the main body of the bag
- adjacent to the appliance adhesive or peristomal wafer.

The skin care they use in each location must both protect their skin and enable adequate adherence of their appliance. For example, moisturising cream used adjacent to the appliance should not cause it to lift by seeping beneath the adhesive area.

Several authors' work has been drawn on to establish the following *principles* of skin care during radiotherapy for stoma patients (Boot-Vickers & Eaton 1999, Campbell & Lane 1996, Faithfull 2001, Wells & MacBride 2003):

- Possible alterations to radiation delivery and skin sparing which could arise through use of stoma care products in treatment areas (generally or to promote healing of damaged skin) must be assessed prior to use, particularly if they are bulky.
- Scattering of the radiation beam should be avoided by not using soaps, creams, powders or stomal equipment which contain metal within the treatment area.
- Mild (e.g. baby) soap can be used to cleanse peristomal skin of effluent while ensuring treatment marks are not washed off.
- Abrasion of the skin should be avoided through patting the skin dry or using a hairdryer on a cool setting, rather than rubbing it dry. If shaving is necessary an electric or battery operated razor

should be used as this is less likely to damage the skin.
- Where skin is broken normal saline should be used for cleansing rather than antiseptics (which may interfere with healing).
- As radiotherapy tends to dry the skin, substances that may further dry it should generally be avoided (e.g. talcum powder). Cotton clothing aids comfort.
- Possibilities for infection occurring should be minimised (e.g. use of cotton bag covers to reduce sweating if bags lie on top of skin within the treatment area).
- Use of moisturising creams to hydrate the skin generally, and increase comfort if erythema or dry desquamation occurs, must be compatible with adherence of stomal equipment. When used, they should be washed off and not left to build up on the skin.
- Creams that are poorly soluble (e.g. petroleum jelly/Vaseline) or increase sensitivity (e.g. lanolin-based creams/E45) should not be used in treatment areas.
- Steroid creams may be prescribed to reduce itching in dry desquamation. If applied sparingly under stomal equipment adhesion can still be achieved. They can delay healing so should not be used for moist desquamation. Prolonged steroid use should be avoided as it can result in skin thinning.
- Where moist desquamation occurs the goal is to prevent infection. Gentian violet should not be used as it may be carcinogenic and systemic absorption could occur through broken skin or mucous membranes. A light dusting of gelatin-pectin powder to moist areas under appliances may help to reduce moisture while allowing appliance adherence (Blackley 2004).
- Healing can be promoted after radiotherapy completion through use of products which create a warm moist environment and can, if necessary, absorb exudates while meeting criteria for stoma care management.

Many of the problems associated with radiotherapy can be avoided or resolved if patients and their families are given adequate information and if staff regularly take time to enquire about each patient's physical and psychological wellbeing and respond appropriately. This deliberate monitoring is particularly useful for picking up problems or concerns which outpatients may have but only feel able to report when given a specific opportunity to do so.

Many patients find the change from attending hospital for radiotherapy to recovering at home after treatment ends is difficult. Later side effects may occur and some patients feel vulnerable and anxious without their informal access to staff for information and support (Faithfull 2001, Wells 2001). Before treatment is completed patients and their families should therefore be prepared for the first few weeks after radiotherapy. This includes providing information they are likely to need and addressing any concerns. They should be encouraged to identify who could give them various kinds of information and support, and how they could obtain any help they require, in similar ways to those described in Chapters 7–9. Contact with their usual stoma care nurse may be appreciated. Generally, the approaches described in this chapter help patients reduce anxiety and feel informed and supported during and after treatment.

References

Association of Coloproctology of Great Britain and Ireland 2001 Guidelines for the management of colorectal cancer. Association of Coloproctology of Great Britain and Ireland, London

Black P K 2000 Holistic stoma care. Baillière Tindall and RCN, Edinburgh

Blackley P 2004 Practical stoma wound and continence management, 2nd edn. Research Publications, Vermont, Victoria, Australia

Boot-Vickers M, Eaton K 1999 Skin care for patients receiving radiotherapy. Professional Nurse 14(10):706–708

Bridgewater J, Gore M 2001 Developments in cancer treatment. In: Corner J, Bailey C (eds) Cancer nursing: care in context. Blackwell Science, Oxford, p 313–333

Brown V, Sitzia J, Richardson A et al 2001 The development of the Chemotherapy Symptom Assessment Scale (C-SAS): a scale for the routine clinical assessment of the symptom experiences of patients receiving cytotoxic chemotherapy. International Journal of Nursing Studies 38:497–510

Campbell J, Lane C 1996 Developing a skin-care protocol in radiotherapy. Professional Nurse 12(2):105–108

Deeny K, McGuigan M 1999 The value of the nurse-patient relationship in the care of cancer patients. Nursing Standard 13(33):45–47

Dikken C 2003 Benefits of using a chemotherapy symptom assessment scale. Nursing Times 99(39):50–51

Dougherty L 1996 Scalp cooling to prevent hair loss in chemotherapy. Professional Nurse 11(8):507–509

Dougherty L, Bailey C 2001 Chemotherapy. In: Corner J, Bailey C (eds) Cancer nursing: care in context. Blackwell Science, Oxford, p 179–221

Downing J 2001 Surgery. In: Corner J, Bailey C (eds) Cancer nursing: care in context. Blackwell Science, Oxford, p 156–178

Drum D 1996 Making the chemotherapy decision. Lowell House, Los Angeles

Dryden H 2003 Body image. In: Faithfull S, Wells M (eds) Supportive care in radiotherapy. Churchill Livingstone, Edinburgh, p 320–336

Eckert R 2001 Understanding anticipatory nausea. Oncology Nursing Forum 28:1553–1558

Faithfull S 2001 Radiotherapy. In: Corner J, Bailey C (eds) Cancer nursing: care in context. Blackwell Science, Oxford, p 222–261

Faithfull S 2003a Fatigue and radiotherapy. In: Faithfull S, Wells M (eds) Supportive care in radiotherapy. Churchill Livingstone, Edinburgh, p 118–134

Faithfull S 2003b Gastrointestinal effects of radiotherapy. In: Faithfull S, Wells M (eds) Supportive care in radiotherapy. Churchill Livingstone, Edinburgh, p 247–267

Faithfull S, Wells M 2003 Supportive care in radiotherapy. Churchill Livingstone, Edinburgh

Fenwick E 2004 Urological cancers. In: Fillingham S, Douglas J Urological nursing, 3rd edn. Churchill Livingstone, Edinburgh, p 185–225

Foster R 2002 Fertility issues in patients with cancer. Cancer nursing practice 1(1):26–30

Heggie D E, Everingham L F, Stevens G 1997 The incidence of radiation side-effects for individuals with an ostomy requiring nursing considerations. World Council of Enterostomal Therapists Journal 17(2):6–12

Ireland J, Wells M 2003 The effects of radiotherapy on nutritional status. In: Faithfull S, Wells M (eds) Supportive care in radiotherapy. Churchill Livingstone, Edinburgh, p 204–226

Jansson J M 1992 Peristomal skin reactions to chemotherapy and radiation in ostomy patients. In: World Council of Enterostomal Therapists congress proceedings. Hollister, Libertyville, IL, p 198–199

Keane P F, Kelly J D, McAlear J J A 2001 Genitourinary malignancies. In: Spence R A J, Johnston P G (eds) Oncology. Oxford University Press, Oxford, p 257–282

Krishnasamy M 2001a Nausea and vomiting. In: Corner J, Bailey C (eds) Cancer nursing: care in context. Blackwell Science, Oxford, p 350–357

Krishnasamy M 2001b Fatigue. In: Corner J, Bailey C (eds) Cancer nursing: care in context. Blackwell Science, Oxford, p 358–366

Lanceley A 2001 Therapeutic strategies in cancer care. In: Corner J, and Bailey C (eds) Cancer nursing: care in context. Blackwell Science, Oxford, p 120–138

Midgley R S J, Kerr D J 2001 Adjuvant therapy. In: Kerr D J, Young A M, Hobbs F D R (eds) ABC of colorectal cancer. BMJ Books, London, p 22–25

National Institute for Clinical Excellence 2002a Guidance on the use of irinotecan, oxaliplatin and raltitrexed for the treatment of advanced colorectal cancer. Technology appraisal guidance no: 33. NICE, London

National Institute for Clinical Excellence 2002b Improving outcomes in urological cancers. NICE, London

National Institute for Clinical Excellence 2003 Guidance on the use of capecitabine and tegefur with uracil for metastatic colorectal cancer. Technology appraisal no: 61. NICE, London

National Institute for Clinical Excellence 2004 Improving outcomes in colorectal cancers. NICE, London

Northover J, Taylor C, Gold D 2002 Carcinoma of the rectum. In: Williams J (ed) The essentials of pouch care nursing. Whurr Publishers, London, p 43–67

Plant H 2001 The impact of cancer on the family. In: Corner J, Bailey C (eds) Cancer nursing: care in context. Blackwell Science, Oxford, p 86–99

Quinn B 2003 Sexual health in cancer care. Nursing Times 99(4):32–34

Ream E, Richardson A, Alexander-Dann C 1997 Patients' sensory experiences before, during, and immediately following the administration of intravenous chemotherapy. Journal of Cancer Nursing 1(1):25–31

Rushworth C 1994 Making a difference in cancer care. Souvenir Press (E & A), London

Stubbs L 1989 Taste changes in cancer patients. Nursing Times 85(18):49–50

Tanghe A, Evers G, Paridaens R 1998 Nurses' assessments of symptom occurrence and symptom distress in chemotherapy patients. European Journal of Oncology Nursing 2(1):14–26

Taylor C 1997 Nausea and vomiting. In: Bruce L, Finlay T (eds) Nursing in gastroenterology. Churchill Livingstone, New York, p 1–25

Tobias J, Souhami R L 2003 Cancer and its management, 4th edn. Blackwell Science, Oxford

Topping A 1991 Nursing patients with tumours of the gastrointestinal tract In: Tiffany R (ed) Oncology for nurses and health care professionals, Volume 3, 2nd edn. Harper Collins, London, p 261–308

Wells M 2001 The impact of cancer. In: Corner J, Bailey C (eds) Cancer nursing: care in context. Blackwell Science, Oxford, p 63–85

Wells M 2003 The treatment trajectory. In: Faithfull S, Wells M (eds) Supportive care in radiotherapy. Churchill Livingstone, Edinburgh, p 39–59

Wells M, MacBride S 2003 Radiation skin reactions. In: Faithfull S, Wells M (eds) Supportive care in radiotherapy. Churchill Livingstone, Edinburgh, p 135–159

White I, Faithfull S 2003 Sexuality and fertility. In: Faithfull S, Wells M (eds) Supportive care in radiotherapy. Churchill Livingstone, Edinburgh, p 303–319

Young A M, Rea D 2001 Treatment of advanced disease. In: Kerr D J, Young A M, Hobbs F D R (eds) ABC of colorectal cancer. BMJ Books, London, p 26–29

SECTION 4

Broader aspects of psychosocial care

Chapter **19**

The patient's background

Brigid Breckman

The essence of successful stoma care is knowing, valuing and working with each patient as an individual human being. Their physical and psychological needs, goals, capabilities and resources can then be used to help them to move from feeling and acting as a 'stoma patient' to being a person engaged in their normal lifestyle who happens to have a stoma. However, we also need relevant background information to help us generally make sense of the experiences and concerns patients and their families have before and after stoma surgery. Such information is therefore provided in this chapter and the next, while the *patient scenarios* throughout the book indicate ways in which it can be used.

People are conditioned from childhood to accept certain beliefs, ways of living and attitudes depending on their social, cultural and religious background. Therefore any care that is given must be planned and provided in ways that are congruent with the patient's cultural and religious background and needs as well as their medical and nursing needs and treatment. Likewise, evaluation of care must entail consideration of whether that care is appropriate in the context of that particular patient's social, cultural and religious background *and* the context of their medical condition, treatment and the care which would normally be required (Ross 1994).

The culture of each patient and their family will be a mixture of beliefs and behaviours prescribed generally by their religion, ethnic background and the society in which they live and work coupled with those beliefs and behaviours that are viewed as normal, right or appropriate in their particular family. Awareness of beliefs that people of different cultures and religions generally hold is useful. It helps us understand and follow the principles underlying requests that care should be provided in particular ways. However, we should not assume people with particular cultural or religious backgrounds must automatically be provided with care that complies with those approaches. This can lead to care being imposed which has little relevance to particular patients' individual lifestyles and beliefs (Neuberger 1998).

AGE AND 'TIME OF LIFE'

Age is often used to create expectations about people: what their needs, capabilities, interests and priorities are likely to be, or should be, and how these will be demonstrated as individuals and members of society as a whole. Expectations of how people should function in childhood, adolescence, adulthood and old age are reinforced by legislation, custom and practice. Assumptions about the ages at which particular life stages occur vary in different countries and communities, for example the ages at which people are deemed to pass from childhood to adulthood, or be suitable for 'work' or 'retirement'.

Where events and activities are not linked to specific ages there may be a general consensus of the age range within which they will usually occur. Examples include acquiring a (marriage) partner, and becoming a parent or grandparent. In such instances social perception of the ages people will generally be when they trigger a need for particular resources can aid planning and provision of relevant health, educational and social systems. However, it is important to consider whether automatically assuming people's requirements according to their age is appropriate for their care. Bailey (2001) reports that patients over the age of 65 with colorectal cancer have been found to be less likely to receive chemotherapy for colorectal cancer. He suggests attitudes towards older people can lead to differential treatments which are not necessarily based on the extent of individuals' diseases and their physical and mental capabilities.

In his thoughtful review of the needs of older people Bailey (2001) also pinpoints the issue of whether people have supportive networks. Family and friends can make a considerable difference to any patient's recovery from stoma surgery. However, patients' ages should not lead us to presume supportive networks will be available or absent. For example, greater longevity and improved health care in some countries may mean a patient's network includes older relatives with variable self-care and supportive abilities. As people have children at younger and older ages, and/or change partners, these factors can increase the variations in what constitutes 'their family' and the types and levels of support available.

Concepts of age and cognitive development are usually helpful when working with children. They help us tailor explanations so they match and keep pace with children's changing abilities to understand and engage in stoma care (see Ch. 13; Fitzpatrick et al 2003).

In many instances the traditional concept that people go through consecutive life stages no longer matches people's experiences of themselves and their lifestyle. Our perceptions and responses to age must therefore become flexible tools rather than sources of stereotyping. A useful starting point can be to treat each person's age as *a cue to enquire* about their goals and needs 'at this time of your life'. Coupled with this we need to regularly monitor whether we, or our colleagues, are using age as a cue to impose inappropriate age-based predictions or assumptions on patients and their families via the treatment and care they are offered or denied.

ATTITUDES TOWARDS ILLNESS AND THE PROVISION OF CARE

The concepts that a patient and his family have of his disease or condition, how treatment for it should be provided, how they should respond to illness generally and in the current situation will influence both what they do and what they expect of others (Chamberlain 1996). For example, many families with an Asian or Middle Eastern background expect to spend considerable time with the patient while he is in hospital, helping to support and care for him (Henley & Schott 1999, Ross 1994). The patient is likely to adopt a sick role that allows him to focus on what he is experiencing, express feelings, and be cared for by others. Both the patient and his family may have difficulty in understanding or accepting the strategy of teaching him how to manage his own stoma care before he leaves hospital if they view him as still occupying a to-be-cared-for patient role. In contrast, many families with an Anglo-Saxon British background will expect only relatives and close friends to visit the patient while he is in hospital, and such visitors generally provide relatively little physical care. The patient is more likely to adopt a sick role in which he and his family expect him to make the best of things, or minimise concerns and difficulties. Likewise the family may minimise or avoid discussing difficulties they are experiencing in an effort to make things easier for the patient. This can make it harder for difficulties to be recognised and resolved.

Expectations of the role which staff should play may also be influenced by cultural beliefs. For example, many patients with a British background believe medical staff will routinely tell them all they need to know. They find requesting information difficult or unacceptable because it may be viewed as unreasonable or critical of the patient's care. Class differences still have their effect on the degree to which British patients seek information or understand explanations when they are provided. It is important that this point is considered when care or treatment is being provided by one specific caregiver, for example a stoma care nurse or a family doctor, particularly if there appear to be difficulties in the giver and receiver of care understanding each other's information and points of view.

Many Asians will consult a doctor privately, or register with an Asian GP, seeking the kind of personal attention which they would thereby get in their country of origin. The NHS hospital system of once or twice weekly visits from the consultant, and frequent changes in the doctors who see them in the wards or outpatients department, can be both alien and distressing to Asian patients who expect a more personal style of care (Henley & Schott 1999). Difficulty with this style of care is certainly not confined to Asian patients, and all patients should be informed of the system through which medical care is provided.

Some patients require stoma surgery because they have cancer. Attitudes towards cancer may be derived from cultural as well as individual ideas and experiences. Patients, their relatives, and members of staff may have differing beliefs as to:

- what a diagnosis of cancer means
- whether cancer can be cured or controlled
- who should be told the diagnosis and be involved in discussions about treatment and prognosis
- which medical and complementary treatments and other approaches are viewed as likely to be curative and/or beneficial
- which side effects are likely to arise from various cancer treatments.

Learning what people of particular cultures generally believe and do in response to investigations and treatment for cancer is beneficial. It increases our awareness of different viewpoints and helps us make sense of actions that patients and their families may wish to take or avoid. It alerts us to the possibility that actions we may take with the best of intentions might be compatible with our beliefs but not those of a particular patient or relative.

For example, in the UK, as in many other countries, it is now commonly believed that patients have a right to be told their diagnosis. Likewise 'good practice' is assumed to usually include giving patients information about possible benefits and side effects of potential treatments. This might lead us to insist patients are given such information if we hold these beliefs. However, Thomas (2001, p 509) reports that Afro-Caribbeans, Chinese, Asians, Italians and Japanese may associate a cancer diagnosis with death. Jewish colleagues have told me of similar beliefs. Patients, relatives and healthcare teams from these cultures may believe that 'good practice' entails preserving patients' rights *not* to have knowledge of their diagnosis imposed on them. Patients may not be told they have cancer as it is thought they would lose all hope. These beliefs could lead us to curtail the levels of information offered to patients about their diagnosis, treatment and prognosis. Neither approach is going to be helpful for all patients.

In my experience it is useful to specifically tell patients that people like varying amounts of information about their situation, condition and treatment, and that it would be helpful for them to tell us what would be right for them. Such statements give patients permission to ask for approaches relevant to their unique mixture of cultural and personal beliefs. Questions to help them do so could include:

- How much information about your condition and treatment do you think it would be helpful for you to have?
- Is there anyone else who you would like to be involved when your situation and treatment are being discussed? Do you think they will want to be involved?
- Is there anyone who will expect to be involved when your situation is being discussed or decisions are being made about the best way forward for you?
- Given this information, is there anything you want us to do now, or avoid doing, so we are looking after you in the best way for you?

The answers to these questions often give us considerable information about patients' cultural assumptions and ways in which they want care given. Acknowledging how useful such information is, and acting on it, gives clear messages that we respect and value their beliefs. Paying attention to patients' needs and opinions in this way helps them become familiar with being asked for such information. It becomes 'normal' to help staff learn about them so that care can be tailored to their needs.

Having this kind of collaborative approach up and running is particularly useful when patients ask questions and we are unsure about what they want to know. The responses they want as individuals may not be those we assume people with their background will be seeking. They may, for example, ask us about their diagnosis.

Some people ask because they hope they will be assured they do not have cancer. Others may want to be told if they do have it. If we have sufficient knowledge and expertise we can give them opportunities to indicate what is in their mind more fully. *For example*, asking someone what 'having cancer' would mean to them, if they did have it, can encourage them to express their particular attitudes, fears and feelings. These can then be taken into account both when their original question is answered and whenever subsequent medical and nursing care is given.

ATTITUDES TOWARDS PAIN AND ITS MANAGEMENT

The length of time during which patients experience pain after stoma surgery is often longer than many people realise. Wade (1989) found 35.8% of patients were experiencing pain one year after stoma surgery. Pringle & Swan (2001) found 40.4% of patients reported pain one year after their bowel surgery. The presence of pain has substantial implications for patients' wellbeing and rehabilitation. Most people's ability to concentrate on and retain information is lessened when they are in pain. It can therefore reduce patients' ability to learn stoma care and retain information about living with a stoma which they will need when they go home. Pain can also affect patients' long-term rehabilitation. Levels of fatigue can be higher and their resumption of, and comfort with, normal activities may be reduced.

Developing a broad understanding of factors that affect the ways pain is perceived, expressed and handled helps us consider and respond to patients' needs more effectively. Relevant factors include:

- the patient's experience of pain
- the patient's perception of how they should respond to that pain and/or pain in general
- the cues/actions with which the patient indicates the presence of pain
- the nurse's level of awareness/recognition of cues which may indicate that the patient has pain
- the inferences or conclusions the nurse draws from the cues which the patient demonstrates
- the assumptions the nurse makes from her knowledge of the patient's background and situation
- the nurse's previous personal experience of pain
- the nurse's perception of how pain should be expressed and dealt with
- the strategies for pain management which the nurse and patient each perceive as available to them to use
- the acceptability of specific strategies for achieving pain control to the patient and nurse
- the perception of desirable goals of pain management which patients and nurses hold, seek to achieve, and use as criteria to judge whether the management of that pain is being appropriately achieved (e.g. eradication of pain; dulling of pain; reduction or absence of pain as long as the patient remains mentally alert).

Most if not all of these factors are influenced by the cultural background of patients and nurses, and the latter are also likely to be influenced by beliefs acquired during their professional training and experience (professional culture).

For example, patients with an Anglo-Saxon background (e.g. many British, Americans and Canadians) may maintain a 'stiff upper lip' approach towards pain, keeping expressions of pain to a minimum because such behaviour is highly valued in their culture. A nurse who comes from a cultural background where people freely express pain may assume that if a patient does not clearly indicate he is in pain, he must be experiencing little or no pain. Likewise accurate assessment of pain can be influenced by nurses' ability to 'read' the cues patients do offer. Davitz & Davitz (1981, p 78) give examples of Westerners assessing Japanese patients as generally having less pain in comparison to the assessments made by Japanese nurses of pain levels in

Japanese patients. Jewish patients, who express pain and psychological distress fairly readily, are apparently assumed to have more pain generally by non-Jewish nurses than, for example, when Israeli patients are being assessed by Israeli nurses. Presumption of the likely levels of pain and the misinterpretation of patients' cues may hinder effective pain management (Krishnasamy 2001, p 339–340).

Davitz & Davitz (1981, p 75) also studied the responses of nurses from 13 countries to the same descriptions of patients' situations, where respondents were asked to assess the levels of physical pain and psychological distress that those patients would be likely to have. British nurses inferred or assumed that a lower rate of physical pain and psychological distress would occur for the patients in these situations compared with nurses from most of the other countries. It may therefore be particularly wise for nurses with a British background to enquire specifically about each patient's experience of pain and use measures like pain charts to help in the identification and management of pain (Thomas 1997, p 71–92). Pain charts that depict faces or naked bodies may be offensive to Muslims and other patients for whom making images of people is forbidden (Henley & Schott 1999).

The importance of effective pain management should be explained to patients, coupled with encouragement to take part in the assessment and management of their pain by providing staff with information about any pain they have and the results of pain-relieving activities. Overviews of pain management covering many of the points raised here more extensively are available (Middleton 2004, Thomas 1997). The use of guided imagery in management of pain and anxiety is also being explored (Dean 1998) and, hopefully, could aid patient comfort without producing the constipatory side effects of analgesics.

ROLES AND RELATIONSHIPS

People undergoing stoma surgery step into the role of 'patient' as part of that experience. How that role is experienced and carried out will vary from person to person. It will be influenced by the expectations and behaviour of staff as well as the roles and expectations each person usually fulfils in their life as a whole. Generally, while the patient is in hospital most of his attention will be directed towards re-

sponding to the demands and experiences of this context. This includes coping with tests, treatment, and the routines of how and when care is provided. However, awareness of his usual roles, the implications and effects of his absence from them at that time, and the implications of how those roles might be affected in the future are also likely to be concerns in the back of his mind. In addition, access to people with whom the patient enjoys some kind of relationship may be dependent on his fulfilling a role; for example, friends with whom he shares hobbies or activities as their main way of relating to each other; colleagues with whom he enjoys planning and achieving goals at work or meeting during meal breaks.

Stoma surgery may have implications for the roles and relationships within the family. For example, the patient may fulfil the role of main (or only) breadwinner. The time needed for that patient to undergo surgery and rehabilitate, and thus be away from work, can have major financial implications. It can also affect how the family (including the patient) view themselves and each other, and the roles they could or should be undertaking. Lowering of self-esteem because of inability to earn wages or provide financial security is not uncommon.

People who are expected to be the decision-makers or the chief providers of support and comfort in their family may feel very guilty or distressed if they are unable to cope with their own experiences as a patient and their usual role. They may not know how to ask for, or how to accept, support from others and may assume it will not be given even if they ask for it. Sometimes this belief is accurate, if family members are unwilling or have not learned how to behave in supportive ways. However, the resources and willingness to help are often present within the family and close friends and all concerned can be helped to change their relationships and allow new roles and abilities to develop.

Patients may have been ill for a considerable time before they undergo stoma surgery, for example some patients with inflammatory bowel conditions or those who have had bladder cancer treated with cystoscopies and resection of localised tumour. These people may have been living a very curtailed lifestyle for months or years in an attempt to handle the effects of their condition. As each person rehabilitates their improved health will give them the opportunity to develop a more extended lifestyle. However, families and friends may have grown accustomed to viewing that person as occupying a sick role, and relate to them accordingly. Sometimes the patient, family members, or friends may find it difficult to let go of any benefits they have experienced from the roles they occupied during the patient's illness. Friends who enjoyed helping with shopping or other tasks may find it difficult to relinquish these tasks to a person who is now able to do them for himself. The patient, family and friends may all need to learn to think of that person as someone who is now able to be included in activities and engagements outside the home, instead of making plans which assume they will only be able to play a minor role in them, or take part if their condition allows it. Discussion and help to plan activities so a more normal lifestyle can be gradually built up as the patient rehabilitates is normally beneficial. Advice on pacing activities to gain adequate rest can be given in tandem with support and encouragement to meet friends or take more part in family and work activities. Patients who have found their needs are usually considered only when they are ill may need to learn how to ask for what they want assertively without relapsing into a sick role. This in turn may challenge other roles generally adopted by family, friends or work colleagues and the patient (and others) may need help to find new and acceptable ways of interacting and getting their needs met.

PERCEPTIONS OF ACCEPTABILITY IN SOCIAL AND WORK CONTEXTS

Anyone who acquires a stoma is likely to have to deal with a variety of assumptions made by friends, colleagues and family as to what the presence of that stoma does to them as a person. Assuring a patient that it will, or should, make no difference to how they are viewed is often inappropriate, as sometimes people's assumptions lead to actions which have serious implications for that patient. It is therefore generally more appropriate to enquire whether the patient thinks having a stoma will make people see him, or act towards him, any differently, or whether they might make assumptions about what he can or cannot do now he has a stoma. This will give him the opportunity to discuss any fears or problems he has, or thinks he will have, and begin to identify ways of dealing with them. Providing him with realistic and factual information about living with a stoma as part of such discussions will also help the patient revise any inaccurate assumptions he is making about his acceptability as a person and colleague, friend, or family member.

For example, assumptions may be (wrongly) made that the patient will no longer be able to work with food, or handle particular machinery or tasks at work. Arranging for a letter from the consultant to be sent to the employer, or for the stoma care nurse to speak to the occupational health officer for that company, can enable misconceptions about the patient's ability to work to be corrected at an early stage. Such action will also help the patient to view himself as someone who continues to have the abilities he had before his surgery, and to accept a staged resumption of work activities as a sensible aid to his rehabilitation and not assume it indicates a permanent lack of abilities.

It can be particularly helpful to encourage patients to differentiate between facts and opinions or beliefs. *For example*, friends or family members may believe that someone with a stoma can no longer travel to other countries. If the patient also believes this he may think it is a fact. However, many people with stomas travel regularly on holiday or as part of their work. Providing such information, and then encouraging the patient to realistically consider what his capabilities for travel are likely to be as he rehabilitates, will help him feel more confident in himself and more able to question the accuracy of his own and other people's beliefs.

Advice regarding a patient's resumption of social or other activities is often given because of the nature of the surgery or its likely short-term effects on the patient's capabilities. However, unless a patient is told why the advice is given he may assume it is because of the presence of the stoma, particularly if it matches his own beliefs about what someone with a stoma can or cannot do. If the stoma is permanent this can result in the patient following the advice permanently. For example, many patients are advised not to drive a car in the early postoperative period. This is because their abilities to concentrate and react quickly in an emergency are likely to be reduced after major surgery or if they are taking painkillers. As they recover so will their abilities to concentrate and react appropriately while driving, and the return of those abilities should be monitored as part of their follow-up care. Unless they have been given the reason for this temporary embargo, patients may assume it is because they have a stoma. This can give rise to much anxiety if the patient needs to drive in order to work or fulfil family or social engagements.

Likewise, advice on resumption of full sexual activity should be clearly linked to the wisdom of first allowing sufficient time for adequate healing of wounds and regaining of energy, or the patient and/or their partner may assume that people with stomas should not want or have sex, particularly if this is a belief that they, or people they know, already hold. Specific permission to continue with their other usual forms of contact with partners, family and friends should be given at the same time as this advice (e.g. to touch, hug, share a bed).

In some cultures the presence of a stoma in one family member can mean that not only is that person viewed as unmarriageable but other family members will also be perceived as ineligible for marriage, or open to divorce proceedings being taken against them. This can lead to the patient and family desperately trying to conceal the presence of the stoma, or seeking to have the stoma reversed when a child reaches marriageable age. Particular problems can arise when the family (who may expect to arrange marriages) hold these traditional views while the younger generation (which may include the person with the stoma) believe in a more Westernised tradition of freedom to choose and be chosen in marriage. It can be hard for the person with a stoma to consider themselves socially and sexually acceptable and desirable in such circumstances. Swan (1999) reports that the numbers of people from ethnic minorities having stoma surgery is increasing. It is becoming easier to find people who are successfully living with a stoma who will visit new patients with a similar background to their own. Such role models demonstrate social acceptance and rehabilitation is possible with a stoma. They encourage patients to believe they too can accommodate a stoma within their lifestyle and develop a sense of themselves as acceptable human beings.

It can also be hard for staff to help patients in situations where their own cultural backgrounds and viewpoints differ considerably from those of the patient and his family. Generally, advice-giving is best kept to a minimum when such differences occur as opinions tend to be flavoured by the cultural assumptions of the advice-giver. The prime need is for the patient and family to express their feelings and concerns and find ways of handling their situation that are acceptable to all concerned.

This is more likely to occur if staff use a counselling approach that is supportive and aims to help the patient and his family identify their own solutions (see Chs 7 and 20).

RELIGIOUS CONSIDERATIONS

It is important for us to acquire some knowledge of the concepts and beliefs upon which the major religions and their rules are based. Information is available both from religious centres and in general publications (Henley & Schott 1999, Neuberger 1998, Clarke 1993). Such information gives us a starting point from which to enquire about patients' individual religious beliefs and requirements, and plan and provide care that meets the spirit as well as the letter of those requirements.

Most people who have religious beliefs put them into practice in their own individual way. Although this may include following the major rules and activities laid down by their own particular religion this is not always the case, and people's interpretation of how those rules and activities should be fulfilled may also differ. It is therefore appropriate when planning care to ask patients what kind of care will be congruent with their beliefs and best help them follow any religious practices they wish to make (Neuberger 1998).

People who have religious beliefs and practices and a stoma may find these affect each other in several ways (Black, 2000). These can include:

- the effect of their religious beliefs on the way in which they carry out physical care of the stoma and appliance
- the effects which the presence and action of the stoma have on them when they wish to engage in religious practices
- the effects of religious practices on the stoma and its actions.

It is therefore usually helpful to ask patients who follow a religion whether they think any of their beliefs, or ways in which they carry out their religious practices, are likely to be affected by the presence and/or action of their stoma. This information can then be used in conjunction with that provided in the following section, and other literature (e.g. Black, 2000), to enable care to be given that will help each patient follow their chosen religious practices as part of their rehabilitated lifestyle.

Personal cleanliness is often linked to spiritual purity in Asian cultures, and cleanliness of the body and clothes for religious observance is a requirement in some religions. For example, Muslims are required to carry out a ritual cleansing before each of their five daily sessions of prayer. This involves washing of the face, from the elbows to the hands, and from the knees to the feet. Birkbeck (2001) reports that a Fatwa ruling about the wearing of pouches during prayer is available, including on the internet at www.ostomyinternational.org/Fatwa.html. In accordance with this Fatwa, Muslims are likely to require a clean appliance for each of their five daily prayer sessions. A two-piece appliance is generally more suitable as it allows application of clean bags to the same base on several occasions, whereas removal of a one-piece bag several times a day could result in more skin damage.

Most Hindus and Sikhs also bath before formal prayer (Neuberger 1998). Washing with running water is preferred and therefore use of a shower or bidet may be more acceptable for care of perineal wounds than sitting in a bath.

The concept that personal cleanliness can be aided by using the right hand for 'clean' activities such as eating, picking things up, and greetings, and the left hand for other activities (such as cleaning the anal and pubic areas) is common in Hindu, Jain, Sikh and Buddhist cultures as well as being a religious requirement for Muslims (Henley & Schott 1999). It is therefore wise to enquire whether people from these cultures wish to follow this practice when carrying out their stoma care. If so, they can be taught to use both hands as necessary to prepare and apply their clean stomal equipment, but use their left hand only for removal of their used appliance and cleansing of the peristomal area.

Observers of the Jewish faith, particularly those following the more stringent orthodox lifestyle, may have some difficulties in reconciling their religious requirements and the presence and activities of the stoma. For example, changing of stomal equipment on the Sabbath (from sunset on Friday until sunset on Saturday) may be viewed as unacceptable because the Sabbath is required to be a day of rest. It may be appropriate to avoid asking patients to do practice changes of their equipment on the Sabbath, as they may well regard these as non-essential activities and therefore forbidden. However, Jewish patients may find it helpful to discuss how they will manage stoma care on the Sabbath once they return home. Release from religious observances is allowed for people who are sick, but once the person has recovered generally from their surgery they may not wish to be regarded as sick. Some people with colostomies find irrigation on alternate days allows them to avoid stoma care on the Sabbath (Yaffe 1984).

Orthodox Jewish women have to take a ritual bath (Mikveh) after each menstrual period as a precondition for the resumption of sexual intercourse. The woman has to be completely nude, with no clothes or stoma bag separating her body from the water in the pool. This may not present too many difficulties for the person with a colostomy, but the more frequent actions of an ileostomy may make fulfilment of this ritual difficult for some people (Yaffe 1984). The presence of a urinary stoma, dripping urine every few seconds, has in at least one instance known to me created a total barrier to completion of the ritual bath and resumption of sexual intercourse by the couple concerned.

People's eating habits may also be influenced by their religion. The main religious prescriptions regarding diet are described in Chapter 16.

Patient-centred care involves building rapport and encouraging patients and their families to provide information about themselves, their lifestyle, and needs (see Ch. 7). It is enhanced when we draw on relevant background information to help us make the best sense we can of people's descriptions of their circumstances and needs. As with the *patient scenarios* in other chapters, the information given here should not be applied wholesale to all patients but used thoughtfully to work well with individuals.

References

Bailey C 2001 The needs of older people. In: Corner J, Bailey C (eds) Cancer nursing: care in context. Blackwell Science, Oxford, p 496–507

Birkbeck J W 2001 Fatwa about preparation for prayer for Muslim ostomates. World Council of Enterostomal Therapists Journal 21(1):32

Black P K 2000 Holistic stoma care. Baillière Tindall and RCN, Edinburgh

Chamberlain J 1996 Cultural, racial, environmental and spiritual influences on stoma patients in South Africa. In: World Council of Enterostomal Therapists congress proceedings. Hollister, Libertyville, IL, p 178–181

Clarke P B (ed) 1993 The world's religions. Reader's Digest Association, New York/Montreal

Davitz J R, Davitz L L 1981 Inferences of patients' pain and psychological distress. Springer, New York

Dean J 1998 Postoperative recovery following guided imagery relaxation therapy - a randomised controlled pilot study. In: World Council of Enterostomal Therapists congress proceedings. Horton Print Group, Bradford, West Yorkshire, p 222–224

Fitzpatrick G, Stammers C, Taylor P 2003 The influence of age on patients' problems. In: Elcoat C Stoma care nursing, 2nd edn. Hollister, Wokingham, Berks, p 75–87

Henley A, Schott J 1999 Culture, religion and patient care in a multi-ethnic society. Age Concern England, London

Krishnasamy M 2001 Pain. In: Corner J, Bailey C (eds) Cancer nursing: care in context . Blackwell Science, Oxford, p 339–349

Middleton C 2004 Barriers to the provision of effective pain management. Nursing Times 100(3):42–45

Neuberger J 1998 Introduction to cultural issues in palliative care. In: Doyle D, Hanks G W C, MacDonald N (eds) Oxford textbook of palliative medicine, 2nd edn. Oxford University Press, Oxford, p 777–785

Pringle W, Swan E 2001 Continuing care after discharge from hospital for stoma patients. British Journal of Nursing 10(19):1274–1288

Ross J 1994 Low anterior resection vs. abdomino-perineal excision: what choice? what problems? what quality? In: World Council of Enterostomal Therapists congress proceedings. Hollister, Libertyville, IL, USA, p 124–128

Swan E 1999 Equal care for all. Nursing Standard 13(27):42–44

Thomas V N (ed) 1997 Pain: its nature and management. Baillière Tindall and RCN, London

Thomas V N 2001 The needs of people from minority ethnic groups. In: Corner J, Bailey C (eds) Cancer nursing: care in context. Blackwell Science, Oxford, p 508–516

Wade B 1989 A stoma is for life. Scutari Press, London

Yaffe A 1984 The influence of Jewish religious laws on orthodox Jewish ostomates in Israel. In: World Council of Enterostomal Therapists congress proceedings. Abbott International and Hollister, USA, p 3–4

Additional Reading

Culley L, Dyson S (eds) 2001 Ethnicity and nursing practice. Palgrove, Basingstoke, Hants

Nursing with dignity series 2002 Nursing Times 98(9–17): 28 February to 23 April, 2002 [This series of articles aims to help nurses meet all patients' needs in a multicultural society.]

Williams J 2002 Patients' perspectives In: Williams J (ed) The essentials of pouch care nursing. Whurr Publishers, London, p 218–234

Chapter 20

Responding to loss and change

Brigid Breckman

Stoma surgery can have substantial effects on patients' sense of themselves and how they function physically and psychologically (Kelly 1985, Salter 1983, 1996). Bredin, writing about self-concept, states:

> Changed experience of the body – when it is permanently damaged, mutilated, incomplete, or spoiled – deeply affects one's sense of self. When that essential familiarity and wholeness is stripped away, feelings of difference, isolation, fragmentation, and a loss of self-worth ensue. (Bredin 2001, p 414)

Losses and changes experienced by individual patients vary. However, most stoma patients do report feelings of loss and change and some will experience it as strongly as Bredin describes. Some patients begin to experience symptoms of loss from the time they learn they require stoma surgery. Others may only realise the extent of the changes with which they have to come to terms as they go through surgery and seek to resume their normal lives. Their experiences are similar to the bereavement people have when they lose a person or object of importance to them (Parkes 1998).

The processes that people normally go through when they are bereaved enable them to mourn their loss and then turn their attention and energy towards their future life. Worden (2003) describes these activities as *griefwork*. Ensuring that our care includes strategies to help patients manage loss and change as well as the practicalities of learning to live with a stoma is important. If patients do not come to terms with their losses it will be difficult for them to disengage from their former sense of self in a way that will enable them to build up a new and acceptable sense of themselves. We therefore need to gain enough knowledge and skills to work with patients in ways that are supportive of any ongoing grief-work or, at the very least, do not impede it. There is considerable research describing the major and diverse effects which unresolved grief can have on people's lives (e.g. Parkes 1998, Raphael 1984) and the substantial therapeutic help which may be required if people do not grieve in a helpful manner at the time of their loss.

In this chapter I will outline losses and experiences of them which patients may experience and discuss various helpful responses. I have linked Parkes' (1998) model of bereavement processes with losses and events of stoma surgery. This will help you recognise and respond to patients' experiences in informed and sensitive ways.

BODY IMAGE AND FUNCTION

Body image is the mental picture each individual has of his own body. It begins to develop from birth, when the infant is not aware that he is a separate being from his mother. He learns about various parts of the body: how they function, and how to gain control over them. Use and mastery of the environment, with evaluation of achievement and failure, will in turn be followed by learning to relate to other people of both sexes. Values and attitudes about the acceptability of one's own or other people's bodies will develop through comparison with one's peer group and, increasingly, with people portrayed in advertisements and programmes on television and thus may be culturally or racially biased.

Stoma surgery generally creates changes in self-image which include:

- how the individual visualises his body internally and externally
- how he perceives his ability to function
- what control he believes he has over how he looks and functions.

It can take up to 2 years for many patients to come to terms with their new ways of looking and functioning and acquire a positive self-image, and some people never reach this stage (Cohen & Zierstein 1994, Dryden 2003).

Strategies to help patients develop a new and positive body image can start preoperatively and should be based on information gained from each patient as to the aspects of their body image and function which they view as important and wish to retain or recreate in an acceptable form. *For example,* many patients who value having control over their elimination benefit from being encouraged to view capability in stoma care and appliance management generally as their new, acceptable form of control over their elimination.

The activity of siting the stoma often starkly brings home to patients that they will shortly be having to live with a stoma (Salter 1983). Acknowledgement of patients' fears, feelings and needs is a helpful first step *before* offering realistic information as to how they, and their stoma, are likely to look in the early postoperative period. However, stoma siting also provides a useful opportunity to help patients look beyond this early period and begin to believe that the stoma could fit in with their normal clothes and activities once they have resumed their normal lifestyle. *For example,* checking by both patient and nurse as to how the stoma site and an appliance fit in with particular positions he gets into at work, carrying out hobbies, and wearing swimwear can enable him to start imagining himself as having a body fit to resume these activities. Checking potential stoma sites on a Muslim patient as he adopts the position for prayer (Sujud), coupled with sensitive acknowledgement that this is an important part of his life, is likely to convey the message that inclusion in religious activities will be possible because his altered body appearance and function are acceptable.

People's perceptions may be shaped by their culture, religion and gender. Some Jewish people may find the stoma particularly difficult to accept because body perfection and freedom from mutilation is expected as part of their religion during life as well as at the time of death (Levine 1997). Salter (1997) suggests that the presence of a stoma may have sexual connotations for some patients. Females, especially if they have a protruding stoma, may regard it as a phallic symbol, while men may liken bleeding of the stoma when it is cleaned to menstruation, and thus think of their stoma as having female characteristics.

Some patients are reminded of the condition for which they required surgery whenever they see the stoma, particularly in the early postoperative months. Patients who have had ulcerative colitis may feel more positive about themselves, aware that they have more control over elimination from their stoma through adept appliance management than they did when they had their diseased colon and rectum (Wade 1989). However, it can be more difficult for people with Crohn's disease to come to terms with having a stoma because their surgery is not always curative. They may have to cope with a changed body image not only at the time the stoma is created but also with subsequent changes if the disease recurs and if further treatment is required. People with cancer face similar difficulties in that their surgery may not always cure their disease. In addition, their concept of cancer and their prognosis, actual or imagined, will affect their self-image. Many people still view cancer as a dirty unsocial disease, and fears that it is contagious are sometimes expressed.

Patients whose surgery is curative will usually in time accept their new body image as normal, and believe themselves to be in charge of their stoma and its care. However, patients whose stoma is palliative may find it difficult to perceive their body as anything but one taken over by cancer cells. Stomal action may be classed with rectal or vaginal discharge as visible, uncontrollable reminders of the encroaching cancer, and their body perceived as undesirable and unacceptable socially.

Helping patients view their stoma positively includes helping them handle their initial experiences of seeing it and feeling it act. Some patients find their initial experience of seeing the stoma devastating (Kelly 1985). However, Wade (1989) states that just over half the patients in her study reported positive reactions on seeing their stomas for the first time, with one-third of the patients reporting an extremely negative reaction. More women than men had negative reactions, as did people with urinary compared to bowel stomas, and people with temporary rather than permanent colostomies. Using a counselling approach can help patients explore and come to terms with the implications or assumptions which they make because of the presence of their stoma, and the thoughts and feelings which arise from these experiences (Salter 1998).

Realistic descriptions of how the stoma will look should be given preoperatively. It should look red, similar in colour to the lining of the mouth, and may well make peristaltic movements reminiscent of a wriggling worm. Such a description may make patients anxious preoperatively. However, if they are told it will look very small or like a rosebud beforehand, that then leaves patients to cope with the reality of a newly formed, often quite large and puffy looking stoma. Many patients then conclude (with greater anxiety) that something must have gone wrong as this stoma is unlike that described to them. They may also be less likely to believe assurances that the stoma will shrink to a neater shape or size. Support from a qualified nurse, experienced in stoma care, during the early bag changes when patients can be encouraged to look at and touch the stoma when they feel ready lays a good foundation for acceptance of the stoma and confident self-care to develop in time. Encouragement to voice thoughts, feelings and beliefs about the stoma also helps patients begin to acknowledge the stoma is part of them, and misconceptions and concerns can be addressed.

Acceptance of the stoma may be considerably influenced by people who are significant in the stoma patient's life (McVey et al 2001, Wade 1989). It is not uncommon to find a new patient assuming that his partner will be unable to cope with looking at his stoma. Support enabling him to ask his partner if she would like to see an appliance changed (and thus see the stoma) before he leaves hospital often reveals that the partner is very pleased to accept this invitation. Each couple should be allowed to make their own decision: insistence that the partner must watch an appliance being changed can do more harm than good as the patient may then not really believe his partner does accept the stoma. It must also be remembered that not all couples appear naked in front of each other, and providing the partner with a full abdominal view complete with stoma may violate that couple's normal rules of behaviour. However, in many cases, where it is appropriate, a change of appliance carried out by an informed nurse who answers any questions raised by the patient or partner can do much to start the patient on the road to acceptance of his new body image.

People can have stomas raised at any age from early babyhood through to old age. They will have many of the same concerns with their changing body as any other person does, but the presence of a stoma and its appliance may bring additional concerns about how they look and function (and how others will view them) at various stages in their lives. It is sometimes (wrongly) assumed that the only body image concerns which patients have relate either to the stoma itself or to possible or actual sexual impairment. A wide range of concerns are well described by Salter (1996, 1997) with indications of helpful responses. Sometimes requests for help with body image concerns are hidden in other comments or questions. For example, a teenager's question about whether they can play a sport where body contact occurs may mask a fear they will be rejected by friends who learn he has a stoma.

People's self-image generally includes their perception of their degree of sexual attractiveness both in terms of how they rate themselves and how they think others view them. Likewise most people's self-image includes a concept of how they think they function sexually and how they believe other people perceive their sexual activities, including the experiences that result from them. Stoma surgery can affect all these components of a person's image of themselves as a sexual being. It is therefore important to know how patients see themselves preoperatively, and want to see themselves once they have recovered from their surgery, so that they can be helped to develop a new and satisfactory self-image as they rehabilitate. This kind of information can generally be obtained as part of the process of gathering information about the patient's lifestyle, needs and concerns (Dennison 2001). It is most likely to be forthcoming if patients have found that when they described other aspects of their lifestyle, or expressed other needs and concerns, the response they got indicated that staff were using that information to understand, value and respond to them as individuals. Timing is important, and the rapport built up as we gain information about the patient's work, social, holiday and family activities and concerns will help us introduce topics such as sex more easily.

Physical impairment of sexual activity is often unhelpfully described as being a result of 'the stoma surgery'. In fact impairment is not due to the procedure of creating a stoma, but rather may occur as a result of some surgical procedures used to deal with the disease or condition that is being treated. This is discussed in Chapters 3, 5 and 6. The actual position of each patient regarding their condition or disease, the extent of their surgery, and the likelihood of sexual difficulties or impairment should be discussed with their surgeon. This should enable accurate, relevant and consistent information and advice to be helpfully provided by appropriate members of the healthcare team.

Clarity about medical terminology used to describe sexual impairment coupled with an ability to translate such terms and advice about handling difficulties into everyday language is essential if staff are to provide information helpfully to patients and their partners. Often a combination of providing information and then using a counselling approach to help patients decide what they will do now they have this knowledge is particularly helpful. *For example*, using diagrams to explain to women where the vagina lies in relation to the area of surgery can help them, and their partners, understand that a change of position can reduce or remove pain on intercourse because the thrust of the penis is not heading for scar tissue which is likely to make that part of the vaginal wall more rigid (Topping 1990). Counselling may help the couple give themselves permission to try out different positions as they make love and believe that they, and their new techniques, are acceptable.

Some patients want to discuss possible sexual impairment in detail and express fears and feelings preoperatively. Others may say they are not overly concerned with the ability to function sexually, particularly if this has been minimal before they come for surgery. Many need to recover from their surgery and resume most aspects of their normal lifestyle before they want to consider their sexual situation or divulge concerns and feelings related to their sexual attractiveness or abilities. General advice about the need to allow body tissues time to heal, and the importance of having sufficient rest, sleep and freedom from pain and anxiety to enable levels of energy and libido to build up is appropriate for most patients (Topping 1990, White 1997). This can be linked to information that many patients find they only want to discuss sexual issues some months or even years after their surgery. Patients and partners should be given explicit permission to make an appointment to have such a discussion in circumstances where privacy is assured if the patient, partner, or both ever wish to do so. Strategies for handling such discussions helpfully are discussed in Chapters 5 and 9.

THE EXPERIENCE OF LOSS

It is essential that patients, their families, and staff understand that it is normal for people to undergo an experience of psychological as well as physical adjustment during and after stoma surgery. This includes learning to manage their stoma adeptly and confidently, but capability in stoma care is not the same as achieving rehabilitation. Parkes (1998) suggests that people whose body image and/or function changes, for example through surgery, are likely to have similar reactions to people bereaved of family or friends. In other words, they *lose a part of themselves* and react accordingly. Such experiences often include three phases:

- an initial numbness
- pining and disorganisation
- reorganisation.

Many patients benefit from a simple explanation that they are likely to go through an experience of bereavement similar to losing someone who is important to them, because they are losing how they used to look and function and will need time to get used to and accept their new selves. Telling patients that they may (rather than will) initially find themselves disorganised and unable to concentrate as well as usual, and may experience changes in mood and feelings for no obvious reason, will help both patient and family view such occurrences as part of recovery rather than as an indication that they are 'falling apart' mentally or physically, either temporarily or permanently. This explanation must be linked to discussion about how the patient and family can help themselves, and obtain support and help from others, in order to cope with their experiences effectively, and move on to physical and psychological rehabilitation (Dryden 2003, Salter 1998; see also Chs 8, 9, 22).

This kind of discussion is important for three main reasons. Firstly, it enables patients and their families to feel more confident that they will know what to do in those early weeks at home. Secondly, it encourages patients and their families to believe that staff are interested in their psychological well-being as well as their physical condition, and so they are more likely to explicitly report, or seek help with, psychological and social concerns as well as physical ones. This increases the possibility that problems such as severe depression or abnormal grief reactions will be identified more quickly, enabling earlier referral for extra psychological support (White 1998). Thirdly, it appears that the families or significant others of some patients experience two periods of high anxiety and stress: one when the patient is in hospital and the second about 3–6 months after discharge (Oberst & Scott 1988). If the family have felt well supported in the hospitalisation period they may find it easier to ask for and accept help and support later on, particularly if they are told this is acceptable and appropriate behaviour. Research is needed to establish whether there is a link between this second period of anxiety in relatives and some patients' emerging concern over their sexual abilities at about the same length of time following surgery. It could well be that it is all part of the overall process of increasing

awareness of the implications and results of surgery which patients and families go through during their recovery from the whole experience.

Loss following stoma surgery is not always a totally bad experience. Ileostomists who have lost the need to continually seek and use toilets because of frequent bowel actions often express relief and appreciation of the more flexible lifestyle they can now develop. Likewise patients losing the experience of painful, and/or frequent micturition as a result of removal of their bladder and gaining a urostomy may find it easier to come to terms with their overall losses because there are also some definite gains in daily living resulting from their surgery. Such patients may have a considerably shorter period of feeling bereaved than others whose 'gains' seem less tangible. Sadly, some patients do not have sufficient time to complete their bereavement process following their stoma surgery before having to deal with recurrent disease and more treatment, or the physical and psychological experiences of dying (Breckman 1982). These bring further experiences of loss to the patient and to those close to them.

It is important to remember that patients who have stomas, or are coming for stoma surgery, may be experiencing loss from other life events. Unresolved grief can be compounded by the losses arising from stoma surgery. Equally, other losses occurring soon after stoma surgery may also be experienced with more grief because of their proximity and require higher levels of support than for a single loss. Worden's (2003) model of the tasks of grieving is a useful aid to recognising and responding to different stages of loss. This may be through direct care, such as in the *scenario* in Chapter 22 (Patient scenario 22.2), or through referral to a more skilled or specialist source of help.

SUPPORTING LOSS, GRIEF AND CHANGE

Much of the care required and described below falls into the categories described by Nichols (2003) as informational care, emotional care and basic counselling. These are often provided as combined elements of care, but it can be useful when planning and reviewing our care to consider whether we are providing enough of each category, and whether more or less of each of them would be helpful given the needs and situation of the individual patient concerned.

People experiencing loss often seek to make sense of what has happened, or is happening, to them.

They may need to recount their experiences several times until their initial shock or *numbness* reduces and they can begin to accept the reality of their situation. Each patient should be given the chance to talk about what they think and feel their situation to be, and what they understand about their operation. As they tell their story patients generally get a more concrete sense of their situation and concerns, particularly if the nurse uses rapport-building and clarifying skills (see Ch. 7). When patients experience themselves as accurately understood they often report a decrease in the amount of shock or numbness they have experienced since learning they must have this type of surgery. The result is likely to be that the patient's grieving process begins to move forward *and* they feel more capable of taking in some of the information they will need to acquire.

Like someone bereaved of a close friend or relative patients can experience a *yearning or pining* for the person they were before they became ill and/or had stoma surgery with the various losses and changes this entails. The conceptual understanding of the need for surgery may do little to diminish feelings such as sadness, anger, guilt, anxiety and fear of how the surgery and resultant stoma might affect their lives. Indeed efforts by family and staff to prematurely reassure the patient of the benefits of surgery can leave them with two problems (firstly they have the feelings and then they get messages implying they should not have them). Staff, family and friends may need support as the patient may attribute the cause of these feelings to the actions or omissions of others around them rather than the surgery and its effects, and blame them accordingly. This can be confusing and distressing if it is very different from the patient's normal behaviour. All concerned can benefit from information that people's feelings and moods can be unusually changeable in situations such as the patient is going through and that, generally, expressing fears and feelings is helpful. It enables information and support that is needed to be identified and provided.

The majority of patients will not require formal ongoing counselling sessions in order to come to terms with their changed sense of themselves and their situation. However, they will benefit from care which helps them express feelings and concerns, clarify their situation, and decide how to manage it. This type of care is often called 'a counselling approach' or 'basic counselling' (Nichols 2003). When using it our focus is on helping people help themselves in accordance with their particular needs, values, lifestyle and goals. This is different from giving advice. When advising our focus is more on clarifying our sense of patients' situations and needs in order to express our opinion of the best ways of responding to them. These approaches, and the skills enabling their use, are described in Chapter 7 in conjunction with a definition of counselling.

Many bereaved people seem to cope with all the decisions and activities which need to take place in the early period after a death before the reality of their loss is fully experienced. As the numbness decreases so their difficulties in thinking clearly, making decisions, and managing changeable feelings increase. Parkes (1998) describes this as a period of *disorganisation*. Patients also often seem to cope with the surgery and gaining sufficient knowledge and skills in stoma care to enable them to go home, and then find they too experience many of the symptoms of disorganisation in addition to all the physical effects which major surgery has on the body (McVey et al 2001, Pringle & Swan 2001, Wade 1990). If patients and their families are not appropriately prepared for this reaction they are likely to fear that something has gone wrong, thus adding to their difficulties. Reassurance that this kind of experience is normal in the early period and will not be a permanent state of affairs may not be believed if it is only given once patient and family report problems rather than as part of the pre-discharge information.

Preparation for possible disorganisation can be through giving the kind of information and care described earlier to patients and relevant family or friends. They can also be helped to plan a structure for the early weeks at home through which a gradual increase in physical and social activities can take place, such as those described in Chapters 8 and 9. Such discussion enables the role which, for example, community nurses could play in providing some of the required care and support to be clarified and referrals made in sufficient time and detail to enable hospital and community care to dovetail adequately.

During surgery and early rehabilitation it is particularly likely that the patient's situation will also cause changes in the lives of family and friends. For example, close family and friends may curtail aspects of their own lives in order to provide care and support for them. Workmates and more distant friends or family may be deprived of their usual meetings or activities with the patient who is not yet fit enough to resume the work or social engagements through which their normal interaction occurs. Changes in role, and expectations about the priority that should be given to meeting the patient's needs, can create substantial problems for those concerned, particularly if the situation continues for a lengthy period.

Nichols (2003) suggests that psychological care includes *acting as agent on behalf of the patient*. In stoma care this may entail also acting on behalf of the patient's family and friends who are closely involved in his support by encouraging them to explicitly plan ways in which any losses and changes arising from the patient's situation could be most helpfully managed. One way of achieving this which I have found to be very effective is to teach patient and family to use the concept of strokes and stroke balance when making their plans (Hay 1992). In transactional analysis (TA) a *stroke* is a unit of recognition or acknowledgement. We give and receive strokes in any interaction through the behaviour which acknowledges the presence of the people concerned. Strokes can be:

- verbal or non-verbal
- positive or negative
- conditional (related to what one does or does not do)
- unconditional (related to what one is).

Berne (1964) suggested that people hunger for mental and physical stimulation and recognition, and that strokes are the system through which those needs are met. As we grow up we learn which behaviours get attention, praise or criticism (i.e. different kinds of strokes) and adapt our behaviour accordingly. Stewart & Joines (1987) make the point that strokes are necessary for our survival and, rather than risk getting no strokes, people will unconsciously seek negative strokes. As we grow up we become accustomed to receiving certain types of stroke, and/or strokes for particular attributes or behaviours. In British culture male children may get praise for being 'big brave boys who don't cry when they are hurt'. Repeated strokes like this may encourage children to learn not to notice or express sadness and they may subsequently have difficulty expressing grief appropriately such as when bereaved. Help may be needed to change this pattern.

As we give and receive strokes in all our interactions so we experience an internal stroke bank or *stroke balance* derived from incoming and outgoing strokes. Over time each person becomes comfortable with a certain level of strokes, above or

below which they may feel discomfort. If our stroke balance is sufficiently depleted there is a risk that we may unconsciously choose to top it up by behaving in ways that will attract negative strokes. These tend to have a greater emotional intensity than positive strokes and thus restore our normal stroke balance with greater speed, albeit greater negative experiences as well. When patients, their family and friends are in a position where their usual ways of giving and getting strokes are altered or curtailed it is highly likely that their stroke balance will also be affected.

For example, patients who get strokes from workmates whom they only meet at lunchtime may become deprived of strokes when this activity stops while they are away from work. Close family or friends who give such priority to meeting the patient's physical or psychological needs that they stop engaging in activities where they usually get strokes may find their stroke balance is depleted as a result. It is also highly likely that they are giving extra positive strokes to the patient in the form of care and support, thus altering their own stroke balance further. Once patients and their families understand the concept of strokes and stroke balance they are usually willing to give time and attention to setting up ways of getting positive strokes both to help themselves feel valued and cherished and as a means of avoiding triggering negative strokes and additional stress. It is important to encourage each person to identify strokes which *they* experience as positive, as attention that is pleasurable to one person may be unacceptable to others. The *scenarios* of Nurse Beech's work with the Earls and Mrs Reid's work with Mrs Jones in Chapter 8 show how these concepts can be used as part of normal care (Patient scenarios 8.5 and 8.6).

PROMOTING SELF-EFFICACY

Patients need to go further than coming to terms with loss and change. They also need to acquire a sense of *self-efficacy*: an expectation that they will manage their stoma and live with it successfully. Bekkers et al (1996) found that patients who expected to be able to take care of their stoma had fewer psychosocial problems in the first postoperative year. McVey et al (2001) asked patients undergoing stoma surgery for cancer about their experiences before and after surgery. The key theme to emerge from patients' descriptions was lowered personal control, coupled with fear preoperatively. They suggested that provision of physical and emotional support was important. Where (medical) information was perceived by patients to be incomplete or curtailed this lowered patients' sense of control over the questions and input they could contribute to these interactions. Help from stoma care nurses and partners was reported as important in enabling patients to become more proactive in stoma care, resuming normal activities, and becoming more positive in their thinking.

Patients' growing use of the internet to acquire information and check the accuracy of advice they have been given indicates their informational needs are not always being met (Ziebland et al 2004). There is some evidence that giving patients audiotapes of consultations when diagnosis and treatment options are discussed is helpful, with patients and their families reporting tapes aided recall and understanding of what was said (Gent et al 2003). Research is needed to establish whether offering patients this facility would increase self-efficacy.

The strategy of linking information and skills to patients' lifestyles described throughout this book should help patients gain a sense of self-efficacy. It is important patients gain sufficient self-care skills before discharge to promote competence and confidence (Metcalf 1999). Learning to use knowledge and skills in pursuit of their goals fosters patients' sense of control over their lives.

Nichols (2003) suggests that, as well as monitoring patients' psychological states, we may need to refer them on for additional or more in-depth care. It is possible for the majority of qualified staff engaged in stoma care to gain and use the knowledge and skills described in this book if they are willing to do so and have access to suitable learning opportunities. However, it is likely that in some situations there will be a gap between the level of knowledge and care required by patients and their families and the expertise of staff usually providing their care (Benner et al 1996, Breckman, 1983). Fulfilment of our professional responsibilities includes monitoring the degree to which patients' needs are being met by the care provided collectively by the healthcare team, and promoting referral to colleagues with greater expertise where this is needed. This should be seen as part of good practice rather than failure in the staff concerned, particularly where advanced knowledge and skills are required. This will be further discussed in Chapters 22 and 23.

References

Bekkers M J, van Knippenberg F C, van den Borne H W, van Berge-Henegouwen G P 1996 Prospective evaluation of psychosocial adaptation to stoma surgery: the role of self-efficacy. Psychosomatic Medicine 58(2):183–191

Benner P, Tanner C A, Chesla C A 1996 Expertise in nursing practice. Springer, New York

Berne E 1964 Games people play. Penguin Books, London

Breckman B 1982 The special needs of terminal patients. Journal of Community Nursing 5(8):4–5

Breckman B 1983 Referrals - whose problem, whose responsibility? Nursing Times 79(42):58–60

Bredin M 2001. Altered self-concept. In: Corner J, Bailey C (eds) Cancer nursing: care in context. Blackwell Science, Oxford, p 414–419

Cohen A, Zierstein R 1994 Drawing your body image. In: World Council of Enterostomal Therapists congress proceedings. Hollister, Libertyville, IL, p 170–171

Dennison S 2001 Sexuality and cancer. In: Corner J, Bailey C (eds) Cancer nursing: care in context. Blackwell Science, Oxford, p 420–427

Dryden H 2003 Body image. In: Faithfull S, Wells M (eds) Supportive care in radiotherapy. Churchill Livingstone, Edinburgh, p 320–336

Gent C, Blackshaw G, Lewis W 2003 Taped consultations enhance patients' memories and perceptions of treatment. Gastrointestinal Nursing 1(9):29–32

Hay J 1992 Transactional analysis for trainers. McGraw Hill, London

Kelly M P 1985. Loss and grief reactions as responses to surgery. Journal of Advanced Nursing 10(6):517–525

Levine E 1997 Jewish views and customs in death. In: Parkes C M, Laungani P, Young B (eds) Death and bereavement across cultures. Brunner-Routledge, Hove, p 98–130

McVey J, Madill A, Fielding D 2001 The relevance of lowered personal control for patients who have stoma surgery to treat cancer. British Journal of Clinical Psychology 40:337–360

Metcalf C 1999 Stoma care: empowering patients through teaching practical skills. British Journal of Nursing 8(9):593–600

Nichols K 2003 Psychological care for ill and injured people. Open University Press, Maidenhead, Berks

Oberst M T, Scott D W 1988 Post-discharge distress in surgically treated cancer patients and their spouses. Research in Nursing and Health 11:223–233

Parkes C M 1998 Bereavement: studies of grief in adult life, 3rd edn. Penguin Books, London

Pringle W, Swan E 2001 Continuing care after discharge from hospital for stoma patients. British Journal of Nursing 10(19):1274–1288

Raphael R 1984 The anatomy of bereavement. Routledge, London

Salter M 1983 Towards a healthy body image. Nursing Mirror, Clinical Forum 8, 157(11): ii–vi

Salter M 1996 Sexuality and the stoma patient. In: Myers C (ed) Stoma care nursing. Arnold, London, p 203–219

Salter M 1997 Altered body image: the nurse's role. 2nd edn. Baillière Tindall, London

Salter M 1998 If you can help somebody … nursing interventions to facilitate adaptation to an altered body image. In: World Council of Enterostomal Therapists congress proceedings. Horton Print Group, Bradford, West Yorkshire, p 229–235

Stewart I, Joines V 1987 TA today. Lifespace Publishing, Nottingham and Chapel Hill

Topping A 1990 Sexual activity and the stoma patient. Nursing Standard 4(41):24–6

Wade B 1989 A stoma is for life. Scutari Press, London

Wade B 1990 Continuity of care and the stoma therapist. Senior Nurse 10(5):11–12

White C A 1997 Living with a stoma. Sheldon Press, London

White C 1998 Psychological management of stoma-related concerns. Nursing Standard 12(36):35–38

Worden J W 2003 Grief counselling and grief therapy, 3rd edn. Brunner-Routledge, Hove

Ziebland S, Chapple S, Damelow C et al 2004 How the internet affects patients' experience of cancer: a qualitative study. British Medical Journal 328(7439):564–567

Additional Reading

Henley A, Schott J 1999 Culture, religion and patient care in a multi-ethnic society. Age Concern England, London

Parkes C M, Laungani P, Young B 1997 Death and bereavement across cultures. Brunner-Routledge, Hove

Price B 1999 Altered body image. Nursing Times monographs no: 29. Emap Healthcare, London

Salter M 2002 Sexual aspects of internal pouch surgery. In: Williams J (ed) The essentials of pouch care nursing. Whurr Publishers, London, p 180–198

SECTION 5

Problems and developments

Chapter 21

Problems in stomal management

Brigid Breckman

In this chapter the term 'problem' includes:

- practical difficulties in managing the stoma, peristomal skin, or equipment
- stoma and skin conditions which indicate an abnormality may be present
- deviations from normal stoma and skin conditions which can create complications.

The focus is on ways of managing physical problems effectively. The various products mentioned, and the general principles whereby they are chosen and used in normal stoma care are described in Chapter 4.

ASSESSMENT

SITUATIONS WHERE A PROBLEM IS THOUGHT TO BE PRESENT

In many instances problems are initially described as a single problem relating to:

- the stoma itself
- the peristomal skin
- stomal function
- stomal equipment.

Once an adequate assessment of the patient's situation has been carried out 'the problem' is often found to be made up of several components. Each component contributes to the overall problem, and thus each needs to be considered before suitable advice and help can be given. A comprehensive description of the patient's situation should be built up. Useful questions include:

1. *What seems to be the problem?* This encourages patients to describe aspects of their situation which they find problematic.
2. *When did this problem start?*
3. *Does this problem occur at any particular **time** or when you are in a particular **place** or **position**?* Questions about the time when a problem occurs may elicit information that links it to other occurrences or specific situations. For example, some women report their equipment adheres less well during their menstrual period. Patients may connect it to times when they let their bag get overfull, such as during lengthy meetings or car journeys.

   Questions about the place or position people are in when problems arise may indicate their body shape in that position contributes to the problem. A history of leakage of urostomy bags at night often indicates that night drainage equipment is incorrectly set up (see later).
4. *When the problem started were there any particular **changes** or **events** happening around that time?* These might include changes to a new box or brand of stomal equipment, or soap used to clean the peristomal area. Patients may report they started a hobby or activity which placed extra strain on their stomal equipment. This question can also elicit information about stressful events such as starting a new job, bereavement, family problems. Some people find their equipment lifts more readily if they are stressed.
5. *What do you think caused the problem?* People may have ideas as to the cause of the problem. For example, some patients think a parastomal hernia indicates that they have a recurrence of their cancer.
6. *What measures (if any) have you tried out so far to resolve the problem? What happened as a result?* It is often helpful to first state that discussing the problem with the healthcare professional is an appropriate measure to resolve the problem. We should then ask if patients have tried other remedies, as the original problem may be masked by strategies they have followed to resolve it.
7. *What effects does this problem have on you and your usual way of life?* This elicits information about the degree to which the problem affects the patient, and sometimes other people as well. It may also signal that individuals might get some 'benefits' from the situation such as time off work, extra attention from friends and family, an excuse not to engage in social or sexual activities. However, we should not assume such connections exist, or

insist that patients accept this is the case, as this can be unhelpful and distressing for patients.
8. *Is there any other information which you or your family think might be relevant, or which you might like to mention?* This open question gives patients the opportunity to express any concerns or ideas if they want to do so.

Once this background information has been obtained patients' stoma, peristomal skin, equipment and needs can be specifically assessed.

The aim of a full assessment is to identify:

- any conditions or symptoms that warrant further investigation or treatment
- any actual or potential causes of problems in stomal management
- the criteria stomal equipment must fulfil in order to suit the patient's situation and needs
- equipment that will match those criteria and thus suit the patient and prevent or minimise problems.

A two-step process can be repeated systematically to fulfil the first three aims:

- gather information through assessing an aspect of the patient's situation
- identify criteria that should be met because of the information gained and its implications for stomal management.

The clarification thus gained (see steps a to g below) enables the final step (h) to then be taken and the fourth aim achieved.

*(a) **Assess the stomal equipment:*** both when it is attached to the patient and after removal. This can reveal a place where the adhesive flange tends to lift, indicating a likely source of strain on equipment there. Observation of the undersurface of a peristomal wafer (i.e. the side once attached to the patient) can reveal melting of a peristomal wafer in a particular area or along a line which may indicate that a dip or crease in abdominal contours is occurring some or all or the time, and that effluent is pooling in those areas. This kind of information provides cues as to which areas should receive particular attention during the rest of the assessment.

*(b) **Assess stomal effluent:*** its consistency, amount generally passed per action, and frequency of action.

- With bowel stomas, also estimate the amount the bag 'blows up' when flatus is passed as this will also need to be accommodated in the stoma bag.

- With urostomies, estimate the weight and amount of urine collected in 2 hours.

  Identify *criteria* that the bag should fulfil, e.g.

- appliance capacity
- style (e.g. drainable/closed bowel; connectable to night drainage for urostomy)
- need for a watertight adhesive.

(c) Assess the stoma generally: its colour, and any signs of bleeding, pressure, epithelialisation etc., as these may warrant further attention (see later). Note the stoma size, and whether this alters or is fairly constant, its degree of protrusion or flushness with skin level.

Identify criteria about the size of gasket/bag opening required; whether an expandable gasket is required (e.g. to accommodate a prolapsing stoma) or a rigid faceplate (e.g. to enable the stoma to stand out more from the surrounding abdomen); what depth of appliance gasket will enable effluent to pass from the stoma right into the bag rather than pool around it.

(d) Assess the patient's abdomen: its general contours near the stoma; presence/absence of bony prominences, scars, creases, drain sites; its visibility to the patient. These all need to be assessed with patients standing, lying down, sitting in an upright chair, easy chair, and (if used) wheelchair. The position clothes occupy on the abdomen (e.g. waistbands) also needs identification.

If patients report that problems arise when they are in a particular position or carrying out specific activities it is generally useful to ask them to demonstrate this while observing the abdomen for changes in shape which may put pressure or strain on the equipment or create bulges or gullies which reduce good flange adherence.

Identify criteria regarding the kind of bag adhesive required (e.g. flexible to go round bones and bulges); any need for materials to fill in creases and create a level surface onto which the bag can adhere; any need for a belt or rigid faceplate (e.g. to push back abdominal bulges overhanging the stoma); the shape of bag that will best fit in with the patient's body contours and clothes.

(e) Assess the patient's skin protective requirements: ask whether there is any history of skin disease, diabetes, reaction to plaster/surgical tape or plastic, burning easily with minimal exposure to the sun.

These all indicate a substantial skin protective such as a hydrocolloid adhesive will probably be required. Note any signs of skin redness, damage, or undue dryness or sogginess, which may indicate reactions to particular equipment or effluent coming in contact with the skin.

(f) Assess the patient's capabilities for using the style of equipment currently in use or likely to be needed: this may include their manual dexterity and ability to: use taps/clips; cut openings in peristomal wafers; apply paste to fill in any abdominal creases present; use a belt.

(g) Assess the patient's preferences and lifestyle: their activities at work, socially, and at home, and whether they will necessitate particular requirements (e.g. a secure enough adhesive to stay in place during sports or when grandchildren climb on a lap; a large enough bag to contain the effluent passed in lengthy meetings at work).

From the information gained in steps e, f and g, *summarise criteria* about the style of appliance and skin care aids that should suit this particular patient.

(h) Assess the appliances and skin care aids available: identify those which meet most or all of the criteria developed as a result of the above assessments: The appliance and aids then chosen by patient and nurse should allow fulfilment of the aims of the assessment, whether this is through a major change in equipment or a relatively minor adjustment to their normal equipment and stoma care.

When we show patients what is being assessed, why and how, they learn how to assess their situation and needs more accurately if further adjustments to their stoma care are required or if problems arise at a later date. This usually helps them feel more confident that problems can be dealt with effectively.

SITUATIONS WHERE PROBLEMS HAVE NOT BEEN IDENTIFIED

Potential or actual problems may not be identified for several reasons, including:

- changes in patients' conditions and abilities to manage self-care occurring too slowly to be recognised as problematic or in need of review
- lack of medical or nursing follow-up where stomal management could have been monitored

- lack of awareness in patients or staff that treatments and equipment to resolve problems exist
- lack of awareness of the significance of changes in appearance or function of the stoma, skin or equipment. Appropriate investigations or treatment may therefore not be sought or offered.

People with stomas should learn how to recognise the normal appearance and function of their stoma, skin and equipment, and when alterations in these warrant further investigation and treatment. Some of this information should be acquired when they learn stoma care at the time of their surgery (see Ch. 4) and more will be gained as a result of living with their stoma. In the early months after stoma formation monitoring of the stoma, skin and equipment should take place through appointments with the stoma care nurse on home or clinic visits, during medical check-ups, or while receiving care from their district nurse. As patients' stomas settle down and become relatively trouble-free, monitoring can be reduced in frequency until an annual or alternate year assessment can be made.

Routine monitoring usually includes four components:

1. Examination of the stoma, peristomal skin, and equipment.
2. Confirmation to patients of satisfactory elements such as the stoma colour, skin condition etc., where this is found to be the case. This helps them learn to recognise normality.
3. Specific teaching about aspects of the stoma or skin which patients might not know are normal, and thus need to learn or be reassured about. *For example:*
   - peristaltic or wiggling movements of the stoma
   - minimal bleeding of the stoma during cleansing
   - an initial red flush of the skin when stomal equipment is removed, coupled with the information that this normally fades as they continue their stoma care.
4. Discussion with patients to establish whether they have any concerns or problems about their stoma and its function or management.

Signs of intermittent problems (e.g. skin reactions, leakage, faulty equipment) may not be apparent during routine appointments. It is therefore important to ask patients for their opinion as to how their stoma, peristomal skin, and equipment are performing overall. This helps patients recall and describe intermittent problems which can then be addressed.

DIAGNOSIS AND TREATMENT

PROBLEMS WITH THE STOMA ITSELF

Bleeding from the surface of the stoma

Stomas are formed from a section of everted bowel, which is highly vascular. Minimal spotting of blood on the material used to clean the stoma and surrounding skin may occur, and is sometimes referred to as 'contact bleeding'. This is not normally serious.

Surface bleeding can also occur if the stoma is being traumatised, for example through rubbing on the stoma of too tight or too rigid an appliance flange. Bleeding can be more severe in such circumstances, and an indentation in the stoma, or a ridge or granuloma on it, may also be present, signalling that pressure or friction has occurred over a period of time.

Treatment

The appliance gasket size should be reviewed to ensure it is 3 mm clear of the stoma right down to the base. If the stoma size varies it is advisable to use equipment with a pliable gasket, and make radial slits in the hole of any protective wafer used so it can expand if the stoma does whilst maintaining good skin protection.

Bleeding from the lumen of the stoma

This is potentially more serious and may be due to a variety of causes. These include peptic ulceration, erosion of a blood vessel from malignancy, or Crohn's disease. Simulated bleeding may occur if foodstuffs or drugs which discolour urine or faeces are taken. For example, beetroot may colour urine red (Black 2000, p 180). Other agents that can cause discolouration are indicated in Chapters 6 and 17.

Treatment

Prompt referral to a doctor should be made if bleeding from the stoma lumen occurs so that the cause can be ascertained and treated without delay.

Alterations in colour

The stoma should be a healthy red colour similar to that of the lining of the cheek. A pallid or colourless stoma may indicate patients are anaemic. A dark purple or brownish looking stoma usually indicates the stoma has a poor blood supply.

Treatment

Prompt referral to a doctor should take place, particularly if symptoms of impairment of the blood supply occur in the early postoperative period. Careful and frequent monitoring of the stoma should be maintained and documented so that a clear record of any changes is available to aid decisions about treatment. It is also prudent to check that the stomal equipment is not constricting the stoma in any way since stomas can increase in size and a larger gasket size may be needed.

Sometimes an outer 'skin' sloughs off, leaving a healthy stoma in place. However, on some occasions further surgery may be required. This may entail pulling the bowel further out without re-opening the abdomen, but laparotomy and excision of gangrenous bowel may be necessary.

Occasionally the condition *melanosis coli* is found at surgery. This is a dark brown or black discolouration of the colon caused by the patient taking frequent strong purgatives. This condition must be recorded in the medical notes of both the hospital and family doctor, as well as appropriate nursing notes, to prevent the stoma colour being thought to be due to a poor blood supply at a later date.

Ulceration of the stoma

In each of the three main situations when ulceration may occur the cause is rubbing of the appliance against the stoma. Firstly, if the appliance opening is too small it will slide partially over the stoma and then rub against that section of the stoma where it lodges because it is too tight to go down to the base. This often creates a ridge or scar. Effluent may pool beneath the appliance where it does not rest on the peristomal skin. This situation is therefore often reported as a problem of leakage or damaged skin, and the stomal ulceration only noted on examination.

Secondly, a stoma that becomes larger, such as through prolapse, can result in the appliance opening becoming generally too small if the stoma remains prolapsed, or intermittently too small if the prolapse occurs from time to time.

Thirdly, ulceration may be caused by an appliance that depends on a belt to maintain its position. If the stoma site is unsuitable for such an appliance and/or the belt rides up the patient's abdomen instead of being worn level with the stoma, then the flange can seesaw around the stoma, or be pulled off-centre and rub against the stoma.

Treatment

The stoma should be carefully measured to ensure that the appliance opening is large enough to accommodate the stoma without friction or constraint, and can rest on the peristomal skin at the base of the stoma. Where ulceration is caused by variations in stoma size a flexible flange may be used, and radial slits made in the hole of any protective wafer used, so both can expand if the stoma does.

Use of a two-piece appliance will enable the stoma to be cleansed and pectin/gelatin protective powder applied twice daily to aid healing (Blackley 2004).

Prolapse

In this condition a length of bowel prolapses out onto the exterior of the abdomen. It occurs most often in transverse loop colostomies. Distal loop prolapse is most common although the proximal loop, or both distal and proximal openings, may prolapse. Urostomy or ileostomy prolapses are less common. The degree of bowel protrusion can vary, as can the problems arising from it.

Treatment

Prolapses need to be carefully assessed because of their potential ability to create problems either in themselves or if unsuitable equipment is used. For example, intestinal obstruction can occur if a proximal loop of bowel prolapses and becomes kinked. If patients continue to use their normal (and now too small) gasket size of appliance then this can constrict the blood supply to their stoma, creating ulceration, oedema, or even necrosis. Medical as well as nursing assessment is advisable (McErlain et al 2004).

Black (2000, p 136) suggests that in some instances the prolapse can be reduced when patients are lying flat by wrapping ice in a towel and applying it to the stoma. When the oedema has subsided, the prolapse can be manipulated back through the abdominal wall. A rigid plastic shield can be applied over the stoma bag and kept in place with a belt in order to contain the prolapse. Blackley (2004) reports that some centres manage a sliding prolapse by applying a wide, firm, elasticised belt. If the stoma is temporary then the prolapse is usually dealt with when the stoma is closed. However, if the stoma is likely to be permanent and the prolapse could be, or is, causing more major problems then surgical correction may be necessary.

With a fairly small prolapse an appliance that is large enough to accommodate the stoma and has a suitable style and size of gasket to prevent ulceration (see above) may be used to physically manage it. Patients often find prolapses somewhat alarming, particularly when they first occur, and in the longer term may find them unsightly and difficult to conceal under clothes. This can lead some people to feel less socially and sexually acceptable and, in some instances, to curtail their normal work and social activities. It is therefore important that physical treatment and advice on management of suitable equipment is coupled with psychological support. Advice to report any change in bowel function (which could indicate obstruction) or stoma colour (which could indicate ischaemia) needs to be carefully delivered. Patients should acquire the ability and confidence to monitor their situation and know when to seek help without becoming unduly anxious and constantly checking for problems.

Retraction

This may arise if patients have gained weight since stoma formation, causing the stoma to recede in relation to the surrounding abdomen. Retraction can also occur as a result of tension on the bowel. For example, if insufficient bowel was mobilised when the stoma was created; through insufficient fixing of the bowel to support it generally or when the bridge of a loop stoma is removed; or if spread of malignant disease in the peristomal area tethers the bowel.

Stomas may appear satisfactory when patients are standing but retract when they lie flat. Patients may therefore say they have a problem of leakage under their appliance at night. When the stoma retracts, pooling of effluent around the stoma occurs so an alternative presenting problem voiced by patients may be that they have damaged peristomal skin.

Treatment

Retraction may also lead to stenosis of the stoma (see later) so assessment for both should be carried out. Some patients would benefit from losing weight. They should be given suitable information about eating and exercise to help them achieve weight loss.

The aim of management is to make the stoma stand out more from the abdomen, thus minimising effluent pooling at skin level. This is usually best achieved through use of a convex flange (Fig. 21.1). Convex systems should be fitted and monitored by

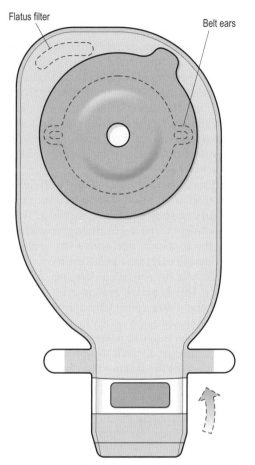

Figure 21.1 Convex flange. Convex area flattens the peristomal area and helps the stoma spout to stand out more.

staff experienced in their use as they can damage the stoma (Black 2000). Extra skin protection with pastes or washers may also be necessary (Blackley 2004, Boyd et al 2004).

If a convex flange cannot be used, then a rigid style of faceplate and a belt can be used with the same goal of making the stoma protrude. Sometimes the stoma site is unsuitable for a belt because it will ride up or down over the patient's body, or be uncomfortable if positioned correctly (i.e. level with the stoma). A third alternative is to use a rigid faceplate or flanged appliance and apply adhesive tape close in to the gasket and over the belt 'ears'. This encourages the stoma to protrude and the abdomen to flatten immediately around the gasket (Fig. 21.2a, b, c). In some instances surgery to refashion and/or reposition the stoma may be required.

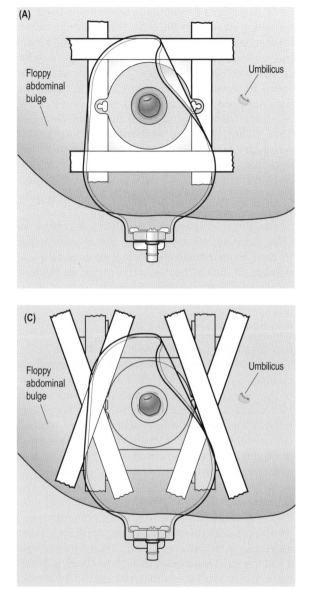

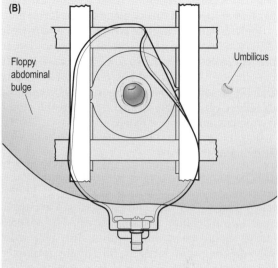

Figure 21.2 Use of adhesive tape to 'weight' belt ears and flatten the peristomal area (splinting). (a) First layer of tape applied around gasket ring and *under* belt ears. (b) Second layer of tape applied vertically across belt ears. (c) Third layer of tape applied diagonally as an X across each belt ear to prevent equipment lifting at the sides.

Stenosis

In this condition the outlet of the stoma becomes narrowed, sometimes almost closed. It can be caused by inappropriate techniques used when creating the stoma, or by formation of scar tissue.

- Patients with urinary stomas may have dark coloured or malodorous urine, loin pain, or recurrent urinary infections.
- Patients with bowel stomas may describe having pain when formed stools pass through the stoma; abdominal cramps; or an intermittent pattern of stomal action.

Treatment

Possible stenosis of urinary stomas must be investigated promptly as this can affect the urinary tract (Blackley 2004).

If stenosis is not severe, gentle stomal dilatation may be prescribed once or twice daily. A gloved lubricated finger can be used or metal dilators, starting with the smallest and moving to a larger one (Black 2000). Dilatation must be done carefully to prevent further tissue damage or scar formation.

Patients with bowel stomas may benefit from dietary advice and stool softening medication to prevent faeces becoming so solid they cannot easily pass through the reduced bowel lumen (see Chs 16 and 17). In some instances surgery may be required to relieve obstruction locally, refashion the stoma completely, and resite it where necessary.

Severing of the stoma

This occasionally occurs as a result of road traffic accidents or if very vigorous activities are undertaken whilst wearing a sliding or seesawing appliance (see ulceration section, above). The severed stoma should be covered with a firm petroleum jelly dressing and medical aid sought promptly. Refashioning of the stoma may be necessary.

Mutilation of the stoma

Occasionally patients may present with severely cut and/or bleeding stomas for which no likely cause is found even after careful assessment and observation of the patient's normal techniques of managing their stoma care. The possibility that the patient is mutilating the stoma should then be considered. Sensitive handling of such a situation is essential.

Treatment

The lack of reports of stoma mutilation in the literature could indicate that this condition is rare. The following suggestions for treatment are based on my experience with only three patients (seen over a period of 12 years in post as a stoma care nurse) where it was thought highly likely that self-mutilation was taking place. *In each case the patient appeared to have no conscious memory of damaging the stoma.* The experience they reported was that they found the stoma damaged, and had not been engaged in any unusual activities or care of the stoma. Their normal style of stoma care was observed, and assessed as appropriate and competent.

In the first case the patient vehemently denied damaging the stoma, and was considerably distressed to discover that staff thought this might be the case. Counselling was provided to enable the patient to deal with a number of concerns and problems, and as these were resolved or minimised, so the cuts and bleeding from the stoma reduced and finally disappeared.

In the light of that first experience I used the following strategy in the other two situations where I believed self-mutilation could be occurring. Firstly, the patients were told that I did not know what caused the stoma damage. Secondly, staff were asked to avoid expressing any opinion that these patients were mutilating their stoma, and not to suggest patients should admit they were doing so. This created a calm supportive atmosphere in which to engage in the third step. Each patient was told that, in my experience, this kind of damage often indicated that the person was involved in a stressful or problematic situation and that dealing with those problems appeared to lead to cessation of the stoma damage. Both patients accepted the offer of counselling sessions and, as they were helped to deal more effectively with their situations, so damage to their stoma ceased. Further research on this aspect of stoma care is desirable.

Additional material on the stoma

Growth of the patient's underlying disease

Occasionally recurrent Crohn's disease or cancer can be found on the stoma itself. This visible reminder of their disease can be distressing. Patients require psychological support to deal with it as well as prompt referral for medical assessment and any relevant treatment. Regular monitoring for possible stenosis is required, and equipment may need to be changed to accommodate both the stoma and growth.

Granuloma

Excess granulated tissue may form, sometimes as a result of friction from an ill-fitting appliance. It can also occur in response to a foreign body, for example a suture, so careful examination to check whether there is any extraneous material should take place (Blackley 2004). Where difficulty in fitting the appliance or persistent bleeding occurs the granuloma can be cauterised using a silver nitrate pencil, obtainable from chemists (Blackley 2004, Porrett & Joels 1996, p 287). Medical consultation to identify other causes or factors for consideration is advisable before cauterisation. For example, some authorities suggest silver nitrate can cause inflammatory responses or metabolic disturbances (Nelson 1999) so long-term use could be inadvisable.

Epithelialisation

This can develop with some urinary stomas and may lead to stomal stenosis. The stoma gains a pearly-white corrugated appearance as the squamous epithelium grows in from the surrounding skin to replace the bowel mucosa, often over a lengthy period of time. Patients should be advised to seek medical help promptly if their normal free passage of urine from their stoma appears to be lessening. A silver nitrate pencil can be used to remove excess tissue but, as indicated above, this may now be deemed inappropriate for frequent or ongoing use.

Phosphate deposits

The normal pH of urine is 6.5 (slightly acid) but infected urine tends to become alkaline, encouraging the growth of phosphate crystals on and around the stoma. These deposits can cause friction and bleeding from the stoma with subsequent ulceration and infection. Substantial growth can also impede stomal action, so monitoring that output is freely flowing is important.

Treatment Acidification can help to reduce infection and deposits, and also the blue discolouration of peristomal skin and appliances which some patients report. This can be achieved either by bathing the affected area at least twice daily using a 5% acetic acid solution, or through application of acetic acid in a gel base such as Aci-Jel. This is discussed in Chapter 6, as is the use of ascorbic acid and cranberry juice.

Patients should preferably wear a two-piece appliance so that the deposits are easily accessible through removal of the bag. Flange removal is minimised, helping preserve skin integrity. This treatment is often slow to show results, and patients should be periodically encouraged to persist with it.

SKIN AND PERISTOMAL PROBLEMS

Mucocutaneous separation

This disruption to the suture line between stoma and skin sometimes occurs in the early postoperative period. Various causes include tension on the suture line, sometimes associated with difficulties exteriorising the stoma (Blackley 2004); infection; and delayed healing (Boyd-Carson et al 2004). The ensuing cavity may be wide and deep, with exudate creating infection and difficulties in appliance adhesion.

Treatment

Small clean areas can be irrigated with warmed normal saline and then protected with pectin/gelatin paste. Use of two-piece appliances enables observa-

tion, cleansing and replacement of protective paste to foster healing while minimising skin damage from frequent bag changes.

Larger areas, particularly where sloughy tissue is present, can also be irrigated with saline. This should be warmed to body temperature to prevent wound cooling, which reduces effective healing (Boyd-Carson et al 2004). The opening in the appliance flange should be cut large enough to ensure that the base will adhere to intact peristomal skin, and allow desloughing agents to be used in the cavity as appropriate (Blackley 2004).

Herniation

Parastomal hernias can arise if there is a weakness in the abdominal wall. They are more common around colostomies than ileostomies or urostomies (Blackley 2004, p 201). Pringle & Swan (2001) reported that a year after surgery one in five of the surviving colostomists in their study had an abdominal hernia. The majority of hernias, even sizeable ones, can be treated conservatively. However, symptoms of acute pain, nausea and vomiting may indicate that the herniated loop of bowel is becoming strangulated and the blood supply could be cut off. Patients should be clearly told to seek medical advice promptly if these symptoms occur.

The problems patients generally report include:

- a persistent dull ache due to the weight of the hernia dragging on the abdominal wall
- difficulty in appliance adherence to the bulging hernia contours, resulting in equipment lifting and possible leakage
- anxiety and distress at this additional alteration to their body image and concern that this bulge could be cancerous.

Treatment

Medical assessment is advisable to establish whether surgical repair is appropriate, and to rule out any underlying complications. Repeat herniation after surgery can occur, particularly in patients with lax abdominal muscles. Patients are (understandably) often keener to have surgical repair than doctors are to provide it, as a large hernia can substantially reduce their quality of life.

The weight of a substantial hernia dragging constantly on the abdominal wall is sometimes likened to being permanently pregnant and can be equally tiring. It creates a bulge that makes wearing normal clothes difficult. Special corsets can be obtained on prescription from several companies, individually fitted to provide support and accommodate the patient's stomal equipment. Black (2000, p 136) suggests patients should put their corset on first thing on waking, so maximum support is applied before the hernia starts to protrude.

Stomal equipment should be reviewed regularly as changes in hernia size and shape may necessitate changes in the equipment and how it is used. The adhesive area may need to be increased, for example, by using a larger peristomal wafer or additional tape. Increased moulding to the bulge can be achieved by making small radial slits around the outer edges of flange/wafer. Change from a substantial or rigid faceplate to a more flexible one can increase adherence and thus reduce leakage, as may a change to a more flexible peristomal wafer.

Patients' lifestyles should also be reviewed. A counselling approach is generally more helpful than blanket advice-giving as patients will need support to face up to the likelihood that changes in their body image and lifestyle (e.g. to avoid lifting anything heavy) are probably going to be permanent. Counselling may also elicit fears of underlying disease, enabling appropriate information and reassurance to be given (Blackley 2004).

Skin damage

Patients with damaged skin should seek help promptly. Initially damage is often localised and its position can help identify possible causes. These can be loosely divided into three areas:

- reaction to stoma care products
- use of inappropriate stomal equipment or stoma care processes
- exacerbation of a skin condition which the patient already has.

Reaction to stoma care products

Modern hypoallergenic equipment has reduced the numbers of patients reacting to stoma products. However, Lyon (2001) found 85% of patients attending a dermatology/stoma care clinic felt their skin reactions were due to product allergies. Tests revealed few were allergic. Where reactions do occur their shape often matches that of the product causing it, particularly in the early stages. If left untreated, reactions can become more widespread, creating more difficulties in treatment and much discomfort for patients.

Treatment

Where reaction to the bag flange occurs assessment should establish whether the patient should continue with the same appliance (e.g. because the style particularly suits them), or change to an appliance with a different adhesive type. Often a peristomal wafer can be used beneath the usual appliance to prevent contact between skin and bag adhesive. Any overlap of flange plaster beyond the wafer should be removed.

If skin damage is minor a lesser degree of protection may be adequate. A non-greasy cream (e.g. E45) or a skin-forming wipe (e.g. Cavilon) can be applied sparingly to the skin beneath the flange. These products can also be used if the flange or peristomal wafer adheres so firmly to the skin that removal of it during equipment changes creates damage. This can occur if equipment is changed rather frequently, perhaps because of leakage/ lifting at one point whilst the rest of the equipment remains firmly stuck down.

Some patients have problems where the bag itself is in contact with their body. Use of an appliance with a fabric backing may prevent sweating or skin reactions, but a cotton bag-cover which encompasses the whole bag may be more effective.

Use of inappropriate stomal equipment or stoma care processes

Completing a full assessment as described earlier will normally identify whether stomal equipment being used is inappropriate and likely to be contributing to skin damage. *For example:* someone with a sigmoid colostomy may be using a colostomy bag with a small area of light adhesive suitable for adherence when stomal action is fairly solid. If their stomal effluent becomes fluid the bag will probably lift frequently, and/or allow seepage of effluent under the adhesive, creating skin damage both from leakage and frequent bag changes. The area of skin damaged may be fairly generalised around the stoma. Use of appropriate equipment, plus revision of the patient's diet, medication and medical situation, should take place to establish the cause of the more fluid effluent and treatment required.

When no obvious cause of skin damage is found it is useful to review patients' stoma care more widely. *For example:*

- the specific procedure whereby the patient changes their appliance (preferably watching a change being done)

- agents used to clean the stoma and peristomal skin (a) at home, (b) away from home, and whether these could affect the skin condition or appliance adhesion
- the frequency with which equipment is changed, and whether this is more or less often than would provide good skin protection
- whether there are any difficulties changing equipment when it needs changing (e.g. awaiting assistance from family or healthcare team)
- whether the patient has psychological difficulties coping with (a) effluent in their bag or (b) carrying out stoma care, which could affect their stoma care management.

Where alterations in patients' usual stoma care should be made in order to prevent skin damage it is helpful to first identify their goals when carrying out their current system. This enables alternatives to be suggested which are compatible with those goals.

For example: a patient who believes the only way he will not smell (his goal) is to have an empty bag may believe he has to endure sore skin as the price for changing bags immediately after stomal action. Information about the odour-containing nature of modern equipment reducing the need for frequent changes may have no effect on what he does. However, he may be willing to change from a one-piece to a two-piece appliance, or from a closed to a drainable bag, so that he can change the bag but not the base, or rinse out the drainable bag after emptying it, thus reducing the number of times equipment is removed from his skin. This alteration in his stoma care is congruent with his goals of not smelling, and feeling socially clean. Depending on the amount of bowel he has left to function above his stoma diversion, this patient might also be eligible to use colostomy plugs (see Ch. 4) or irrigation (see Ch. 15).

Lyon (2001) reports the prevalence of different causes of skin conditions in his study:

- irritant reactions from effluent leakage: 40%
- infections: 11%
- allergic contact dermatitis: 0.4%
- pre-existing skin diseases, particularly psoriasis and eczema: 20%
- pyoderma gangrenosum: 0.6%.

Certain *patterns* of skin damage indicate the first three of these causes could be present, including the four patterns described below.

(1) A red, sore, or soggy-looking area of skin immediately around the stoma

The likely cause is lack of skin protection due to the opening in the flange/peristomal wafer being so large that effluent can collect on that area of skin. This may be because an inappropriate size of flange or wafer hole is being used. However, it can be due to equipment being left on so long that the skin protective melts away. Effluent can collect there and damage skin.

Treatment   The stoma should be measured and the gasket size and/or the hole being cut in the adhesive revised to ensure they will fit properly and protect the skin from effluent. It is also important to check that equipment openings are large enough as, if not, they can lodge part of the way down the stoma instead of around the base, which enables effluent to pool underneath them. Hydrocolloid adhesives should fit snugly around the base of the stoma at skin level. If a stoma changes size or shape (e.g. due to gut motility or prolapse) then radial slits can be cut in the opening, creating some flexibility if the stoma expands or contracts. Appliances should leave about 3 mm gap around the stoma, particularly those with rigid gaskets. Filler paste or a peristomal washer can be used to give extra skin protection if needed.

On removing used equipment its undersurface should be examined to ascertain where and to what degree it has disintegrated since application. This helps establish the frequency of changes required to prevent exposure of the underlying skin and whether there may be abdominal dips and gullies requiring additional filling in to create a level surface for the equipment.

A similar pattern of skin damage and/or equipment disintegration can also be found where stomas retract, as described earlier. It is therefore important to observe the stoma and abdomen to see if this is occurring, and also to assess whether abdominal dips and gullies (signalled as possibly present by hydrocolloid disintegration) are actually there and needing attention.

(2) A semi-circle of damaged skin immediately below the stoma

This pattern of skin damage is often found if the stoma is tilted and effluent becomes directed downwards onto the skin below it rather than outwards into the appliance. On examination (particularly when patients are standing) their abdomen often bulges out above the stoma but not below it. When

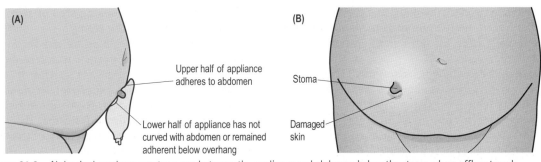

Figure 21.3   Abdominal overhang creates a gap between the appliance and abdomen below the stoma where effluent pools, particularly if stoma tilts downwards. (a) Effects of an overhang are usually best seen from side view when patients are standing. (b) Skin damage typically occurs below the stoma where effluent is pooling. Overhang and gap between equipment and abdomen may not be visible from front view, particularly if patients are lying down.

equipment is applied it rests on the overhang above the stoma but leaves a gap under the stoma into which effluent pools (Fig. 21.3a and b).

Treatment   The aim is to create a level peristomal area, thus preventing stoma tilt and enabling all round equipment adherence. A convex flange, or a rigid faceplate and belt, or supportive tape, can be used as described earlier for retraction. Alternatively, the area under the stoma can be built up by application of half a peristomal ring or wafer. This creates a level abdomen all around the stoma onto which the usual appliance can be fitted. Initially the build-up may be fitted separately in order to judge the amount required. Once this is known some patients prefer to stick the building-up material to the undersurface of their flange first, then apply it as an all-in-one system. This is particularly helpful if stomal action is frequent or unpredictable and speedy application of new equipment is desirable.

(3) Patches of damaged skin beside the stoma

These often indicate the presence of an abdominal dip or gully into which effluent is leaking beneath the appliance. Patients may report that leakage occurs or the appliance lifts in that area. Examination of the undersurface of the appliance/wafer will often reveal it has melted just where that pooled effluent occurs. Examination of patients (particularly when sitting) usually reveals the gullies.

Treatment   A level peristomal area should be created to prevent pooling, leakage and skin damage. Either the abdomen can be flattened using a convex flange or rigid faceplate, or small amounts of filler paste or pieces of peristomal ring/wafer can be used to fill in the gully. A peristomal wafer will then usually be

applied over these fillers, creating a level surface. An appliance that has an integral hydrocolloid flange can be used, or a wafer can be applied under a bag with a less substantial adhesive.

(4) Shiny, tightly–stretched looking skin, often bright red

This type of skin damage may occur under part or all of the appliance adhesive, and can be a skin reaction to that adhesive. However, bacterial and fungal infections can also create similar skin appearances, which look rather like an early sunburn reaction.

Treatment   Lyon (2001) reports that routine swabbing is advisable as the appearance of fungal and bacterial infections under appliances may be atypical. Where treatment is necessary the agents used must be compatible with appliance usage. Peristomal wafers will generally adhere over sprays, lotions and powders. The stoma should be covered whilst applying treatment to prevent absorption through the stomal mucosa.

Blackley (2004) suggests patients may be more at risk of fungal infections (e.g. *Candida albicans*) if they have moist denuded skin and may be immunosuppressed because they are taking corticosteroids or antibiotics. She suggests:

- apply antifungal lotion or powder sparingly for 3 weeks to eliminate the infection and avert potential recurrence
- use an appliance system which can adhere to the skin for several days whilst enabling effluent to be discarded (e.g. two-piece, enabling bag changes, or drainable appliances).

Routine use of antibacterial agents for skin protection is inadvisable as it could reduce their effectiveness in dealing with future local or systemic infections. Steps to reduce potential problems include:

- shaving of intact hairy peristomal skin (to minimise warm moist conditions conducive to infection)
- use of a hairdryer on a low setting to help dry skin gently but thoroughly following cleansing.

Exacerbation of skin conditions which patients already have

Patients with known skin conditions, allergies and sensitivities (e.g. to plasters, make-up, sun) will usually have been patch-tested prior to surgery. However, if problems arise further tests can be conducted to identify the nature of the problem and suitable treatment and equipment to resolve it. Joint appointments with a dermatologist and stoma care nurse enable assessment to be holistic and treatments to be prescribed in a format compatible with appliance usage. Possible peristomal problems include:

- manifestation of pre-existing skin conditions
- pyoderma gangrenosum
- sensitivity to particular substances
- skin-related reactions to situations.

Management in each of these situations involves minimising trauma to the peristomal skin coupled with treatment to resolve the problem and subsequently prevent its recurrence. Trauma to peristomal skin is minimised by achieving a balance between:

- changing stomal equipment often enough to prevent skin protectives melting and leaving skin exposed to effluent, *and*
- peeling equipment off peristomal skin infrequently enough to avoid skin damage.

Generally this balance is achieved by using equipment with a hydrocolloid adhesive. Two-piece equipment enables the base to remain in situ whilst bags are changed more frequently. Alternatively, a drainable bag can be used to allow effluent disposal whilst leaving the bag in place.

Psoriasis and eczema appear to be the most common *pre-existing skin conditions* perhaps due to an association between them and inflammatory bowel disease (Lyon 2001). Treatment with moderate strength corticosteroids in lotion form enables stomal equipment adhesion to be maintained. Lyon (2001) suggests that, because topical steroids can result in skin damage and systemic absorption, continuous treatment should be restricted to 4 weeks, and occasional treatments to a maximum of once every 10–14 days.

If oily topical treatment has to be used a large semi-permeable film dressing can be used to cover the treated peristomal skin and provide a surface for appliance adherence (Blackley 2004).

Pyoderma gangrenosum is an inflammatory skin disorder associated with inflammatory bowel disease as well as other conditions (Burch 2004). It can present as painful ulcerations which exude purulent or serosanguineous fluid and fail to heal. Lesions have dusky blue margins and an erythematous halo (Blackley 2004). Lyon (2001) found more than half the patients with recurrent pyoderma gangrenosum used convex appliances. He suggests that they can cause pressure to the skin, which then precipitates this condition in predisposed patients.

Systemic treatment of the underlying condition is usually required as well as local treatment and equipment review (Burton 2003). Small ulcers can be treated with corticosteroid lotions. Pain relief may be required before treatment of larger ulcerations, either with oral analgesics or with a topical anaesthetic gel (Blackley 2004). Lyon (2001) reports that treatment with topical tacrolimus in a carmellose sodium paste to allow bag adherence has given a 75% success rate.

Where possible when patients appear to have a *sensitivity to stomal equipment* the cause should be ascertained and treated. Some patients develop dermatitis through contact with an appliance over time. This could be due to ongoing occlusion of the peristomal skin or ingredients used in stoma care. In some instances patients may need to change equipment each time this occurs. Short-term use of topical steroids before using the different equipment can help reduce immediate inflammatory responses (Blackley 2004).

Some patients have *conditions that are problematic and appear to be skin-related*. For example, they may report that appliances seem to stick less well or for shorter times under certain circumstances, or when stressed. The need to cope with unpredictable or extra bag changes can itself be stressful, creating a self-perpetuating cycle of stress production. A careful history needs to be taken to establish whether there are recognisable factors which either need to be dealt with because they trigger stress, or need to be taken account of because their presence makes it more likely the problem will occur. For example, women who find equipment lifts more often during menstruation may benefit from accepting as normal the need to accommodate extra monitoring and changes of equipment within their usual lifestyle at such times. Likewise, people who are experiencing stressful situations can be encouraged both to deal with the cause of the stress (to reduce its effect on appliance adherence), and to manage their time so extra bag changes can be easily included in their schedule if needed.

Some patients report peristomal skin irritation which may or may not be linked to damaged skin. Calamine lotion can act as a soothing agent, and peristomal wafers will usually adhere on top of the dried lotion. Where there is a persistent sense of skin irritation but the skin appears normal and intact, it is advisable to consider whether the patient is stressed or trying to express a need for help.

For example: a patient reported persistent itchy peristomal skin soon after formation of her urostomy. Examination on several occasions had revealed no skin damage. She was told that I had no doubt she was experiencing irritation, and substantial discomfort from it. I then told her such circumstances sometimes occurred when people were stressed or having problems either generally or because they were coming to terms with having a stoma. In response she began to talk about two bereavements she had suffered at the time of her surgery. The focus moved to identifying sources of help where she could get acceptable support to deal with these losses and her new body image. She was assured that she could continue to have her peristomal area and equipment checked, and ready access to the stoma care service. She found this acceptance and the bereavement counselling she subsequently obtained helpful. Her skin remained intact and the irritation disappeared.

PROBLEMS IN STOMAL FUNCTION – BOWEL STOMAS

Patients can become constipated or have diarrhoea just like other people. However, the implications of such altered bowel function can be more significant for them both in terms of what could be causing the constipation or diarrhoea (e.g. recurrent cancer or Crohn's disease) and in the effects it can have on someone with a shortened bowel pathway and no anal sphincter.

Since the terms 'constipation' and 'diarrhoea' are used to describe a wide range of stomal actions the first step is to get a specific description of the effluent from the patient, including:

- consistency and colour of effluent
- frequency and amount of stomal action per 24 hours
- whether there is any other material being passed, e.g. excess mucus or wind, any blood or undigested food
- whether there is *an alternating pattern* of constipation and diarrhoea, which could signal constipation with overflow is occurring
- length of time the problem has been occurring.

It is also useful to ask in what way the changed stomal action is of concern/problematic to them. This helps establish the interpretation patients are putting on their situation and the size of the problem as they experience it. Sometimes all someone needs is further information. *For example:* now that they are eating normal-sized meals instead of the small light meals taken postoperatively the move to two larger semi-solid actions from their sigmoid colostomy per day is normal and does not constitute diarrhoea.

A fuller assessment would normally include:

1. A review of their medical and surgical history, to ascertain:
   - the type of stoma and extent of previous surgery
   - the degree of bowel function likely to be available given the position of the stoma along the bowel pathway and any resections of bowel above the stoma
   - the condition which necessitated stoma surgery and whether it is currently thought to be present or absent
   - the presence of any other medical conditions
   - any medication, treatments and/or special diet being taken.
2. Further information from the patient in addition to that obtained earlier to ascertain:
   - their normal diet and eating patterns, and any changes in these which occurred before or during the period of changed stomal action
   - any changes in medication/treatment/lifestyle/patterns of exercise that have occurred before or during the period of changed stomal action
   - any other symptoms/possible causes the patient or family have noticed (including problems, sources of stress/concern).

The above information helps elicit factors which can affect bowel action but which the patient may not be aware do so, or has not linked to the current situation (Thompson et al 2003).

3. Examination of the patient's abdomen and peristomal area to ascertain:
   - whether there are signs of abdominal distension, tenderness, faecal impaction etc., for which medical aid should be sought.

Digital examination of the stoma may be necessary and should be carried out by staff trained to do so.

Dietary surveys

Careful assessment will often pinpoint causes of problems with enough certainty for relevant information and treatment to be given, and their effects subsequently reviewed. In some instances further information is needed to clarify the problem or to increase patients' understanding of what they can do, or stop doing, in order to minimise difficulties. These patients should be asked to keep a record of their intake and output for 1–2 weeks. This is generally sufficient time for intermittent patterns and interrelated factors to be identifiable. Clear guidance on what to record and why is necessary. Many patients are unaware that their bodies make adjustments in their bowel and urinary functions in order to rebalance their overall body system, so the need to record both should be explained. Suggest patients use black ink so their records can be photocopied as required whilst they retain original documents.

Intake: ask patients to record all:

- food
- snacks
- sweets
- fluids (including alcohol)
- medications.

These need not be measured, but it is helpful to indicate the amount of fluid (e.g. cup, mug) and food portion size (e.g. large, small) which they actually ate and drank and the time taken.

Output: ask patients to record approximate times and amounts of:

- urinary output (e.g. large, small amount)
- faecal output, plus colour and consistency (e.g. few small brown knobs; large amount, soup-like consistency)

- any unusual amounts or timing of flatus or mucus being passed
- any vomiting.

The information thus gained should be carefully reviewed with patients. It helps clarify:

- whether referral to specialist colleagues is advisable
- whether further tests, information and/or treatment are required
- whether adjustments to diet, medication and lifestyle are advisable
- what patients could do to help avoid or minimise difficulties, and whether they need help to do so.

Constipation

This is rarely found in patients with an ascending or transverse colostomy as effluent is diverted from the body before fluid reabsorption in the colon can produce it, but can occur where most of the colon is functioning (e.g. with a sigmoid colostomy). People with ileostomies rarely become constipated, but may report reduced or absent stomal action due to food blockage (see later).

Treatment

A twin-track approach is generally required in order to:

- reduce or remove the causes(s), to prevent re-occurrence
- remove constipated material, relieving the current situation.

Increasing fluid and fibre intake may be sufficient to promote passage of constipated faeces (see Ch. 16). Medication may also be necessary (see Ch. 17, and below). Eating, drinking and exercise patterns should be reviewed (Thompson et al 2003). Thompson et al suggest that twenty minutes of moderate exercise 3–5 times weekly aids peristalsis.

Sometimes lubrication and mechanical stimulation of the bowel via the stoma is also required. Treatment will depend on the cause, how near the stomal opening the faeces lie, and whether the presence of a bowel anastomosis and/or disease in or around the bowel (e.g. cancer) make substantial bowel stimulation inadvisable. These aspects should be discussed with the patient's doctor so that suitable treatment can be identified and coordinated. Due to the lack of a sphincter retention of suppositories is difficult but an irrigation can be used (see Ch. 15). Enemas can be used for faecal removal via an *end* colostomy. If oil is used patients should be asked beforehand whether they are allergic to nuts so nut-containing oils (e.g. arachis) are avoided.

Breckman (1998) suggests the following procedure:

1. Examine the stoma digitally to identify the direction of the colon and rule out the presence of local tumour. Clean the stoma and peristomal skin as usual.
2. Insert a medium-sized Foley catheter well into the stoma and inflate the balloon to 5 ml so it will aid retention of the oil or enema.
3. Apply a drainable bag over the stoma and pass the catheter into the bag so it can be reached through its outlet. Ensure a bag clip and catheter clamp are within easy reach. Instil the warmed oil retention enema gently, then clamp the catheter, tuck it into the bag and apply its clip. (Bag application prior to oil instillation prevents difficulties in adhesion from oil seeping onto the skin.)
4. After 10 minutes (if oil alone is being given) let down the balloon and remove the catheter; reclamp the bag and make the patient comfortable. Remind the patient that faeces may take some time to be passed even with this additional lubrication.

If an enema that will attract fluid by osmosis is also to be given (e.g. sodium phosphate enema, or sodium citrate micro-enema) this should be given after the initial 10 minutes for the oil, and the re-clamped catheter left in situ for a further 10 minutes before removal.

Constipation with overflow

This occurs when faecal fluid passes and impacted faeces is present. The patient may report only diarrhoea or constipation so it is always wise to ask whether an alternating pattern of fluid followed by rock-like faeces is occurring. Digital stomal examination often reveals the impaction but it can occur higher up the colon.

Treatment

Impacted faeces will require removal as described above. Aperients may also be needed to clear impaction higher up the bowel. It is essential for patients to understand the rationale for treatment, particularly if they present the problem as having diarrhoea, or they will not accept the need to stimulate faecal action rather than reduce it.

Ileostomy obstruction

Food blockage is a potential problem for people with ileostomies because the narrow lumen of ileum may not allow passage of undigested foods, particularly high fibre and stringy foods (Meadows 1997). This problem can present as:

- *Partial blockage*: watery explosive stomal actions, which may be intermittent, occur. Abdominal distension and pain, and swelling of the stoma may also be present. Nausea and vomiting are usually absent.
- *Complete blockage*: there is no stomal action; nausea and vomiting are occurring; and the stoma may be discoloured as well as swollen.

Treatment

This generally depends on whether blockage is partial or complete, but if in any doubt patients should seek medical advice promptly.

Partial blockage: if some stomal action is occurring Blackley (2004, p 182) suggests ileostomists can be given the following advice:

- Apply heat from a shower, bath or hot water bottle to relax abdominal muscles.
- Lie on right side massaging the peristomal area towards the stoma to dislodge the food bolus. Change of position to knee chest position with massage may prove successful.
- Ensure the pouch does not constrict the stoma, which may swell. Replace it with a pouch that is cut to fit the oedematous stoma.
- Avoid solids. Maintain intake of oral fluids if some stool is draining from the ileostomy.
- Take nothing orally if no stool has drained recently.
- If no stool has drained for 6 hours seek assistance from the doctor or stoma care nurse.

Complete blockage: if no stool is draining and patients are nauseated and vomiting they should be advised not to take food or drink and to obtain medical advice promptly. Hospitalisation may be necessary, particularly if dehydration and/or electrolyte imbalance occur.

Once problems have been resolved it is advisable to review any guidelines patients have for minimising such problems (see Ch. 16) to ensure they are relevant and are being used appropriately.

Potential constipation due to effects of regular medication

Some drugs, particularly analgesics that are opiate derivatives, reduce gut motility and secretions and thus make constipation likely (see Ch. 17). Patients requiring ongoing pain control require routine medication to prevent constipation as well as their regular analgesic regime, and will need a clear explanation so they accept the need to maintain this dual regime. Constipation may need mechanical clearance as described above. A softener such as lactulose which acts osmotically, principally in the small bowel, to retain fluid may also be needed initially. However, a combination of stimulant and softener may then be useful for maintenance of soft faeces (Sykes 1998).

Diarrhoea

Patients require a realistic sense of the solidity of faeces which their remaining bowel will produce in order to differentiate between this consistency and diarrhoea. Explanations that link the potential consistency with bowel function which may be present/absent (due to their specific surgery and stoma position on the bowel pathway) help patients to recognise when their body is functioning normally or abnormally.

Following standard types of resection and diversion (see Chs 2–5) these consistencies would generally be expected:

- *Ileostomy*: a toothpaste-like consistency, requiring a drainable bag which can be emptied several times daily.
- *Right-sided or transverse colostomies*: a semi-solid or more fluid consistency, usually requiring a drainable bag. If a high fibre diet is taken and a firmer less frequent stool produced this may enable management with a closed bag. A two-piece system may be desirable to allow sufficient bag changes but minimal skin damage through less frequent flange changes.
- *Left-sided colostomy*: a formed or semi-formed consistency with 1–3 daily actions, allowing use of a one- or two-piece bag.

Diarrhoea is the frequent passage of a more watery bowel effluent. Full assessment to identify the cause of diarrhoea should take place as described earlier. In particular the significance of diarrhoea for patients with ileostomies should be recognised: dehydration and electrolyte imbalance can occur rapidly, requiring urgent treatment. Signs of these include dry mouth, decreased urinary output with a darker colour, lethargy, weakness, nausea and vomiting (Blackley 2004).

Causes of diarrhoea can include:

- *Diet*: e.g. oranges, figs, prunes, chocolate, beer, although many people have little problem with small amounts (see also Ch. 16). Blackley (2004, p 182–183) suggests excessive intake of alcohol or fresh fruits with a high sorbitol content (peaches, plums, grapes) are likely to cause fluid stools.
- *Medication*: including some antibiotics and anti-cancer treatments; drugs which increase gut motility (see also Chs 17, 18).
- *Disease and/or obstruction*: e.g. Crohn's disease, cancer, and their effects such as subacute obstruction. Ileostomy obstruction due to food is discussed above.
- Other causes can include infection, electrolyte imbalance, malabsorption and anxiety (Blackley 2004).

Treatment

Stomal equipment may need to be adapted or a different style used which will enable containment of the more fluid faeces, promote good skin protection and prevent leakage. Generally a drainable bag will be required as this provides adequate capacity and enables emptying of effluent without frequent bag changes.

Other treatment will depend upon the cause of the diarrhoea. Medication can be used to reduce gut motility, giving bowel contents a longer transit time in which fluid reabsorption can take place (e.g. loperamide, co-phenotrope, codeine phosphate).

Medication that will 'mop up' intestinal fluid can be given, creating a more bulky stool (e.g. methylcellulose (Celevac) or ispaghula husk (Fybogel)). Patients should be given specific instructions as to how to take these bulkers, which can be prescribed for both constipation and diarrhoea. When given *with plenty of fluid* they create a softer, bulkier (less constipated) stool. For the patient with diarrhoea they should be given *with a small amount of fluid* so they mop up the excess fluid in the bowel, reducing it to more bulky faeces. Patients who are nauseated may find large tablets or granules difficult to take, and prefer smaller-sized medication for reducing gut motility.

Patients should also be advised regarding oral fluid replacements and any electrolyte requirements, particularly if they have an ileostomy (see Ch. 16; Blackley 2004).

PROBLEMS IN STOMAL FUNCTION – URINARY STOMAS

Epithelialisation and phosphate deposits have been discussed earlier. Other problems that arise are often due to the conduit itself being made from bowel, usually ileum, which retains the ability to reabsorb elements from the urine passing through it. Normally the length and construction of the conduit enables urine to flow freely through it, minimising reabsorption. However, if the bowel segment is too long urine can pool in it, giving time for electrolytes to be reabsorbed instead of excreted. Stagnating urine can also become infected. These side effects can, over time, affect the urinary tract thus increasing the likelihood of kidney damage, so monitoring and treatment of recurrent problems is advisable. Mechanical causes of obstruction such as kinking or stenosis of the conduit may require surgery.

Specimens of urine obtained to ascertain the presence of infection *must be obtained from the stoma itself and not from the stoma bag* (see Ch. 6). It is the presence of infection in urine that is within the urinary tract which is important to identify, rather than that which often occurs in the urine collecting in the appliance after elimination. Infected urine often has a pungent offensive odour which is distressing and socially unacceptable to patients. It may also have an alkaline pH instead of the usual acid pH.

Treatment

Antibiotics may be used to deal with substantial infection but should not be routinely prescribed. Patients should maintain a high fluid intake (e.g. a glass or mug of fluid each hour of the day they are awake, with fluids available by their bed to take if they wake during the night). Stott (2000) suggests cranberries help to break up mucus, making it easier to pass, as well as helping to prevent urine becoming alkaline which is linked to urinary infections and calculi. She encourages all individuals with continent urinary diversions and ileal conduits to take cranberries but suggests diabetics should take cranberry tablets rather than the (sweet) juice. However, cranberries should be recommended with caution if patients are taking warfarin as there is

some evidence of interaction between the two (Suvarna et al 2003).

Acidification of urine in the stoma bag by adding two teaspoons of vinegar when the bag is emptied or changed appears to help many patients reduce offensive odour from their urine.

Reabsorption from the ileal conduit

Diabetics may have sugar in their urine reabsorbed from the ileal conduit, so their urine can test negative even when blood sugar levels are raised. As most diabetics now use blood testing this is less likely to cause monitoring difficulties than when urinalysis was used. However, it is important to discuss this possibility with them, so they are aware of it as well as medical and nursing staff involved in their care.

Where patients are receiving anti-cancer drugs which are excreted via the kidneys it is advisable to consider whether reabsorption from the stoma could occur, leading them to be recycled rather than eliminated at the normal rate. For example, some patients whose tests for excretory function were adequate before administration of methotrexate subsequently experienced substantial mouth ulceration of a level usually only found when excretion of the drug is delayed. In these instances the dose of methotrexate given in later courses was considerably reduced in order to minimise tissue damage as it was thought reabsorption of methotrexate via the ileal conduit was taking place, thus prolonging its action.

PROBLEMS WITH STOMAL EQUIPMENT

Faulty equipment

Manufacturers' use of sophisticated systematic quality control systems has minimised the number of faulty appliances supplied to patients. However, it is prudent for patients to habitually test taps on urostomy bags and clips on drainable bags to ensure they can readily open and close their newly applied equipment, especially if they do not carry a spare set of equipment as they go about their usual activities.

Patients should be advised that where two or three appliances in a batch are faulty the used bags, washed clean of effluent, should be returned to the manufacturer (not the chemist), with the batch slip or code number if possible, and details of the fault found. Return of a couple of unused bags may also help manufacturers' investigations.

Patients may describe difficulties with effluent containment or skin reactions as being problems with their equipment. Often the equipment itself is not faulty, but has become unsuitable for use in their changed situation. Use of the assessment procedures described earlier will elicit patients' current situation and the styles of equipment that will now best suit them.

Difficulties with night drainage equipment

Most patients with urinary stomas pass a greater volume of urine overnight than can be contained in their urostomy bag. Some patients choose to wake and empty their bags during the night but the majority connect their stoma bag to night drainage equipment. Some patients use leg bags, particularly if they change their position frequently while sleeping. A history of urostomy bags lifting or leaking at night even though someone is using a night drainage system almost always indicates that urine is not flowing adequately from the stoma bag into the secondary bag. Patients should be taught to pay particular attention to two points in the system when setting it up, and if drainage does not readily occur.

(1) The connection between urostomy bag and night drainage bag tubing

Boxes of urostomy bags usually contain connector taps or tubing for use with night drainage and leg bags. Connectors may need to be kept and cleansed when the bags are discarded so patients always have sufficient connecting equipment. Where manufacturers do not supply secondary drainage equipment with their stoma bags it is essential to check that the connector is of a size and type that is fully compatible with both stoma and night drainage equipment.

Patients must ensure there is no twisting of their stoma bag, for example from tension in the way the equipment is set up, as that can prevent urine flowing from one to the other. A small amount of urine can be left in the urostomy bag so that, following connection to the night drainage system, patients can observe whether it empties freely into the secondary bag before they go to sleep.

(2) The connection between the night drainage tubing and secondary drainage bag

Kinks in the section where the tubing joins the secondary drainage bag opening prevent urine flowing into the bag. The resultant collection of urine in tubing and stoma bag is the commonest cause of leakage from urostomy equipment at night. Correct use of a night drainage hanger (Fig. 21.4) should enable this connecting area to be kept straight, so urine flows into the secondary drainage bag, leaving the urostomy bag reasonably empty (Fig. 21.5).

Demonstration of how, exactly, patients set up their night equipment may reveal they are hanging the secondary equipment too high for their bed height (so urine has to go uphill in the tubing before entering the night drainage bag). They may be lying the night drainage bag on the floor in order to let urine drain down into it, but in so doing kinking the tubing to bag section, or allowing it to twist, creating a blockage. Patients who do not wish to use a hanger may use two safety pins to pin the drainage bag to the bottom bed sheet using the hanger holes. A third safety pin can then be pinned across the tubing just above its connection with the bag to prevent kinking at the join.

Curtailment of fluids during the evening so that less urine is passed overnight should be discouraged. Fluid intake spread over patients' waking hours should be sufficient to produce an output of 1000–1800 ml urine in 24 hours in order to reduce the risk of urinary infection or stone formation.

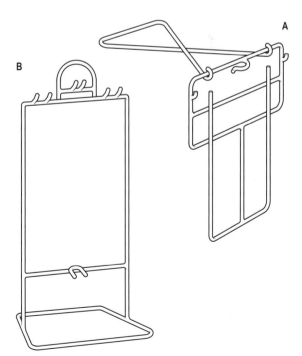

Figure 21.4 Night drainage hangers (a) for attachment to the bed, (b) free standing.

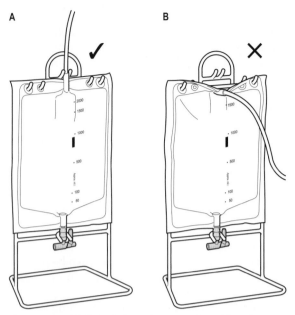

Figure 21.5 (a) Night drainage bag correctly positioned on stand. (b) *Incorrectly* positioned bag, with a kink in the section of tubing where it joins the night drainage bag.

CONCLUSION

Although a wide range of physical problems can occur, these can usually be resolved or substantially reduced. However, when they do occur the degree to which they disrupt and impair patients' lives should not be underestimated (Wade 1989, Pringle & Swan 2001). Systematic assessment coupled with knowledge of, and access to, a range of stomal equipment will enable nurses and patients to pinpoint the likely causes and solutions of problems speedily and effectively.

References

Black P K 2000 Holistic stoma care. Baillière Tindall and RCN, Edinburgh

Blackley P 2004 Practical stoma wound and continence management, 2nd edn. Research Publications, Vermont, Victoria, Australia

Boyd K, Thompson M J, Boyd-Carson W, Trainer B 2004 Use of convex appliances. Nursing Standard 18(20):37–38

Boyd-Carson W, Thompson M J, Boyd K 2004 Mucocutaneous separation. Nursing Standard 18(17):41–42

Breckman B 1998 Stoma management. In: Doyle D, Hanks G W C, MacDonald N (eds) Oxford textbook of palliative medicine, 2nd edn. Oxford University Press: Oxford, p 839–845

Burch J 2004 Pyoderma gangrenosum: a literature review. Gastrointestinal Nursing 2(2):33–38

Burton J 2003 Stories from the bedside: a care study on pyoderma gangrenosum. World Council of Enterostomal Therapists Journal 23(3):35–38

Lyon C L 2001 The skin disorders of abdominal stomas. World Council of Enterostomal Therapists Journal 21(3):40–42

McErlain D, Kane M, McGrogan M 2004 Prolapsed stoma. Nursing Standard 18(18):41–42

Meadows C 1997 Stoma and fistula care. In: Bruce L, Finlay T M D (eds) Nursing in gastroenterology. Churchill Livingstone, New York, p 85–118

Nelson L 1999 Points of friction. Nursing Times 95(34):72–75

Porrett T, Joels J 1996 Continuing care in the community. In: Myers C (ed) Stoma care nursing. Arnold, London, p 283–294

Pringle W, Swan E 2001 Continuing care after discharge from hospital for stoma patients. British Journal of Nursing 10(19):1274–1288

Stott C A 2000 Management of patients with urinary diversions. In: World Council of Enterostomal Therapists congress proceedings. Hollister International, Libertyville, IL, p 22–26

Suvarna R, Pirmohamed L, Henderson L 2003 Possible interaction between warfarin and cranberry juice. British Medical Journal 327:1454

Sykes N P 1998 Constipation and diarrhoea. In: Doyle D, Hanks G W C, MacDonald N (eds) Oxford textbook of palliative medicine, 2nd edn. Oxford University Press, Oxford, p 513–526

Thompson M J, Boyd-Carson W, Trainer B, Boyd K 2003 Management of constipation. Nursing Standard 18(14):41–42

Wade B 1989 A stoma is for life. Scutari Press, Harrow, Middlesex

Chapter 22

Problems in rehabilitation

Brigid Breckman

The dividing line between what constitutes 'normal or general stoma care' and what is classed as 'care to be provided if problems occur' is changing. More has become known about difficulties which patients often experience in the first couple of years after surgery. Therefore management of such problems is now being included in the general stoma care taught to patients and healthcare staff. This is reflected in the material included in Chapters 1–7 in which research has been used to identify common difficulties (e.g. Pringle & Swan 2001, Wade 1989, White 1998) and ways in which they can be effectively managed. Useful ways of generally promoting patients' psychological recovery have been included in Chapters 1 and 7–9, and you can use those approaches in conjunction with the skills and strategies described in this chapter.

Some patients require additional help to achieve the maximum rehabilitation of which they are capable. As indicated in Chapter 1, the third stage of patients' rehabilitation involves integration of the stoma and its management, and other changes arising from their condition and treatment, into their self-image and style of living.

In this chapter the main focus is on helping patients deal with difficulties preventing their achievement of this third stage. The approaches can be used to monitor patients' progress towards rehabilitation as well as problem-solving strategies. They are particularly helpful when working with patients whose rehabilitation is difficult. Some of the processes discussed here may require more advanced levels of practice than you or your colleagues have acquired. As these approaches are described consider which ones you can use now, and which you have yet to learn. You may also like to discuss how they can be learned and used with your supervisor and other colleagues.

The five processes are:

1. accurate identification of patients' current experiences and needs
2. identification of the experience of 'being rehabilitated' which patients seek, and criteria they can use to monitor their progress
3. promotion of goals that enable patients to achieve and maintain their desired levels of rehabilitation
4. monitoring of patients' progress in completing the tasks of grieving for any losses they may be experiencing in order to identify where help with such task completion may be required
5. provision of help which enables patients to complete the tasks of grieving where necessary and thus become freer to focus on present and future needs and goals.

ACCURATE IDENTIFICATION OF PATIENTS' CURRENT EXPERIENCES AND NEEDS

This process can be considered from two perspectives:

(a) monitoring for any effects of past experiences on patients' current wellbeing, so needs arising from them can be identified
(b) clarification of experiences and needs expressed by patients.

Three areas where there is now evidence that past experience is likely to affect stoma patients' subsequent wellbeing are:

- previous experience of loss (see later section on tasks of grieving)
- previous psychological problems
- experience of there being a mismatch between the level of information which the patient wanted when undergoing surgery and that which was provided.

White (1998, 1999) reports that patients who have previously had psychological problems are at risk of experiencing greater levels of psychological difficulty after stoma surgery, particularly anxiety and depressive disorders. Preoperative identification of such experience enables patients' psycho-

logical state to be assessed at that time, providing a baseline with which to compare their present and subsequent wellbeing and identify any help they may need. White (1999) also suggests that knowledge of the features of these disorders will help staff differentiate between reactions that are part of normal adjustment and rehabilitation and the presence of clinically significant mental disorders such as:

- *Anxiety disorders:* characterised by frequent, intense and lasting experience of anxiety, worry and apprehension. Avoidance, ritual acts and repetitive thoughts are often developed as a means of protecting the sufferer from experiencing the anxiety.
- *Depressive disorders:* characterised by depressed mood and a markedly diminished interest and pleasure in everyday activities. The mood state is distinctly different to the patient's normal mood state.

Awareness of potential problems can help us recognise when they could be occurring, and thus promote early provision of extra or more specialised help in order to minimise patients' difficulties.

Research has shown a strong association between stoma patients' dissatisfaction with the information they received and postoperative depression (Pringle & Swan 2001, Wade 1989). Key problems seemed to be that:

- there was a mismatch between the *levels* of information these patients thought they wanted and had received (i.e. it was more *or* less than they wanted)
- they had difficulty understanding the information they were given.

When monitoring patients' current experience of rehabilitation it is therefore important to ask patients what their experience of gaining information about their situation and treatment has been like. This kind of open question encourages patients to let us know whether they had any difficulties gaining or understanding the information they wanted, enabling us to respond to any problems at an early stage. Where the levels or type of information that was given, or the manner in which it was provided, are perceived as unhelpful by the patient or family member then giving them time and help to recount their experience and express their feelings can be beneficial. Ways of providing information helpfully, and enabling patients to understand and use it, are discussed in Chapter 7.

Patients may initially mention concerns to nurses either to obtain direct information and help or to ascertain whether their difficulty warrants medical attention. As with the stoma problems described in Chapter 21, people often describe problems as separate concerns whereas they may well be interrelated. The communication approaches described in Chapter 7 can be used to build up a detailed description of the symptoms and problems which will need to be considered within the 'context' of that particular patient: their individual condition; surgery; curative or palliative situation; and their social and psychological environment. Nurses can use these skills to help patients become more specific about their problems and how and when they occur. This will enable the nature, cause and urgency of the problem to be better understood as long as it is assessed by sufficiently experienced members of the healthcare team.

For example: experienced stoma care nurses would automatically carry out the kind of broad assessment of the patient's stomal function and appliance needs and management described in Chapter 21. Their combination of knowledge, skills and previous experience would tell them that any interrelated factors need to be identified and dealt with in addition to what may have initially appeared to be a single presenting problem. Less experienced or knowledgeable colleagues might not know what information to collect or, having acquired a broad description of the problem, which factors are the crucial ones to which they should respond (Benner et al 1996).

Helping patients clarify their concerns or problems as a first step is a useful activity as it enables them to provide a more detailed description of them. Even if referral will subsequently be required they are often then able to give a second, more concise yet specific account of the problem as a result of the initial clarifying interaction. This preparation prior to medical assessment can be crucial in the context of a busy GP surgery or outpatients department where time and medical help are in short supply, and attention may only be given to the information that is first presented by the patient.

This kind of clarification also helps patients understand they need to move from focusing on the problem to identifying what needs to be achieved, and how this could be done, if problems are to be resolved. The approaches described in the following two sections below can be used to resolve individual problems as well as to promote rehabilitation generally.

IDENTIFICATION OF THE EXPERIENCE OF 'BEING REHABILITATED'

Patients differentiate between the experiences of 'resuming normal lifestyle activities' and 'feeling myself again', with the latter more integrated sense of themselves being identified as the real goal of rehabilitation. Therefore when patients are identifying rehabilitative goals it can be more useful to start by focusing on the kind of *experience of being rehabilitated* which an individual wants, and then consider which activities might help them gain their desired experience. With this approach engaging in an activity is often the means to an end (a strategy) rather than a goal in itself.

For example: in Patient scenario 8.5 in Chapter 8 Mr Earl tells Nurse Beech that the purpose of seeing his friends who normally stay overnight with the Earls is to have the *experiences* of (a) sharing common interests and hobbies and (b) feeling he is getting back to his normal world. Once these experiences becomes the goal (rather than how to cope with the activity of friends coming to stay) it is then possible for Nurse Beech to help Mr Earl identify alternative strategies (such as prearranged phone calls) through which he could gain a similar experience in a less tiring way.

IDENTIFYING THE STRUCTURE OF EXPERIENCE

When we want to know about someone's experience we tend to informally ask what it was like. However, this often only elicits part of the picture, depending on what the person reports and what elements we enquire about. Cameron-Bandler (1985) provides us with a model of 'an experience' which enables us to gather relevant information systematically and obtain a more holistic understanding. In this *model of the structure of subjective experience* she suggests:

- any experience is made up of the same components, so these constitute *what* the structure of experience entails
- *how* these structural components interrelate generates experience
- *how* these components are experienced (separately or in combination) will differ depending on the person and their circumstances (see Patient scenario 22.1, below).

In Cameron-Bandler's (1985) model the structural components of experience are:

(a) *Context.* This is the setting in which the situation being discussed (present or future) takes place.

(b) *External behaviours.* These are behaviours that can be observed: what someone does on the outside.

(c) *Internal state.* The person's internal sense of their experience in that context, including feelings and body sensations.

(d) *Internal computations.* The person's internal ways of making sense of a situation through hearing and making pictures or representations of it (past, present or future).

(e) *Cause-effect.* Relationships may exist, or be perceived as existing, between experiences, occurrences and situations (e.g. between a behaviour and an internal state). Thus the expression or occurrence of one leads to the occurrence of the other.

(f) *Criteria and criterial equivalences.* Criteria relate to a person's values: the standards through which they measure or evaluate an experience and its meaning to them. They may be expressed as what is important to them, or what having the particular experience will give them. Someone holding or using a criterion will have a set of particular experiences and behaviours they need to *see*, *hear* and *feel* in any given situation in order to know whether that criterion is being met. This set of cues is called a *criterial equivalence*.

This model is particularly useful because it includes people's thoughts, feelings and beliefs as specific components. These are elements of their inner world that patients often experience as problematic even when they are carrying out activities competently. The model can be used to identify:

- what someone's *current* experience is like (e.g. to clarify which aspects of it are satisfactory or problematic)
- what someone's *desired* state would be like (e.g. the experience they might want to have in a specific situation, or of 'being rehabilitated' generally)
- what the differences are between that person's current and desired experiences, so goals can be identified which are most likely to reduce or remove problems, or put in place more helpful alternatives
- what criteria or cues an individual uses to judge whether their experience is satisfactory or not.

This model can therefore be used in all healthcare settings both to identify and to record the

rehabilitative experience a patient wants or is having. Once a desired state or experience has been identified the degree to which it is being achieved can be recognised, and which elements of that experience a person needs to alter or further develop. This is easier to do in the context of rehabilitation as a whole if patients have identified rehabilitative goals which include how they will inwardly think, feel and see things (including themselves) in different contexts (e.g. at work; on holiday; in bed with a partner) as well as what they will be doing (e.g. carrying out specific tasks at home; going abroad on holiday; making love without their bag becoming dislodged).

When we use this model with someone it is best used as part of a larger interaction, as shown in Appendix 22.1. Many of the skills described in Chapter 7 can be used to create the level of rapport with which we can then help the individual to identify the particular experiences and goals they want, and the strategies with which to achieve them. Overall, the steps of this larger goal-achievement process which need completion are the same but the *order* in which individuals can most readily use the processes of identifying desired experiences and setting goals may differ. Some people find it easier to first identify the kind of experiences they want to have in particular situations and, secondly, set goals which will help them achieve those experiences. Other people may start by identifying goals or outcomes they want to achieve, and then consider what their experience will be like when those outcomes have been achieved.

When we ask questions to elicit the structure of someone's experience they tell us (verbally and nonverbally) how they experience a situation and how they produce that experience. As they are talking they re-experience some of it, and provide us with *observable cues* that this is taking place (e.g. through their physiological posture, breathing, facial expression, voice tonality, use of representational systems). As you will know from conversations with friends and family, as well as patients, there are differences between when someone experiences their situation as problematic and when they experience it as satisfactory. We can use these different cues to monitor their progress towards thinking of, and acting in that situation in ways that will meet their needs and goals and thus produce their desired state or experience (see Patient scenario 22.1, below).

Maintenance of rapport is important as some of the questions asked may make individuals aware for the first time of processes they use, such as representational system usage (see Ch. 7), or beliefs on which they act. They will be more able to use this information if they feel accepted and supported while they are providing it. Matching and pacing are useful skills (see Ch. 7) but the questions used must be open enough for that person's processes to be elicited and for us to avoid leading them into thinking they use our processes. Similar questions can be used to identify someone's current experience of a situation and what that experience will be like once they have achieved their goal or outcome (desired state). It is important to start with *context* questions to identify the setting of the experience. Some people suggest that the order used in this next *scenario* is the most helpful to use when eliciting someone's present state or experience (Whitney 1988).

PATIENT SCENARIO 22.1   Ruth Goldsmith is a 43-year-old ileostomist who had surgery 6 months ago. Mrs Reid remembers that Ruth led a very curtailed existence prior to surgery because of the effects of her Crohn's disease. She is having difficulty extending her social activities now she is physically well enough to do so, but would like to rejoin a women's social group she enjoyed before she became ill.

Mrs Reid uses a series of questions (Q), in conjunction with other communication skills, to help Ruth identify her desired experience (A). (Examples of helpful questions are given here. Other similar questions could have been used to elicit Ruth's answers.)

Context
Q: what will be happening in this situation?
A: I will be going to the group's meetings most months for lunch and afternoon activities.

External behaviour
Q: what, specifically, will you be doing?
A: I will be talking to people I know and choosing suitable food and drink at the communal lunch.

Internal state
Q: How will you be feeling as you are there?
A: I will feel relaxed and confident and will be enjoying myself.

Internal computations
Q: What will you be thinking inside yourself during the meeting? How will you be seeing yourself?
A: I will think I look all right and that my bag is secure. I will see myself as looking attractive and approachable. I will know what to say to people.

Cause–effect
Q: What will help you to be OK there?
A: I will go with Naomi and she will make me join in instead of sitting in a corner or leaving early, so I will be all right.

Criteria
Q: What is important to you about being at these meetings in this kind of way?
A: The women will make me feel welcome so I will know it is the right kind of place for me to make friends.

Criterial equivalences
Q: How will you know that you are welcome? What will let you know you could make friends there?
A: People will smile at me and listen to what I say. They will include me in their conversation.

Ruth has now got a more specific idea of the experience she wants. She can use this to consider whether the goals implicit in her description are achievable (see later) and to compare what she wants with her current experiences and capabilities. While she was describing her difficulties in socialising initially, and then what her desired experience in the group would be like, Mrs Reid was noticing how, physiologically, Ruth was demonstrating the state she was in during each experience. She will use this information to monitor whether, when Ruth sets goals and strategies for achieving them and imagines these in action, her physiology is matching that of her desired state.

PROMOTION OF GOALS THAT ENABLE PATIENTS TO ACHIEVE AND MAINTAIN DESIRED LEVELS OF REHABILITATION

Goals or desired outcomes need to have certain characteristics if they are to be achievable. In neuro-linguistic programming (NLP) this is known as having *well-formed outcomes* (Cameron-Bandler 1985, O'Connor & McDermott 1996). We can help people ensure they are setting goals that have a likelihood of success when we encourage them to consider whether their goal meets these characteristics or criteria by asking:

1. *Is it stated positively*, as the outcome the person wants (rather than does not want)?
2. *Is it appropriately contextualised: and specified*: when, where, with whom is their outcome wanted?

3. *Is it demonstrable in sensory experience*, so it is measurable or verifiable, so its achievement can be recognised?
4. *Is it initiated and maintained by the goal-setter(s)*, so they have the power/control needed to achieve it and/or realistically elicit help from others?
5. *Is it preserving any positive by-products of the current situation/state?* (so these are not lost, although they may need to be obtained by an alternative route).
6. *Is it in keeping with the goal-setter's values*, in terms of the outcomes and consequences arising from them?
7. *Is it worthwhile*, given the time, effort, resources used to achieve it?

These criteria can be used to shape new goals or outcomes being planned or to review goals someone is having problems achieving, as they may not have been identified or pursued in ways which make it likely they can be achieved.

For example, Mrs Reid notices that Ruth has said other people will be causing her to join in the group's activities, and provide evidence through their behaviour that the group is the right kind of place for her to socialise and make friends. This is not necessarily in her control to set up (e.g. Naomi may not be willing to go with her or behave in this way), and she may also need help to reshape her outcomes so they include criterial equivalences related to her own experience (e.g. what, specifically, does she need to see, hear and feel, in order to know she is confident? relaxed? has a secure bag?) Once Ruth's outcomes are well formed it will be easier for her to identify strategies through which she can promote these outcomes.

As you can see from the flowchart in Appendix 22.1, even once outcomes are clearly defined people may need help to access resources and solutions or strategies that will support goal achievement. It can be helpful to encourage people to interpret the term 'resources' widely. It could include relevant skills or information, help obtained from others, an increased ability to create and maintain a helpful state.

Once resources and strategies have been identified it is very useful to encourage the person to 'future pace' (O'Connor & Seymour 1993). This is a system of encouraging the person to step into the future in their imagination and mentally rehearse the outcome/desired experience in action, for example, the next time they will be in that situation. As they do this they can identify whether this is the experience they want. Meanwhile, we can observe whether they maintain the physiology and other characteristics of their desired state, or whether they exhibit the cues which they had shown earlier when describing their problem state/experience. If they revert to the problem state it is an indication that more help is needed, either with us or through referral. It is important to remember to direct the person to return to the present time after they have used 'future pacing'.

When we use these approaches to help people with problems we can give them information about the models and how they can be used to achieve desired outcomes generally as well as in the situation being considered at that time. In this way they will gain tools for more resourceful living.

MONITORING OF PATIENTS' PROGRESS IN COMPLETING THE TASKS OF GRIEVING FOR LOSS

The majority of patients whose surgery includes stoma formation do experience some form of loss. Even if they are not consciously grieving for a specific loss the symptoms they describe are often similar to those that bereaved people experience. For example, Parkes (1998) found in his various research studies of people experiencing loss of a partner, home or limb that the grieving processes they went through were similar. Feelings commonly experienced in these mourning phases are summarised in Table 22.1.

Parkes (1998) also found that factors of stigma and deprivation help determine people's overall reaction to bereavement. Stoma patients often express concern as to whether they will be socially acceptable now they eliminate urine or faeces in a different manner and this can signal they are experiencing stigmatisation, or a change of attitude towards their acceptability, in themselves or in other people. They may also experience deprivation if they perceive their disease, operation and/or stoma as depriving them of elements of their normal lifestyle as well as altering their body image and function. Some of the concerns, problems and experiences reported in both Wade's (1989) and Pringle & Swan's (2001) research with patients during their first year after surgery are congruent with the phases and feelings listed above as grief reactions and described by researchers of bereavement (Parkes 1998, Worden

Table 22.1   Phases of adult mourning and related feelings (from Lendrum & Syme 2004 (Table 4.2), with permission of Thomson Publishing Services)

Phase	Related feeling
Numbness	Shock
	Disbelief
Yearning	Reminiscence
	Searching
	Hallucination
	Anger
	Guilt
Disorganisation and despair	Anxiety
	Loneliness
	Ambivalence
	Hopelessness
	Helplessness
Reorganisation	Acceptance
	Relief

2003). Providing a style of stoma care which would help people deal with loss if they so wished can therefore be an important part of enabling them to rehabilitate fully.

Worden (2003) suggests that after someone sustains a loss there are certain tasks that must be accomplished for equilibrium to be re-established and for the process of mourning (adaptation to the loss) to be completed. These *tasks of mourning* are to:

1. accept the reality of the loss
2. work through to the pain of grief
3. adjust to an environment in which the deceased is missing
4. emotionally relocate the deceased and move on with life.

When these tasks are not completed considerable difficulties can arise which, if not resolved, can affect many aspects of people's lives. It therefore makes sense for us to offer a style of rehabilitative stoma care which promotes completion of these mourning tasks so that problems can be minimised and dealt with as early as possible. Since many bereaved people take about 2 years to complete these tasks it is advisable to monitor patients' progress for at least this period of time after their surgery. It is equally important not to expect patients to fit into a specific timeframe or all experience the same levels of grief. The meaning they attribute to their experiences, and any loss and changes they feel, will be individual.

Worden (2003) suggests a number of *principles* of bereavement counselling. I have adapted these below for use as part of normal stoma care.

1. *Ensure staff, patients and relatives have appropriate information about the possibility that experiences of loss and grief will occur, and the nature and importance of 'normal' grief expression.*

It is important to get a balance between giving sufficient information to be helpful but not such an amount or prescriptive type of information that it creates anxiety. It is generally helpful to first ask if the patient and family have experienced major loss or bereavement and, if so, what that was like. The information they give in response can then be used to identify the amount and type of information that is now likely to be helpful to them. People who have experienced major change or loss within recent years prior to surgery (e.g. death; divorce; redundancy) may take longer to complete tasks of mourning related to their surgery if they are still coming to terms with previous loss(es). Some individuals welcome being given this kind of information and an opportunity to discuss how they can get support as part of their preparation for discharge home. Other people may want less specific loss information but may benefit from explicit permission to contact their stoma care nurse or family doctor if they are having symptoms (which could be loss-related) such as difficulty in sleeping, undue emotional mood swings, unusual levels of sadness, anger or anxiety. Family members whose lives and roles have been significantly affected by the patient's situation may also need to work through these processes.

2. *Help patients actualise their losses.*

Many patients find the timespan between experiencing themselves at their normal level of health, discovering they have a condition which necessitates substantial surgery, and undergoing that surgery and any adjuvant treatment is quite short. They report feeling dazed or shell-shocked, and that these events and the resultant changed body appearance and function seem unreal. They may need to recount the whole series of events a number of times in order for the nature and permanence of their situation and inherent losses to become real to them. Staff and family may need to be told that this kind of repetition over the first few months serves a useful purpose and that they can aid long-term recovery by giving the person time and attention while they tell their story, rather than seeking to prevent them from repeating it. *For example,* community nurses visiting patients at home regularly to provide perineal wound care can also provide opportunities for patients and families to describe their experiences.

3. *Help the patient to identify and express feelings.*

The feelings associated with the patient's losses do not occur in isolation: they take place in the context of them also undergoing major surgery. Surviving tests, surgery, difficulties such as pain, lack of sleep, food and privacy, and learning sufficient stoma care to cope on discharge are more than enough to initially occupy the thoughts and feelings of most people. As recovery goes on, many people become more aware of their feelings. They may need help to experience them *to the degree they need to be felt in order to bring about an effective resolution.* Patients and their families may feel guilty that they feel sad or angry rather than grateful for the care and treatment provided. Anxiety that they may be labelled 'bad' patients if they express their feelings strongly may be present, as may concern that such expression could upset their family.

Staff as well as friends and relatives may be uncomfortable in the presence of strongly expressed emotions or continuing distress, and may act on their beliefs that it will be better if the patient is discouraged from showing them. Denial that feelings exist and/or avoidance of their expression have been found to leave people with substantial pain, often involving some form of depression (Bowlby 1980, p 158). Systems for helping patients and their families handle feelings which are likely to arise 3–12 months after surgery need to be set in place so that their feelings can be experienced with the intensity needed for completion of the second task of mourning. This includes ensuring they have alternatives to dampening down feelings with inappropriate use of drugs or alcohol, which only put off the time when those feelings will need to be expressed.

Although approaches and skills for aiding emotional expression have been clearly described and can be learned (e.g. Lendrum & Syme 2004, Worden 2003) it is unfortunately also true that relatively few healthcare staff have the requisite training, time and support with which to help patients and families feel and work through the pain of loss and grief at the level they may need. Gentle enquiries can establish whether there is a potential or actual mismatch between the level of emotional expression in which the patient is likely to engage and the ability, willingness and availability of family, friends and staff to support such expression. Processes such as match-pace-lead can be used to help people move from awareness that emotional expression is a normal part of recovery to considering whether, if they needed to, they might use support from local sources such as religious personnel; the Samaritans; bereavement support agencies such as Cruse. Qualified counsellors may also be available via the GP or through organisations such as the British Association for Counselling and Psychotherapy (BACP). Knowing that additional support could be gained if necessary can help patients, their families and friends feel less alone in their efforts to deal with the emotional ups and downs of psychological recovery.

4. *Assist patients and their family to develop a structure within which emotional recovery can take place.*

Resolution of grief following major loss quite often takes a couple of years. Much of patients' grief work therefore takes place when they will be having little contact with healthcare staff if physical recovery is satisfactory. The need to plan and pace physical activities to fit in with physiological healing and recovery of strength is usually recognised. Patients and their families may not know it is also advisable to plan for, and pace, activities to promote emotional recovery (which includes completion of the tasks of mourning). *For example,* patients and their families may need help to learn how to negotiate who fulfils which roles and responsibilities, and how to adapt these to be in step with changing levels of psychological and physical recovery. They may also need encouragement to assess whether proposed activities and normal styles of celebration are congruent with the patient's emotional as well as physical ability to enjoy them at that time.

Ensuring help is easily accessible, through channels that patients and their families will actually use, is particularly important because of patients' potential risk of depression. People with depression often find it difficult to seek or utilise help. As indicated earlier, depression may arise from previous experiences but it can also be a symptom of unresolved grief (Worden 2003). Some people suggest that encouraging patients and their families to face the possibility of grief reactions and plan strategies for enabling them to take place are likely to create distress and anxiety but this is rare *when discussion is knowledgeable and skilled.* Sensitive, appropriate preparation carries with it the hope and vision of emotional healing and movement towards a better future. It gives people a map with which to make sense of their experiences and progress, and strategies for avoiding or minimising unresolved loss reactions such as depression.

5. *Facilitate movement of patients' emotional investment from the person they used to be into the person they have become as a result of their experiences.*

Worden (2003) suggests that mourners need not 'give up' a dead person but rather find a suitable place for the dead person in their emotional lives which acknowledges that person's importance but enables survivors to reinvest their emotional energy in living and in other relationships. Likewise, patients can acknowledge the person they were and reinvest their emotional energy in the person they have now become through their various experiences. This is normally essential if full psychological as well as physical rehabilitation is to take place. It is easy to see the relevance of these processes for patients whose situation and capabilities are perceived as diminished by their operation. However, patients who have apparently gained much from their surgery (e.g. an ileostomist's ability to eat a more varied diet) and only lost problems (e.g. a urostomist's pain and frequency of elimination now absent) also have losses to mourn and changes in body image and function to accommodate. They too should be given the help they need to do so.

PROVISION OF HELP THAT ENABLES PATIENTS TO COMPLETE THE TASKS OF GRIEVING

Dilts (1990, p 209–212) suggests that we function at different logical levels which are related and operate as an internal hierarchy in which each level is progressively more psychologically encompassing and impactful. We can use this model to assess a patient's progress in completion of task (5) above (like Worden's task 4 – described earlier) or rehabilitation generally and also to plan and provide help if difficulties are occurring.

These **logical levels** (from lowest to highest) are:

environment: *where and when*; any external constraints; people we are with
behaviours: *what* we do, our specific conscious thoughts and actions

capabilities: *how* we do things; our use of skills, strategies, mental maps
beliefs and values: *why* we act; what we believe to be true, permissible, possible or not, important to us
identity: *who* we are, core beliefs and values, our mission in life
spiritual: *our* connections and influences beyond individual identity, our humanness.

Identifying which level someone is using when they experience problems is important because continuing to use that same logical level to resolve them generally maintains rather than solves the problem. We can help people operate more effectively by working with them at a different logical level (O'Connor & McDermott 1996). In this next *patient scenario* Mrs Reid is using some of the *skills* described in Chapter 7 in combination with Dilts' **logical levels**.

PATIENT SCENARIO 22.2   John Fletcher has told Mrs Reid he is back working almost full-time now and, in the past, this amount of work has made him tired enough to sleep well. However, now he is waking early but does not feel rested. He is finding it difficult to recall customers' requirements and other work details at times. Previously he has dealt with worries by focusing on work, keeping his mind on all the details that make a job look good. Mrs Reid recognises that John is using logical levels of **behaviour** and **capability** both when the problems occur and to resolve them. She uses *primary level empathy* to indicate she has understood he likes to do good work. She then asks him **why it is so important to him** (inviting him to **use a higher logical level**). He tells her he has always been able to do high class work and keep the money coming in to support his family. He says he took on the man's role from the age of 17 when his Dad died, and he became the family wage-earner. John's **beliefs** and **sense of identity** are being challenged by his current symptoms and Mrs Reid recognises it is at these levels she and John will need to work. She also knows that sleep disturbances can signal unresolved grief and/or depression. She *matches* John physiologically *to maintain rapport* as she seeks to establish whether John has unresolved grief from this previous loss impinging on his current experience. She uses *linked statements* to make a gentle enquiry:

> So when your Dad died you had to step into his shoes right away and be the breadwinner ... and now, because you and your friend are self-employed, the pressure is there for you to quickly take on your share of the work so you don't lose orders and the income is kept up for you and Mary and him. I'm wondering what happened to the part of you that maybe needed time to grieve for what you had lost ... and perhaps has feelings now.
>
> John's eyes filled with tears as for the first time he talks about what it was like to push his own needs and feelings to one side in order to meet the expectations that he and his family had about his responsibilities and how he should fulfil them. Afterwards he thanks Mrs Reid, saying he knows he has more sorting out of his current situation to do, but that he feels as if there is less of a weight on his shoulders.
>
> Mrs Reid has used a variety of counselling skills to enable John to express his feelings at some depth, and share some of the pain of that past loss. She decides to discuss this interaction with John with her supervisor. She wants to discuss whether her expertise (gained during her certificate in counselling skills course) is likely to be sufficient to help John complete the other tasks of mourning. In doing so she thinks she will improve her ability to differentiate between situations she can handle competently and those where referral might be more appropriate.

Once the tasks of grieving have been completed patients are usually in a better position to consider the degree to which they are achieving their chosen style of rehabilitation. They may wish to achieve new outcomes and we can use the approaches described earlier in this chapter and in Chapter 7 to help them.

Much of the focus in this chapter has been on patients whose surgery is curative, bringing with it the time and possibility of full rehabilitation. However, as discussed in Chapter 3, some patients' cancer will have spread too far to enable surgery to be curative. Some patients will have conditions which can be contained, or which may recur intermittently such as Crohn's disease, or for which they require palliative care. These patients will also have losses and changes to deal with, situations they want to alter, and experiences and goals they want to achieve. If we are willing to work flexibly with patients and their families then often the main outcomes of a desired goal can be experienced (Breckman 1998, Nichols 2003, Salter 1998). We can use all the approaches described in this chapter to help people with a wide variety of situations and needs to make the most of their capabilities to live life as fully and enjoyably as possible.

APPENDIX 22.1

The following flowchart shows an interaction to help someone achieve goals.

Step 1: enter interaction and establish rapport

↓

Step 2: (or step 3): identify the structure of the person's subjective experience *

↓

Step 3 (or step 2): gather information and set well-formed outcomes *

↓

Step 4: access resources and create solutions

↓

Step 5: 'future pace' to establish that the goal(s) and problem-resolving measures are appropriate and sufficient for the person's purpose

↓

Step 6: close interaction.

* Steps 2 and 3 can be completed in either order.

People who have little idea of specific goals they want may find it easier to start by considering what their current experience is like, and what kind of experience they would prefer to have, and then set goals which would help them achieve it.

People who have identified goals may like to first ensure they are well formed (i.e. likely to be achievable), and then check whether these goals will give them the kind of overall experience they want to achieve.

References

Benner P, Tanner C A, Chesla C A 1996 Expertise in nursing practice. Springer, New York

Bowlby J 1980 Attachment and loss: loss, sadness and depression, Volume 3. Basic Books, New York

Breckman B 1998 Stoma management. In: Doyle D, Hanks G W C, Macdonald N (eds) Oxford textbook of palliative medicine, 2nd edn. Oxford University Press, Oxford, p 839–845

Cameron-Bandler L 1985. Solutions. FuturePace, San Rafael, CA

Dilts R 1990 Changing belief systems with NLP. Meta Publications, Cupertino, CA

Lendrum S, Syme G. 2004 Gift of tears, 2nd edn. Brunner-Routledge, Hove

Nichols K 2003 Psychological care for ill and injured people. Open University Press, Maidenhead, UK

O'Connor J, McDermott I. 1996 Principles of NLP. Thorsons, London

O'Connor J, Seymour J 1993. Introducing neuro-linguistic programming. Aquarian Press, London

Parkes C M 1998 Bereavement: studies of grief in adult life, 3rd edn. Penguin Books, London

Pringle W, Swan E 2001 Continuing care after discharge from hospital for stoma patients. British Journal of Nursing 10(19):1274–1288

Salter M 1998 'If you can help somebody' (nursing interventions to facilitate adaptation to an altered body image). In: World Council of Enterostomal Therapists congress proceedings. Horton Print Group, Bradford, West Yorkshire, p 229–235

Wade B 1989 A stoma is for life. Scutari Press, Harrow, Middlesex

White C 1998 Psychological management of stoma-related concerns. Nursing Standard 12(36):35–38

White C A 1999 Psychological aspects of stoma care. In: Taylor P (ed) Stoma care in the community. Nursing Times Books, London, p 89–109

Whitney B 1988 Handouts, NLP Practitioner Course. UK Training Centre for NLP

Worden J W 2003 Grief counselling and grief therapy, 3rd edn. Routledge, London

Chapter 23

Developing stoma care

Brigid Breckman

The roles and responsibilities of nurses engaged in stoma care are constantly changing as knowledge, care and treatment develop and we respond in various ways. At first glance when a nurse's post gets incorporated into a different team, department or broader role it can appear that the whole role has changed. A closer look often reveals that the nurse can adapt many skills already learned to fulfil the new role. The skills and approaches described in this book are being related to stoma care. However, many can also be used as core skills, for example, by nurses engaging in care of patients with gastro-intestinal, urological, and cancerous conditions who may not have a stoma.

Likewise, new healthcare initiatives and goals can be experienced as triggering major role changes when the requirements to fulfil them first cascade down to clinical nurses. Again, the skills we use to provide a holistic, patient-centred style of stoma care can often be utilised to fulfil changing local and national healthcare goals. In this chapter I will therefore *not* focus discussion on how we fulfil specific roles or healthcare initiatives. These vary depending on the countries and healthcare systems in which we work. Instead I will consider some ways in which we can develop stoma care practice that will also enable us to respond effectively to changing roles and responsibilities. These are:

- creating a framework for development
- promoting acquisition of skills
- promoting evidence-based care and evaluation of practice.

CREATING A FRAMEWORK FOR DEVELOPMENT

In this section I will outline some of the broader processes we can use when developing stoma care practice. They help us structure our plans and activities so development becomes more coherent and less piecemeal. They include:

- managing information flow
- identifying what we could learn
- developing clinical judgement.

MANAGING INFORMATION FLOW

Previous chapters have shown there are many fields from which we can draw information, concepts, skills and strategies to enhance our provision of stoma care. Increasing internet access makes it much easier to find out about developments. However, this wealth of information, the extent to which it is constantly being added, and its availability to public and healthcare professionals has implications.

(a) It raises expectations of the breadth and depth of knowledge, and the level of up-to-dateness which nurses should have. For example, there are expectations that nurses have the ability and equipment to access websites and online journals, engage in literature searches etc., and will acquire relevant information from these and other sources.

(b) The speed with which information becomes available, and is reported as available, is increasing. For example, media coverage of new research, tests or treatments can almost instantly result in patients and their families asking for information and answers to questions.

(c) People's accessibility to sources of information and help is changing. More patients are using the internet and the media to gain information about symptoms, diagnoses and treatments, in addition to discussing their situation with the healthcare team (Ziebland et al 2004). We need to acquire a more global knowledge of reputable sources which we and our patients can use, and the nature, reliability and relevance of their material and services. For example, support services available in one country may be unavailable or of limited use to patients elsewhere. Patients may require help to deal with their feelings if they discover they cannot access treatment available in other countries.

(d) The increasingly vast network of information and sources can lead us to feel overwhelmed rather than enabled by it.

Identifying strategies through which we will systematically seek information can help us deal with all these factors more effectively. *For example,* keeping a record of topics, aspects of care, organisations and websites we want to look up can help us focus and prioritise our search for information. Scheduling time in diaries for gathering that information helps us turn updating plans into action. Such strategies enable us to obtain sufficient information over time to update and expand our knowledge without getting overloaded. As part of this ongoing process you and your colleagues could draw on the useful contacts in Chapter 24.

IDENTIFYING WHAT WE COULD LEARN

O'Connor & Seymour (1993, p 6–8) suggest that there are four stages of learning:

(1) Unconscious incompetence

At this stage we may not know:

- how to do something
- that we do not know how to do something, or how to do it better
- that we are unaware of our effect on others.

(2) Conscious incompetence

This is the stage where we are beginning to realise what we are doing and/or not doing. Although it is an uncomfortable stage it indicates progress: we have realised there is learning to be done.

(3) Conscious competence

At this stage we:

- try out new behaviours to discover what 'works' for us
- can use skills and complete tasks, but need to think about them whilst using them.

(4) Unconscious competence

At this stage we have integrated new options into our behaviour as part of our normal way of being.

As we learn the various components of stoma care we move through these stages. We can have reached stages 3 or 4 in some aspects of stoma care while remaining at stage 1 regarding other elements that we could develop. It is therefore prudent to include strategies for discovering what we do not yet know we need to learn in our plans for developing stoma care. Luckily, strategies that help us manage information flow systematically also enable us to do this. *For example*:

- completing literature searches to find books, articles and journals which can inform us of relevant research, new ideas, and developing or changing practice
- conducting internet searches via reputable websites to expand our awareness of available information, sources of help, courses, and new stoma care products
- identifying treatment options for the various conditions which stoma patients may have, including the changing availability of trials and standard treatments in our own and other countries.

Once we have acquired such information it is important to consider its relevance and likely accuracy. Regularly documenting such professional updating activities and describing what we have learned from them is useful. It helps us clarify and consolidate what we have understood and how we can use it to inform and extend our practice. This kind of reflection can help us build up our abilities to analyse and justify effective care, and question poor practice. It also enables us to pinpoint aspects of practice where we need further input. *For example*, it could help us identify aspects of care we need to learn directly by spending time with a colleague in their clinical setting, and those we could acquire from courses or study days.

Nurses with novice and advanced beginner skill levels need help to identify what care to give and how to recognise priorities in care (Benner et al 1996). Nurses with little experience in stoma care could use the following strategies to help them consider aspects of practice to develop:

- Using descriptions of competencies compiled by expert colleagues to identify core and extended competencies which it is desirable to learn, and help others to learn.
  Examples: RCN (2002a) Standards of care project: colorectal and stoma care nursing; RCN (2002b) Competencies in nursing project: caring for people with colorectal problems.
- Using descriptions of different levels of skill usage in nursing, how these may be acquired, and in what timeframes.
  Example: research by Benner (1984) and Benner et al (1996). (Some of their key findings are outlined in the Introduction to this book as well as utilised throughout it.)
- Using a definition of nursing, its values and characteristics to identify whether the style of stoma care being developed is in step with nursing concepts and practice in the overall healthcare system, and/or leading to enhancements in care.
  Example: RCN (2003) definition of nursing.
- Noticing expertise and opportunities where it can be demonstrated and 'unpacked' to enable learning to occur.
  Examples: situations like: Patient scenario 1.1 in Chapter 1, where multidisciplinary approaches are used to enhance nurses' abilities.
- Learning from people who successfully manage their stoma care and living with a stoma.
  Examples:
  - drawing on the collective expertise of members of the 'patient organisations' to enhance levels of understanding of how to live with, and manage a stoma successfully, and identify care which helps achieve this
  - asking patients and their families to give us feedback so helpful elements of care can be identified and offered to other patients.
- Considering the content of courses in stoma care and related fields, to identify which elements of care are deemed important to include for course participants.
  Examples:
  - modules specifically on stoma care which are offered as stand-alone stoma care courses or as part of degree or diploma pathways
  - topics scheduled in such courses. *For example*, inclusion of genetic information and the help patients may need if their diagnosis could have implications for their family too (Yeomans & Kirk 2004).

DEVELOPING CLINICAL JUDGEMENT

In earlier chapters many skills and care components have been described separately, so that their nature could be portrayed as clearly as possible. However, the core nature and characteristics of nursing as defined by the Royal College of Nursing (2003) remind us that the use of clinical judgement lies at the heart of effective nursing practice.

Part of using clinical judgement involves the capacity to identify the right information and skills to draw on at the right time, and combine them in the best manner to achieve a desirable outcome in the particular circumstances. This is why the *patient scenarios* describe nurses' thoughts as well as their actions in some detail. They indicate how clinical judgement can be used to inform, shape and evaluate care in these situations.

We also need to be able convey to others the rationale on which our care is based. The cluster of skills for doing this could be called 'justification of practice skills'. They include the ability to describe care which is planned and provided in a manner that enables others to recognise the knowledge, choices and decisions on which our practice is based. When we do this well the case for using particular information, skills and strategies to achieve care goals and minimise problems becomes apparent and viewed as justified. Patient scenario 5.1 in Chapter 5, where Nurse Hill is demonstrating how to recognise an appliance needs changing, is an example of clinical judgement being made visible so the patient and a colleague can begin to acquire it too.

As our perception of the complexity of stoma care grows so our awareness of the need to expand our knowledge and skills increases. In many instances we achieve this by noticing *what* care more experienced colleagues plan and provide. We also observe *how* they engage in care themselves, and collaborate with patients and colleagues to ensure appropriate care is given. These activities give us a greater sense of what it is possible to learn and provide in the way of care. However, increasing our abilities in this way is considerably dependent on having access to colleagues with the requisite expertise. Time for expert colleagues to work directly with inexperienced colleagues and actively help them develop expertise may well be limited because of the workload and responsibilities which all concerned are handling. This prompts the question: *what levels of expertise should individual nurses, and the team who collectively provide patients with stoma care, seek to acquire?*

A key element of the care described throughout this book has been the importance of nurses being able to, firstly, recognise the nuances and implications of patients' situations, treatment, and experiences and, secondly, respond appropriately. As Benner et al's (1996) research shows this level of sophisticated care is only demonstrated by nurses who have considerable knowledge and skills in their particular care context. It is therefore arguable that at least one nurse in each patient's team should have acquired expert or proficient level capabilities. Their depth of knowledge can ensure that planning, provision and evaluation of stoma care is well thought out and delivered overall. Their direct engagement in clinical care spearheads the development of expertise in patients and colleagues particularly as, over time, they teach colleagues how to manage problems and more advanced aspects of care.

However, patients usually have a very short pre- and postoperative period of contact with most healthcare staff. During this time they must take in substantial amounts of information, gain basic stoma care skills, and learn how to apply these in their own particular circumstances. Like all learners, patients need to be actively helped to acquire a foundation of novice and then advanced beginner capabilities (Benner 1984). Ways of promoting these are described in Chapter 4. To achieve these goals at least some of the staff planning, providing and evaluating patients' daily care need to have Benner competent level category stoma care abilities.

Utilisation of nurses with these levels of expertise benefits organisations responsible for care provision as well as patients and clinical colleagues. Goals and targets regarding the outcomes to be achieved from healthcare are set by government agencies as well as organisational providers. The greater breadth and depth of knowledge applied by experienced nurses helps them to respond to clinical and managerial goals. For example, they are more likely to be able to specify the goals, results and efficacy of patients' care, and accept the importance of documenting it clearly. This enhances clinical audit completion as well as the team's ability to collaborate and provide relevant care.

A key point brought out in Benner's (1984) research was the degree to which *expertise is contextual*. When we change to looking after patients with a different condition, or ones who are undergoing different treatments to those with which we are familiar, then our competency levels temporarily diminish. This is because our background knowledge, and ability to recognise cues which tell us what is normal and abnormal in this new situation, is less expert than in the old one. As we build up sufficient experience in this new situation, coupled with the necessary background knowledge, so our competencies and clinical judgement levels increase again. It is important that nurses moving between specialisms which may be viewed as similar, such as stoma care, colorectal or urological nursing, are helped to transfer skills and develop their competencies in their new role. Obviously this is important to ensure patients receive good care. In addition, it can be uncomfortable to find that our capacity to make advanced clinical judgements is no longer as automatic and reliable as we had become used to. It is important that nurses are supported and given opportunities to round out their expertise (Sherwood 2003). The strategies discussed in this chapter can help us develop in this way, and help colleagues do likewise.

WAYS OF PROMOTING ACQUISITION OF SKILLS

A skill is a learned capability. We use skills to follow strategies (means to an end) to achieve goals (Egan 1998). Skills are most effective when they are used purposefully in order to achieve particular outcomes. Many of the skills that enable us to help learners (i.e. patients and colleagues) acquire capabilities have already been described earlier in the book so ways of using those approaches to promote skill acquisition are indicated in the following summary.

- Establish rapport with learners and monitor their readiness to learn before beginning to teach them, individually or in groups (see Ch. 7).
- Ask people how they learn most easily and adapt our way of teaching to be congruent with their systems, e.g. provision of pictures or written information; use of audio or video tapes (Fretwell et al 2004).
- Use learners' ways of processing material when we give them information, e.g. use of representational systems in Chapter 7.
- Provide information and demonstrate techniques at a pace that suits the learner, e.g. using the match–pace–lead process (see Ch. 7) with individuals and groups.

- Use learning processes that are appropriate for learners' level of skill acquisition, as discussed in the Introduction.
- Prepare learners for experiences to come so their anxiety levels are reduced and they can assimilate information and handle those experiences more easily, e.g. preparation for surgery (Ch. 1) and managing problems (Ch. 9).
- Make explicit the outcomes that activities are meant to, or could, achieve, e.g. Nurse Ash's work with Mrs Jones in Chapter 8 (Patient scenario 8.1).
- Use *constructive* feedback so learners have confirmation of what they have grasped and what they can do to improve, e.g. Mrs Reid's work with Mr Patel in Chapter 7 (Patient scenario 7.2); when colleagues are engaging in exercises to practise skills in study days.
- Help learners *use* information as soon as possible after they are given it, as this early experience of applying it helps it stick in their minds more readily; e.g. Mrs Reid's discussions with Mr Earl as to ways of obtaining more equipment after discharge (Patient scenario 8.4), and with students on a course (Patient scenario 8.3).
- Help learners develop beliefs/attitudes that will help them use capabilities they are acquiring e.g. Mrs Reid's work with Mrs Jones in Chapter 8 (Patient scenario 8.6).

When we seek to acquire capabilities, or to help colleagues and patients do so, our approaches need to include identification of the thinking which underpins the capability and shapes how it may be or has been used.

USING A 'DEMONSTRATE AND UNPACK' STYLE OF TEACHING AND LEARNING

Capabilities include more than external behaviour. Judgement as to when and why abilities could be used, and how their success in achieving the user's desired outcome will be evaluated, are also involved. Most of this is, of course, in the user's head rather than explicitly available to other people. When we specifically describe or 'unpack' the inner processes we are using (e.g. thoughts, feelings, visual images, mental maps, assumptions/beliefs) and link them with our observable behaviour, then learners can understand and acquire all these elements of the capability more successfully.

Unpacking underlying expertise can take place during or after its demonstration. *For example*, most stoma care nurses describe what they are thinking and why they are doing something as they demonstrate practical stoma care management. However, when demonstrating how to engage in a preoperative visit with a patient (either clinically or in a classroom role play) it may be more useful for learners to observe what such an interaction includes overall first, and discuss it and have questions answered afterwards. Specific aspects of a capability or broader approach and how they relate to the outcomes being sought can then be linked to questions and observations made by the learner(s). Video and audio tapes can also be used as demonstrations with subsequent unpacking of aspects which can be learned from them.

We can use a similar approach of 'try out and unpack' when we are learning skills. This is a common approach when learning communication skills but can also be very useful when learning to provide broader aspects of care such as ways of preparing patients for discharge. Observation of a skilled demonstration can be followed by practice in groups of three, which is then followed by reflection on our own experience of seeking to use the skill/approach before being given constructive feedback from the 'patient' and 'observer'. (Where role play has been used it is important for the 'patient' to be de-roled at this point, even in short exercises, so they do not retain elements of their adopted role.) Such unpacking helps clarify the ways in which we are making sense of, responding to, and evaluating situations internally as well as externally, and whether these are appropriate and effective expressions of the skill/approach being learned.

THROUGH WRITTEN DESCRIPTION AND ANALYSIS OF CLINICAL CARE AND/OR HOW APPROACHES FROM OTHER FIELDS CAN BE UTILISED IN STOMA CARE

This can include strategies to aid personal learning and ones that enable others to learn. As we recall events and knowledge, and concentrate on getting our thoughts and actions down on paper, this can help us become more aware of the ways we do, or could, function and the effects this might have on ourselves and others. *For example*:

- keeping a reflective journal for one's own private development

- completing a case study with specific descriptions of how material learned on a course has been used in a patient's care, and an analysis of the outcomes of its use
- publishing an article or book describing how particular aspects of care have been, or could be, used, including concepts, models, and/or research.

USING CLINICAL SUPERVISION

This is a process in which one person (the supervisee) is helped to describe and reflect on some aspects of their work while supported and facilitated by one or more experienced colleagues (the supervisor(s)).

Although supervision helps us review our practice and manage problems, it is different from other activities which include review and reflection, such as counselling and managerial discussion. Supervisors should not normally also be their supervisee's manager or counsellor. This can create difficulties with overlapping areas of responsibility and how information is used.

Driscoll (2000) and Betts (2003) provide useful accounts of clinical supervision, including definitions and descriptions of what it entails. Key points to consider when arranging to have supervision include:

- the stage of expertise the supervisee has developed so far
- what aspects of practice and levels of competency the supervisee now wants to develop through supervision
- what expertise the supervisor should have in order to help the supervisee improve their practice
- the availability of the supervisor and supervisee to work together, given their overall commitments and activities, and the locations where these take place
- any personal and professional characteristics that the supervisee would prefer their supervisor to have or not have.

The expertise that we want supervisors to have can change as our own practice develops. *For example*, in earlier stages of skill development priority may be given to having a supervisor with considerable expertise in stoma care. Their clinical credibility can increase supervisees' willingness to reflect on patients' needs, and the skills which they could be, or are using to meet them. However, facilitation skills will also be needed by these supervisors so that they enable supervisees to gain the insight and skills to move from advanced beginner to competent levels of practice.

Nurses acquiring competent, proficient and expert levels of competency can have different supervisory needs, particularly when working as specialist nurses. At these stages nurses have good practical stoma care abilities, and growing background knowledge and experience with patients. Development of greater expertise in communication and counselling may now be given higher priority as the need to help patients achieve psychological as well as physical wellbeing is more clearly recognised.

The experiences and issues with which stoma patients need help can be emotionally demanding of staff, as well as very satisfying when patients find our care helpful. Hingley (1992) found that the lack of organisational support and understanding of stoma care nurses' role was the second highest source of their stress, and many comments being made by colleagues today indicate this still holds true. Research has shown that staff who demonstrate good levels of counselling and communication skills on courses stop using them if the environment in which they subsequently work is not supportive in helping them deal with the results of using these skills (Fallowfield & Davis 1991). Therefore, in addition to finding ways in which experienced nurses can expand and consolidate their capabilities, we also need systems that are supportive as we extend our practice. These factors can lead nurses who want to develop advanced levels of practice to view the style of supervision offered to counsellors as more likely to meet their needs. This is sometimes called non-managerial supervision or (as in this book) a 'counselling style' of supervision.

Inskipp & Proctor (2001a, p 1) define supervision as 'a working alliance between a supervisor and a counsellor in which the counsellor can offer an account or recording of her work, reflect on it, receive feedback, and where appropriate, guidance. The object of this alliance is to enable the counsellor to gain in ethical competence, confidence and creativity so as to give her best possible service to her clients'.

The situations that Inskipp & Proctor (2001a, p 2) give as reasons why supervision is needed by even the most experienced and talented practitioners are ones that nurses as well as counsellors may well experience:

- we may be working with people when they are at their most vulnerable, distressed or needy
- we may choose, or be required, to work with clients who leave us puzzled and confused
- we may become case hardened or burnt out without realising it – failing to communicate empathically, respectfully and helpfully
- we will get out of date in such a rapidly developing field, and may need to be reminded about that
- we may develop haphazardly, and not realise we have lost sight of our core values and ideals.
- we may become exploitative of our clients – emotionally, financially, or sexually – without realising it.

Supervision helps us identify information and skills that we could acquire and improve. It also enables us to clarify which elements of our practice are effectively helping patients, their families, and ourselves achieve the outcomes we seek to promote and support. This helps us work more strategically as our clinical judgement develops, improving our ability to monitor the effects of individual elements of care as well as to evaluate situations and care more holistically.

Supervision can be gained through a variety of arrangements including:

- one to one with a supervisor
- within a group led by a supervisor
- within a group of peers, who may work as a whole group and/or in twos and threes
- one to one with a peer, each experienced nurse offering supervision to the other.

Books, audiovisual aids, and courses can be used to gain a more specific understanding of what supervision can entail. The package developed by Inskipp & Proctor (2001a, 2001b) is a useful starting point for considering counselling style supervision as it includes audio tapes and exercises for individual and group use on making the most use of supervision (part 1) and becoming a supervisor (part 2).

It is important to remember that *in supervision* the aim is to help the supervisee reflect and develop through a judicious mixture of support and challenge rather than for the supervisor to provide or prescribe care. Difficulties with roles and responsibilities could arise if the supervisor is also planning and providing clinical care for the same patients as their supervisee. Therefore helping colleagues learn through demonstration, teaching and informal discussion are acceptable when we share patients with them: providing formal supervision with those same colleagues may be inadvisable.

WAYS OF PROMOTING EVIDENCE-BASED CARE AND EVALUATION

USING RESEARCH STUDIES

Traditionally the term 'evidence-based care' has been used to mean care that is based on sizeable research studies whose results are accepted as valid and reliable, and where the relevance of the research to the situations and people with whom it will be applied is deemed acceptable. Stoma surgery impinges on many aspects of patients' lives. This creates numerous areas where research is needed to help us understand and respond to patients' experiences and evaluate whether our care is having the desired outcomes. There are growing amounts of research directly related to stoma surgery and its effects, patients' experiences and concerns, and the effects of nurses' care. These are indicated in references throughout this book. You will also find use of research from other fields such as bereavement and loss (see Chs 20 and 22), communication (e.g. in Chs 7–9), and cancer care (Ch. 18). Tools for assessing patients' needs, abilities, confidence etc. are also increasing (e.g. White 1999). Our care is likely to benefit patients most if we remain flexible in our ideas as to what constitutes 'research which is relevant to stoma care', and which disciplines and fields it may come from.

Benner (1984, p 35) suggests a number of strategies for eliciting more specific information about how expert nurses are operating:

(a) through explicit, systematic documentation of actual clinical performances that record and describe expertise and/or breakdowns in performance
(b) by making systematic efforts to develop a shared, descriptive language and system of comparable and compatible observations amongst experts
(c) study of proficient and expert performances and the resultant patient outcomes, so that the knowledge thus gained can be used to develop nurses to the expert level

(d) the use of expert nurses to provide consultation for other nurses, for example:
  ● to help make a case for further medical intervention when they detect early clinical change
  ● to help competent level nurses develop a sense of 'what is possible', a characteristic present in nurses with proficient and expert levels of skills.

These strategies could all be used in stoma care, and they could be the subject of traditional style research programmes. However, Benner also writes of the difficulty which some expert level nurses can have in describing how they know how to respond to a situation, use a skill etc. because much of their expertise is now operating at an unconscious, intuitive level. This can be understood when we think of the 'conscious competence' model of learning mentioned earlier.

USING MODELLING TO DEFINE SKILLS AND THEIR OUTCOMES

The neurolinguistic programming (NLP) process of *modelling* entails eliciting and describing the structure of the experience which enables someone to generate a specific ability (Gordon & Dawes 1998). It is a more comprehensive way of discovering how people 'do' skills than the informal enquiries we generally make. For example, we can all remember times when someone has described a situation and, if we ask about an aspect of it they had not mentioned, they are then able to recall that information and give it to us. As a result our understanding of that situation changes and we increase our perception of what that experience was like, for them, and how and why they responded in the way they have described. Modelling enables us to find out, in similar but much more systematic ways, what people are doing when they are using a particular capability at, for example, expert or proficient level. This is because we generate or create particular capabilities or skills through having specific experiences. We are able to enquire systematically how experts 'do' a particular capability because every experience has a *structure*: a number of components which interact and thereby create it. These include:

● the context in which the skill is being used
● beliefs (e.g. about what is important; what causes particular effects)

- internal thoughts, feelings, pictures
- external behaviour
- the skill-user's *test*: what they need to see, hear and feel that enables them to know they have the outcome they sought from the particular skill or approach they were using.

When we want to understand how an expert generates a skill we can ask them to specifically describe what each of the above structural components of their experience is like when they are using that skill. Our questions help them recall elements of their situation which they may usually only notice at an unconscious level but, in response to our enquiry, these elements return to conscious recollection and can be described. Gradually we build up an overall map of the experience through which that expert generates the specific skill. If we then ask other people with similar levels of expertise to describe their experience when generating that same skill, enquiring about the same structural components, we will begin to find key patterns that are central to doing or generating that skill. A description or *model* can now be created of the structure of the skill-generating experience (i.e. the key components and patterns which anyone wishing to gain expert ability to use that skill will need to acquire). This model or described mental map is then used by other people to test whether, when they use it to create a similar experience in themselves, they generate the same ability. This system enables concepts and descriptions of 'what an ability entails' to be tested quite robustly and adapted as necessary until an effective model of the ability-generating experience is produced (Dilts 1998).

There are variations in the structural components (jigsaw pieces) of an experience which different people suggest should be elicited in order to make a model of it (e.g. Dilts 1998, Gordon & Dawes 1998). I have listed similar components above to those described in the model of the structure of experience outlined in Chapter 22. Both times I am using the concept that 'an experience' is made up of these particular components. However, it is important to remember that although the structural components are the same *the questions we use to invite people to tell us about their experience will have differences in their purpose and focus.*

- The questions in Chapter 22 were about how to elicit a map of someone's current and desired

experiences for the *purpose* of identifying problems and promoting solutions.
- When we use modelling our *purpose* is to discover how, specifically, someone generates a capability.

This is so that we can, firstly, gain it and/or help others acquire it and, secondly, evaluate the degree to which using the acquired ability leads to achievement of the outcome we wanted. It is not possible to describe modelling in more depth here. There is some additional information in my account of using questions derived from modelling approaches by Cameron-Bandler (1985) and Gordon & Dawes (1998) in order to enable workshop participants to begin modelling the ability 'gaining sufficient background information for use when siting a stoma' (Breckman 1998).

The potential of modelling to help us build up a body of knowledge of the most effective ways of generating different elements of stoma care expertise is considerable. As well as enabling us to pinpoint and transfer expertise between nurses it could also be used to map and aid transfer of skills and strategies patients use to successfully rehabilitate. *For example,* it could help us:

- use the same system of enquiry to elicit from exemplars (colleagues or patients) in different locations how, specifically, they generate specific capabilities so this information can be compared and essential components of those skills identified
- describe abilities in a way which enables other people (colleagues or patients) to understand the key patterns they need to acquire and utilise
- identify different patterns used by people who have acquired various levels of skill acquisition (e.g. those described by Benner (1984)); more specific help can then be given to enable people to move adeptly from one level to the next
- enable nurses and patients engaged in teaching and learning stoma care to focus on the key elements that need to be gained for maximum skill acquisition in the time they have available together
- identify which elements of skill acquisition are proving difficult for someone to acquire and thus where attention needs to be given
- clarify the specific elements we need to utilise in situations where sometimes our skill usage is adept and effective and at other times it is not.

Once we have learned how to model the structure of an exemplar's experience of generating a capability we can use this process to enquire about, describe in detail, and acquire a wide variety of skills and broader approaches. This system can be used by individual nurses. However, it could also be used by groups. *For example*, time could be allocated within or adjacent to national and international conferences during which specific skills used by expert stoma care nurses could be modelled. In time this would create a 'library' of modelled skills which in turn could be used to assist members wishing to extend their expertise, e.g. via journal or Internet publication, workshops, or teleconferencing.

Currently lecture formats are often used as the main system in study days and events such as the World Council of Enterostomal Therapists' (WCET) congresses. Presentations are allocated short time-spans and, understandably, speakers seek to impart as much information to colleagues as they can within their brief session so their speech is often rapid. This disadvantages nurses whose understanding of English is minimal. Nurses whose experience of stoma care is at novice and advanced beginner levels also often find it hard to understand more complex presentations as they have not yet acquired sufficient knowledge with which to make sense of the material presented. Members can end up feeling less skilled, confident, and/or enthusiastic about stoma care as a result of such experiences. The slower paced, focused style of interaction used both to elicit models from exemplars (e.g. in master classes), or to present a model of a skill and help colleagues acquire it, could enable more effective skill transfer to be achieved. Nurses who are relatively new to stoma care may also come from countries, or locations within countries, where there are few expert colleagues readily available to consult. It is therefore particularly important that they get the maximum help to learn effectively when they do get to specialist conferences. Modelling is one way in which this could be achieved more systematically and effectively than is often the case at present. Nurses at competent, proficient, and expert stages of skill acquisition would also benefit as they learned to use a shared conceptual structure and language to define, try out, and evaluate the effects of capabilities that are needed now and in the future in stoma care.

USING DEFINED OUTCOMES TO EVALUATE CARE

When we help patients to specifically define the kind of 'rehabilitation' they want to achieve, we then have a blueprint or guide to help us both plan care that will promote and support its achievement and evaluate with patients the degree to which their actual experiences match those they originally wanted. The model of the structure of subjective experience which is described in Chapter 22 is particularly useful as it gives us a systematic way of helping people describe experiences they are having, want to have, and any gaps between them. It can be used to define and evaluate experiences for as large or as small a span of stoma care provision or time as patient and nurse think would be helpful. *Examples* include experiences of:

- preoperative discussion about living with a stoma
- learning to change stomal equipment
- managing the first week at home after surgery
- enjoying a special event (e.g. holiday, staying with friends, family celebration)
- achieving acceptable levels of pain relief with minimal side effects
- having accepted their new body image
- having achieved the maximum level of rehabilitation.

If stoma care is to be truly patient-centred then their experiences should play a central role in defining what constitutes evidence of appropriate, effective and/or successful care. Regrettably, it is not uncommon to hear patients' descriptions of the results of particular care approaches dismissed as 'only the patients' viewpoint'. However, being rehabilitated is not just the ability to complete tasks (e.g. change stomal equipment) or engage in particular activities (e.g. resume work; go on holiday), although the occurrence of these events may well be easier for outside observers to verify. Rehabilitation also includes patients' thoughts, feelings and beliefs about themselves, their experiences, and what is possible and desirable for them to achieve in their particular situation. That may be living with a chronic condition, being cured of a disease, or requiring palliative care. Whatever their circumstances evidence-based planning, provision and evaluation of care should include comparison of patients' desired and actual experiences. Ultimately, what is important to patients and their families is the relevance of care to their needs, and the quality of their experiences which that care helps them achieve.

In this book we have described a style of stoma care which we believe can make a significant con-tribution to patients' wellbeing and rehabilitation. We hope it serves also as a reminder that stoma care is an exciting and satisfying field in which to work, and one where we can continue to expand the boundaries of what constitutes expert nursing.

References

Benner P 1984 From novice to expert. Addison-Wesley, Menlo Park, CA

Benner P, Tanner C A, Chesla C A 1996 Expertise in nursing practice. Springer, New York

Betts A 2003 Making the most of clinical supervision. In: Ellis R B, Gates B, Kenworthy N (eds) Interpersonal communication in nursing, 2nd edn. Churchill Livingstone, Edinburgh, p 145–161

Breckman B 1998 From novice to expert via NLP modelling. In: World Council of Enterostomal Therapists congress proceedings. Horton Print Group, Bradford, West Yorkshire, p 114–116

Cameron-Bandler L 1985 Solutions. FuturePace, San Rafael, CA

Dilts R B 1998 Modeling with NLP. Meta Publications, Capitola, CA

Driscoll J 2000 Practising clinical supervision. Baillière Tindall and RCN, Edinburgh

Egan G 1998 The skilled helper, 6th edn. Brooks Cole, Pacific Grove, CA

Fallowfield L, Davis H 1991. Organizational and training issues. In: Davis H, Fallowfield L (eds) Counselling and communication in health care. John Wiley, Chichester, p 319–342

Fretwell I, Mallender E, Smith K 2004 Computerised digital photography for stoma and wound management. Gastrointestinal Nursing 2(5):19–24

Gordon D, Dawes G 1998 Modelling Course handout. Metacommunications, London

Hingley P 1992. Occupational stress in stoma nursing. World Council of Enterostomal Therapists' congress proceedings. Hollister. Libertyville, IL, p 76–78

Inskipp F, Proctor B 2001a The art, craft and tasks of counselling supervision. Part 1: making the most of supervision, 2nd edn. Cascade, Twickenham, Middlesex

Inskipp F, Proctor B 2001b The art, craft and tasks of counselling supervision. Part 2: becoming a supervisor, 2nd edn. Cascade, Twickenham, Middlesex

O'Connor J, Seymour J 1993 Introducing neuro-linguistic programming. Aquarian Press, London

Royal College of Nursing 2002a RCN standards of care project: colorectal and stoma care nursing. RCN, London

Royal College of Nursing 2002b RCN competencies in nursing project: caring for people with colorectal problems. RCN, London

Royal College of Nursing 2003 Defining nursing. RCN, London

Sherwood L 2003 Macmillan training fellowship-a year with the colorectal cancer team. Gastrointestinal Nursing 1(7):8–9

White C A 1999 Psychological aspects of stoma care. In: Taylor P (ed) Stoma care in the community. Nursing Times Books, London, p 89–109

Yeomans A, Kirk M 2004 Genetics for beginners. Nursing Standard 18(40):14–17

Ziebland S, Chapple S, Damelow C et al 2004 How the internet affects patients' experience of cancer: a qualitative study. British Medical Journal 328:564–567

Chapter 24

Useful contact information

Brigid Breckman

The purpose of providing brief outlines about some organisations that could be of help to you and your patients is to give you a starting point for identifying useful resources and further information. Many of these organisations have more functions than those described below. The majority are UK based, but some have links to, or knowledge of, similar organisations in other countries.

Appliance manufacturers and suppliers have not been listed as their contact details and product availability varies in different countries. The range of stoma care products now available is considerable (see Ch. 4). Doing an internet search at intervals (using topics such as stoma care products, colostomy, ileostomy or urostomy appliances) will enable you to update your information about the products available and the various manufacturers and suppliers from whom they may be obtained.

Association of Coloproctology of Great Britain and Ireland

at: The Royal College of Surgeons of England
35-43 Lincoln's Inn Fields
London WC2A 3PE
Tel: 020 7973 0307
Fax: 020 7430 9235
Email: acpgbi@acpgbi.org.uk
Web: www.acpgbi.org.uk

Guidelines for the management of colorectal cancer, and other documents available to be downloaded from website. Has links to a range of other websites including medical, nursing and charity organisations.

Association for Spina Bifida and Hydrocephalus (ASBAH)

42 Park Road
Peterborough
Northamptonshire PE1 2UQ
Tel: 01733 555 988
Fax: 01733 555 985
Email: info@asbah.org
Web: www.asbah.org

Has about sixty independent local organisations in the UK. Offers information, support and specialist services for people with these conditions and their families.

Beating Bowel Cancer

39 Crown Road
Twickenham
Middlesex TW1 3EJ
Tel: 020 8892 5256
Fax: 020 8892 1008
Email: info@beatingbowelcancer.org
Web: www.bowelcancer.org

Seeks to raise awareness of bowel cancer in professionals and the public. Supports training in colonoscopy centres. Offers training grants for colorectal nurses.

Bristol Cancer Help Centre

Grove House
Cornwall Grove
Bristol BS8 4PG
Tel: 0117 980 9500 (reception);
0845 123 2310 (helpline)

Fax: 0117 923 9184
Email: info@bristolcancerhelp.org
Web: www.bristolcancerhelp.org

Various complementary therapies and activities utilised in a holistic approach to cancer. Runs residential courses for people with cancer and close family/friends.

Offers courses for healthcare professionals and complementary therapists.

British Association for Counselling and Psychotherapy (BACP)

BACP House
35-37 Albert Street
Rugby
Warwickshire CV21 2SG
Tel: 0870 443 5252
Email: bacp@bacp.co.uk
Web: www.bacp.co.uk

Has directories listing counsellors and supervisors throughout the UK, and training centres for counselling. These indicate therapeutic models and theories used. Range of journals including ones on healthcare counselling and research.

British Colostomy Association (BCA)

15 Station Road
Reading
Berkshire RG1 1LG
Tel: 0118 939 1537; helpline: 0800 328 4257
Fax: 0118 956 9095
Email: sue@bcass.org.uk
Web: www.bcass.org.uk

Offers support and help to people with a colostomy and their families, including literature and half-yearly newsletter.

CancerBacup

3 Bath Place
Rivington Street
London EC22 3JR
Tel: 020 7696 9003;
standard rate UK helpline: 020 7739 2280;
UK freephone helpline: 0808 800 1234
Fax: 020 7696 9002
Email: via website
Web: www.cancerbacup.org.uk

Information on all aspects of cancer plus UK counselling and other resources. Wide range of publications; ability to search for clinical trials available to UK patients, including European trials. Some local cancer centres with specialist cancer nurses. Black and ethnic minorities section, with some bilingual link workers and booklets in Asian and Chinese languages.

Cancer Black Care

16 Dalston Lane
London E8 3AZ
Tel: 020 7249 1097
Fax: 020 7249 0606
Email: cbc@cancerblackcare.org
Web: www.cancerblackcare.org

Support offered through helpline, leaflets, drop-in service, and advocacy/interpreters.

CancerHelpUK

Institute for Cancer Studies
University of Birmingham
Edgbaston
Birmingham B15 2TA
Email: HayleyLW@cancer.bham.ac.uk (secretary);
cancer.info@cancer.org.uk (nurses)
Web: www.cancerhelp.org.uk

Includes information for professionals and patients regarding different trials and who can take part in them.

Cancer Research UK

National Office
PO Box 123 Lincoln's Inn Fields
London WC2A 3PX
Tel: 020 7242 0200 (switchboard);
020 7009 8820 (customer services)
Fax: 020 7269 3100
Web: www.cancerresearchuk.org

Information and statistics on all types of cancer. Includes prevention, screening, treatment and research from the UK's cancer authority. Patients can access descriptions of trials going on for cancers at different sites.

Cascade Publications

4 Duck's Walk
East Twickenham
Middlesex TW1 2DD
Email: weipke@yahoo.com
Web: www.counsellingsupervisiontraining.co.uk

Counselling supervision *package* with two books plus audiocassettes (see Ch. 23) and other items on counselling and supervision available from *postal or email address*.

Information on supervision *training* for counsellors available from website.

Chai Cancer Care

144-146 Great North Way
London NW4 1EH
Tel: 020 8202 2211; Helpline: 0808 808 4567
Fax: 020 8202 2111
Email: info@chaicancercare.org
Web: www.chaicancercare.org

Provides support for Jewish patients and families with home, hospital and hospice visits. Offers counselling, resource library, range of complementary therapies.

Cochrane Collaboration

UK Cochrane Centre
Summertown Pavilion
Middle Way
Oxford OX2 7LG
Tel: 01865 516300
Fax: 01865 516311
Email: general@cochrane.co.uk
Web: www.cochrane.org

Prepares systematic reviews of healthcare interventions. There are Cochrane centres in Asia, Africa, Australia, Europe, North and South America. The various fields reviewed include a Cancer network.

Colon Cancer Concern (CCC)

9 Rickett Street
London SW6 1RU
Tel: 020 7381 9711 (general);
InfoLine Tel: 08708 50 60 50 (nurses)
Fax: 020 7381 5752
Email: info@coloncancer.org.uk
Web: www.coloncancer.org.uk

Offers a range of booklets and factsheets on colorectal cancer and its treatment in addition to information and support from specialist nurses via the infoline. Regional directory accessible via website showing on-site availability of specialist nurses and doctors at UK hospitals.

Continence Foundation

307 Hatton Square
16 Baldwin's Gardens
London EC1N 7RJ

Tel: 0845 345 0165
Email: continence-help@dial.pipex.com
Web: www.continence-foundation.org.uk

Provides factsheets and booklets for people with bowel and bladder problems, plus professional resource packs. Organises annual continence awareness campaign.

Core

3 St Andrew's Place
London NW1 4LB
Tel: 020 7486 0341
Fax: 020 7224 2012
Web: www.corecharity.org.uk

Previously known as Digestive Disorders Foundation. Offers leaflets and factsheets on a range of digestive disorders.

Crohn's in Childhood Research Association (CICRA)

Parkgate House
356 West Barnes Lane
Motspur Park
Surrey KT3 6NB
Tel: 020 8949 6209
Fax: 020 8942 2044
Email: support@cicra.org
Web: www.cicra.org

Seeks to raise awareness and fund research into Crohn's disease. Leaflets available for individuals, parents, teachers and potential donors. Has quarterly newsletter and annual open day.

European Organisation for Research and Treatment of Cancer (EORTC)

Central Office
Avenue E. Mounierlaan, 83/11
B-1200 Brussels
Belgium
Tel: +32 2 774 16 11
Email: eortc@eortc.be
Web: www.eortc.be

Conducts, coordinates and stimulates research in Europe on the experimental and clinical bases of treatment of cancer and related problems. Has some information on complementary and alternative cancer medicine (CAM) in Europe.

FP Sales Ltd

Freepost CF 3963
Rhymney

Gwent NP22 3BF
Tel: 0870 444 5116
Email: sales@fpsales.co.uk
Web: www.fpsales.co.uk

SexWare catalogue describes a range of sexual products which have been reviewed by a medical practitioner. Descriptions of products and books are clear and low-key. They include items for assisting erection and lubrication.

Gay Ostomists Association

Flat 1, Park Court
1 Alexandra Drive
Liverpool L17 8TA
Tel: 0151 726 9019
Email: sydmccaffrey.goa@bushinternet.com

Offers informal help to people with a stoma or permanent urinary catheter who identify as bisexual, gay, lesbian or transgender. Has links and knowledge of gay and gay-friendly organisations.

IBS Network

Northern General Hospital
Sheffield S5 7AU
Tel: 0114 261 1531;
helpline 01543 492 192 weekdays, 6–8 p.m.
Fax: 0114 261 0112
Email: penny@ibsnetwork.org.uk
Web: www.ibsnetwork.org.uk

Offers factsheets on irritable bowel syndrome and helpline support. Lists international websites with information on IBS.

Ileostomy and Internal Pouch Support Group (ia)

ia National Office
Peverill House
1-5 Mill Road
Ballyclare
County Antrim
Northern Ireland BT39 9DR
Tel: 028 9334 4043; Freephone: 0800 0184 724
Fax: 028 9332 4606
Email: info@the-ia.org.uk
Web: www.ileostomypouch.demon.co.uk

Aims to help anyone who has, or is about to have, their colon removed with all aspects of rehabilitation. Has groups throughout the UK and a postal group for overseas members. Publishes booklets, factsheets and quarterly journal.

Institute of Cancer Research (in conjunction with Royal Marsden Hospital)

123 Old Brompton Road
London SW7 3RP
Tel: 020 7352 8133
Fax: 020 7370 5261
Web: http://www.icr.ac.uk

Website includes lists of cancer-related organisations and web addresses.

International Ostomy Association (IOA)

102 Allingham Gardens
Toronto
Ontario ONM3H 1YZ
Canada
Tel: +1 416 633 6783
Fax: +1 416 633 6712
Web: www.ostomyinternational.org

An association of national patient associations, now covering many parts of the world. Has Fatwa about preparation for prayer for Muslims.

International Union Against Cancer (UICC)

3 rue du Conseil General
1205 Geneva
Switzerland
Tel: +41 22 809 1811
Fax: +41 22 809 1810
Web: www.uicc.org

Lists international voluntary cancer leagues, and international directory of cancer institutes and organisations.

Macmillan Cancer Relief

89 Albert Embankment
London SE1 7UQ
Tel: 0808 808 2020; textphone for deaf: 0808 808 0121
Email: cancerline@macmillan.org.uk
Web: www.macmillan.org.uk

Offers information and support. Directory of UK self-help and support groups available.

Marie Curie Cancer Care

89 Albert Embankment
London SE1 7TP
Tel: 020 7599 7777
Email: info@mariecurie.org.uk
Web: www.mariecurie.org.uk

Provides care for UK patients in their own home and in 10 hospices. Funds research. Provides a range of courses, study days, conferences for healthcare professionals.

Medical Research Council

MRC Clinical Trials Unit
(Cancer Division)
222 Euston Road
London NW1 2DA
Email: contact@ctu.mrc.ac.uk
Web: www.ctu.mrc.ac.uk/
Website offers links to useful cancer websites, including a page for patients, and websites with information about trials in different countries.

National Advisory Service for the Parents of Children with a Stoma (NASPCS)

51 Anderson Drive
Valley View Park
Darvel
Ayrshire KA17 0DE
Tel: 01560 322024
Email: john@naspcs.co.uk
Web: www.naspcs.co.uk
Offers introductory leaflet for parents of children with bladder and bowel problems plus leaflets for parents about various birth conditions. Has a genetic interest group. Website has links to other organisations and sources of help.

National Association of Crohn's and Colitis (NACC)

4 Beaumont House
Sutton Road
St Albans
Hertfordshire AL1 5HH
Tel: 0845 130 2233 (information);
NACC in contact support line: 0845 130 3344
Fax: 01727 862550
Web: www.nacc.org.uk
Website includes links to inflammatory bowel disease (IBD) associations around the world.

National Cancer Institute (NCI)

9000 Rockville Pike
Bethesda
Maryland 20892
USA

Tel: +1 800 422 6237 (in USA and its territories)
Email: via website
Web: http://cancer.gov/cancerinformation
Government agency with extensive range of cancer information related to the USA. Publications can be downloaded from website (useful to non-Americans too).

National Electronic Library for Health (NELH)

Web: www.nelh.nhs.uk
Specialist electronic libraries for patients and carers, health professionals, the public. Has links to a range of other useful websites.

National Institute for Health and Clinical Excellence (NICE)

Mid City Place
71 High Holborn
London WC1V 6NA
Tel: 020 7067 5800
Fax: 020 7067 5801
Email: nice@nice.nhs.uk
Web: http://www.nice.org.uk
Information regarding treatment regimes and their appraisal (including their availability under the NHS), available for professionals and the public.

NHS Cancer Screening Programmes

The Manor House
260 Eccleston Road South
Sheffield S11 9PS
Tel: 0114 271 1060
Fax: 0114 271 1089
Email: info@cancerscreening.nhs.uk
Web: www.cancerscreening.nhs.uk
Gives information on pilot and actual screening programmes. Unable to offer advice on specific clinical problems.

Pelican Centre

Pelican Cancer Foundation
The Ark
North Hampshire Hospital
Aldermaston Road
Basingstoke
Hampshire RG24 9NA
Tel: 01256 314746
Fax: 01256 314861
Email: admin@pelicancancer.org
Web: www.pelicancentre.com

Specialises in surgery for pelvic cancers and liver surgery. Offers free second opinion for NHS patients who have GP's referral letter.

Royal College of Nursing of the United Kingdom (RCN)

20 Cavendish Square
London W1M 0AB
Tel: 020 7409 3333
Web: www.rcn.org.uk

RCN members can join the Gastroenterology and Stoma Care Nursing Forum, which has a newsletter and an annual conference. Library stocks some journals and books relevant to stoma care.

Sexual Dysfunction Association (SDA)

Windmill Place Business Centre
2-4 Windmill Lane
Southall
Middlesex UB2 4NJ
Tel: 0870 7743571
Email: info@sda.uk.net
Web: www.sda.uk.net

Seeks to raise awareness of erectile dysfunction in public and medical profession, and help sufferers of impotence. Does not give individual advice but puts callers in touch with specialist practitioners. Website also has section on female dysfunction and treatment.

Smilie's People Network

Chris Corker (secretary)
36 Noble Street
Hoyland
Barnsley S74 9LW
Tel: 01226 744 859
Web: www.smiliespeople.org.uk

Network of individual families who have a child living with inflammatory bowel disease. Members join NACC initially (see above).

Thames Regions Polyposis Registry

St Mark's Hospital
Northwick Park
Watford Road
Harrow
Middlesex HA1 3UJ

Tel: 020 8235 4272
Fax: 020 8235 4278
Email: kneale@netcomuk.co.uk
Web: www.polyposisregistry.org.uk

Registration of people with polyposis living in Thames regions. Provides information and support for patients.

Ulster Cancer Foundation

40-42 Eglantine Avenue
Belfast BT9 6DX
Northern Ireland
Tel: 028 9066 3281; Helpline: 0800 783 3339
Fax: 028 9066 0081
Email: info@ulstercancer.org
Web: www.ulstercancer.org

Offers information and help for people with cancer through helpline, support groups, patient-to-patient contact, funding research.

United Ostomy Association (UOA)

Central Office
19772 MacArthur Boulevard
Suite 200
Irvine
California 92612-2405
USA
Tel: +1 800 826 0826
Fax: +1 949 660 9262
Email: info@uoa.org
Web: www.uoa.org

Has Chapters (branches) throughout the USA, also in Bermuda, Canada, Puerto Rico. Supports people with bowel and urinary stomas. Range of special interest groups includes: continent diversion network, gay and lesbian ostomists, parents of ostomy children, pull-thru network, young adult network, 30+ network.

Urostomy Association (UA)

Hazel Pixley
National Secretary
Central Office
18 Foxglove Avenue
Uttoxeter
Staffordshire ST14 8UN
Tel: 0870 770 7931

Fax: 0870 770 7932
Email: secretary.ua@classmail.co.uk
Web: www.uagbi.org

Supports people who have, or will have a urostomy and their family. Has a number of branches throughout the UK and a postal branch for UK and overseas members. Journal published three times a year.

World Council of Enterostomal Therapists (WCET)

WCET Central Office
PO Box 48099

60 Dundas Street East
Mississauga
Ontario L5A 144
Canada
Tel: +1 905 848 9400
Fax: +1 905 848 9413
Email: info@wcetn.org
Web: www.wcetn.org

International network of nurses involved in stoma care. Biennial conferences. Quarterly journal. List of members updated annually. Supports development of stoma care courses. Some support for members to attend courses and conferences.

Index

Q

R

S